W9-BSV-667

# Handbook of
# Medicine in
# Psychiatry

# Handbook of
# Medicine in
# Psychiatry

Edited by

## Peter Manu, M.D.

*Professor of Clinical Medicine, Psychiatry and Behavioral Sciences,
Albert Einstein College of Medicine; Director, Medical Services,
The Zucker Hillside Hospital, North Shore–Long Island Jewish Health System,
Glen Oaks, New York*

## Raymond E. Suarez, M.D.

*Resident Physician, Department of Psychiatry,
Montefiore Medical Center and Albert Einstein College of Medicine,
Bronx, New York*

## Barbara J. Barnett, M.D.

*Assistant Professor of Emergency Medicine and Medicine,
Albert Einstein College of Medicine; Director,
Emergency Medicine/Internal Medicine Residency Program,
Long Island Jewish Medical Center,
North Shore–Long Island Jewish Health System,
New Hyde Park, New York*

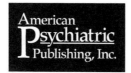

American
Psychiatric
Publishing, Inc.

Washington, DC
London, England

**Note:** The authors have worked to ensure that all information in this book is accurate at the time of publication and consistent with general psychiatric and medical standards, and that information concerning drug dosages, schedules, and routes of administration is accurate at the time of publication and consistent with standards set by the U.S. Food and Drug Administration and the general medical community. As medical research and practice continue to advance, however, therapeutic standards may change. Moreover, specific situations may require a specific therapeutic response not included in this book. For these reasons and because human and mechanical errors sometimes occur, we recommend that readers follow the advice of physicians directly involved in their care or the care of a member of their family.

Copyright © 2006 American Psychiatric Publishing, Inc.
ALL RIGHTS RESERVED

Manufactured in the United States of America on acid-free paper
09   08   07   06        5   4   3   2   1
First Edition

Typeset in Adobe's Palatino, HelveticaNeue, and City.

American Psychiatric Publishing, Inc.
1000 Wilson Boulevard
Arlington, VA 22209-3901
www.appi.org

**Library of Congress Cataloging-in-Publication Data**

Manu, Peter, 1947–
    Handbook of medicine in psychiatry / by Peter Manu, Raymond E. Suarez, Barbara J. Barnett. — 1st ed.
        p. ; cm.
    Includes bibliographical references and index.
    ISBN 1-58562-182-X (pbk. : alk. paper)
    1. Clinical medicine—Handbooks, manuals, etc. 2. Psychiatry—Handbooks, manuals, etc. 3. Mentally ill—Medical care—Handbooks, manuals, etc.
I. Suarez, Raymond E., 1977–   . II. Barnett, Barbara J. III. Title.
    [DNLM: 1. Diagnosis, Differential. 2. Physical  Examination—methods. 3. Medical  History  Taking—methods. 4. Mental  Disorders—complications. 5. Psychiatry—methods. 6. Signs and Symptoms.  WB 141.5 M294h 2005]
RC55.M25 2005
616.89—dc22                                                                              2005017099

**British Library Cataloguing in Publication Data**
A CIP record is available from the British Library.

# Contents

## PART I

### Cardiac Arrest and Airway Obstruction

Jennifer Muneyyirci, M.D.
Barbara J. Barnett, M.D.

Catalina Vazquez, M.D.

Stephanie M. Reynolds, D.O.

## PART II

### Abnormal Vital Signs

Pamela Arsove, M.D.

David Shih, M.D.

## PART III

### Respiratory Distress

Jill Karpel, M.D.
Peter Manu, M.D.

# PART IV

## Pain Symptoms

Kumar Alagappan, M.D.

Lorna Breen, M.D.

Barbara J. Barnett, M.D.

Douglas A. Isaacs, M.D.

Barbara J. Barnett, M.D.

Tom Kuo, M.D.

Michael Bennett, M.D.

Peter Manu, M.D.

# PART V

## Neurological Symptoms

Marc L. Gordon, M.D.

Scott Leibowitz, M.D.

Raymond E. Suarez, M.D.

Sung Wu Sun, M.D.

Giselle P. Wolf-Klein, M.D.

## PART VI

### Gastrointestinal Abnormalities

Nakechand Pooran, M.D.

## PART VII

### Signs of Common Infections

Barbara J. Barnett, M.D.

# PART VIII

## Skin and Soft Tissue Abnormalities

Barbara J. Barnett, M.D.

# PART IX

## Hematological Abnormalities

Dilip Patel, M.D.

# PART X

## Renal and Electrolyte Abnormalities

Hitesh Shah, M.D.

# PART XI

## Endocrine and Metabolic Abnormalities

Harvey L. Katzeff, M.D.

# PART XII

## Electrocardiographic Abnormalities

Gino Farina, M.D.

# Contributors

**Ananea Adamidis, M.D.**
Fellow, Division of Nephrology, North Shore–Long Island Jewish Health System, New Hyde Park, New York

**Kumar Alagappan, M.D.**
Associate Professor of Emergency Medicine, Albert Einstein College of Medicine, Bronx, New York; Associate Chairman, Department of Emergency Medicine, North Shore–Long Island Jewish Health System, New Hyde Park, New York

**Barbara J. Barnett, M.D.**
Assistant Professor of Emergency Medicine and Medicine, Albert Einstein College of Medicine, Bronx, New York; Director, Emergency Medicine/Internal Medicine Residency Program, Long Island Jewish Medical Center, North Shore–Long Island Jewish Health System, New Hyde Park, New York

**Michael Bennett, M.D.**
Resident, Department of Emergency Medicine, North Shore–Long Island Jewish Health System, New Hyde Park, New York

**Michael E. Bernstein, M.D.**
Resident Physician, Combined Emergency Medicine/Internal Medicine, North Shore–Long Island Jewish Health System, New Hyde Park, New York

**Archana Bhargava, M.D.**
Fellow, Division of Hematology/Oncology, North Shore–Long Island Jewish Health System, New Hyde Park, New York

**Madhu C. Bhaskaran, M.D.**
Assistant Professor of Medicine, Albert Einstein College of Medicine, Bronx, New York; Division of Nephrology, North Shore–Long Island Jewish Health System, New Hyde Park, New York

**Lorna Breen, M.D.**
Attending Physician, New York Presbyterian Hospital, New York, New York

**Robert J. Brunner, M.D.**
Fellow, Division of Gastroenterology, North Shore–Long Island Jewish Health System, New Hyde Park, New York

**Juliet Caldwell, M.D.**
Resident, Combined Emergency Medicine/Internal Medicine, New York Presbyterian Weill Cornell Medical Center, New York, New York

**Jerry Chang, M.D.**
Chief Resident, Department of Psychiatry, The Zucker Hillside Hospital, North Shore–Long Island Jewish Health System, Glen Oaks, New York

**Sally S. Chao, M.D.**
Attending Physician, Department of Emergency Medicine, St. Vincent's Hospital, Bridgeport, Connecticut

**Grace Chen, M.D.**
Resident, Department of Emergency Medicine, North Shore–Long Island Jewish Health System, New Hyde Park, New York

**Thomas Doohan, M.D.**
Attending Physician, Department of Emergency Medicine, Huntington Hospital, Huntington, New York

**Gino Farina, M.D.**
Program Director, Emergency Medicine Residency, North Shore–Long Island Jewish Sleep Disorders Center, New Hyde Park, New York

**Angelo M. O. Fernandes, M.D.**
Fellow, Division of Gastroenterology, North Shore–Long Island Jewish Health System, New Hyde Park, New York

**Vicki Figen, M.D.**
Medical Services, The Zucker Hillside Hospital, North Shore–Long Island Jewish Health System, Glen Oaks, New York

**Anne Frederickson, M.D.**
Resident, Department of Psychiatry, The Zucker Hillside Hospital, North Shore–Long Island Jewish Health System, Glen Oaks, New York

**Michael Gitman, M.D.**
Clinical Instructor of Medicine, New York University, New York, New York; Attending Physician, Division of Nephrology, North Shore–Long Island Jewish Sleep Disorders Center, New Hyde Park, New York

**Jakob K. Goertz, M.D.**
Attending Physician, Department of Emergency Medicine, North Shore–Long Island Jewish Health System, New Hyde Park, New York

**Marc L. Gordon, M.D.**
Associate Professor of Clinical Neurology, Clinical Psychiatry and Behavioral Sciences, Albert Einstein College of Medicine, Bronx, New York; Chief of Neurology, The Zucker Hillside Hospital, North Shore–Long Island Jewish Health System, Glen Oaks, New York

**Mark F. Gordon, M.D.**
Attending Physician, Department of Neurology, North Shore–Long Island Jewish Health System, New Hyde Park, New York

**Terry Gray, Ph.D.**
Director, Diabetes Education, North Shore–Long Island Jewish Health System, New Hyde Park, New York

**Harly E. Greenberg, M.D.**
Section Head, Division of Pulmonary Medicine, North Shore–Long Island Jewish Sleep Disorders Center, New Hyde Park, New York

**Howard Hao, M.D.**
Resident, Department of Psychiatry, The Zucker Hillside Hospital, North Shore–Long Island Jewish Health System, Glen Oaks, New York

**Aung Htoo, M.D.**
Chief of Service, Pulmonary, Critical Care, and Sleep Medicine, Southern California Permanente Medical Group, Bakersfield, California

**Douglas A. Isaacs, M.D.**
Resident, Department of Emergency Medicine, North Shore–Long Island
Jewish Health System, New Hyde Park, New York

**Prasun Jalal, M.D.**
Fellow, Division of Gastroenterology, North Shore–Long Island Jewish
Health System, New Hyde Park, New York

**Gnanaraj Joseph, M.D.**
Fellow, Division of Pulmonary and Critical Care Medicine, North Shore
University Hospital, Manhasset, New York

**Edward Kan, M.D.**
Combined Emergency Medicine/Internal Medicine Resident, North
Shore–Long Island Jewish Health System, New Hyde Park, New York

**Harvey L. Katzeff, M.D.**
Chief, Division of Endocrinology, North Shore–Long Island Jewish
Health System, New Hyde Park, New York

**Mansoor Khan, M.D.**
Resident Physician, Combined Emergency Medicine/Internal Medicine,
Long Island Jewish Health System, New Hyde Park, New York

**Brian Koo, M.D.**
Fellow in Sleep Disorders Medicine, Cleveland Clinic Foundation,
Cleveland, Ohio

**Dawne Kort, M.D.**
Attending Physician, Department of Emergency Medicine, North
Shore–Long Island Jewish Health System, New Hyde Park, New York

**Bon S. Ku, M.D.**
Ultrasound Fellow, Department of Emergency Medicine, The Hospital
of the University of Pennsylvania, Philadelphia, Pennsylvania

**Tom Kuo, M.D.**
Resident, Department of Emergency Medicine, North Shore–Long Island
Jewish Health System, New Hyde Park, New York

**Sheron Latcha, M.D.**
Assistant Professor of Medicine, New York University, New York, New York; Physician, Division of Nephrology, North Shore–Long Island Jewish Health System, New Hyde Park, New York

**Scott Leibowitz, M.D.**
Resident Physician, Department of Psychiatry, The Zucker Hillside Hospital, North Shore–Long Island Jewish Health System, Glen Oaks, New York

**Rosanne Leipzig, M.D., Ph.D.**
Vice Chair for Education, Mount Sinai Hospital, Bronx, New York

**Mary C. Mallappallil, M.D.**
Attending Physician, Division of Nephrology and Hypertension, North Shore University Hospital, Great Neck, New York

**Peter Manu, M.D.**
Professor of Clinical Medicine, Psychiatry and Behavioral Sciences, Albert Einstein College of Medicine; Director, Medical Services, The Zucker Hillside Hospital, North Shore–Long Island Jewish Health System, Glen Oaks, New York

**Cinthya Marturano, M.D.**
Geriatric Medical Director, Geriatric Psychiatric Unit, Mount Sinai Hospital, Bronx, New York

**Joseph Mattana, M.D.**
Associate Director, Division of Nephrology, North Shore–Long Island Jewish Health System, New Hyde Park, New York

**Alexandra E. McBride, M.D.**
Assistant Professor of Clinical Neurology, Albert Einstein College of Medicine, Bronx, New York; Attending Neurologist, Long Island Jewish Comprehensive Epilepsy Center, New Hyde Park, New York

**Boris I. Medarov, M.D.**
Fellow, Division of Pulmonary Medicine, North Shore–Long Island Jewish Health System, New Hyde Park, New York

**Stuart Morduchowitz, M.D.**
Director of Medical Education, Division of Endocrinology, North Shore–Long Island Jewish Health System, New Hyde Park, New York

**Jeffrey Nachbar, M.D.**
Resident, Department of Psychiatry, The Zucker Hillside Hospital, North Shore–Long Island Jewish Health System, Glen Oaks, New York

**Sassan Naderi, M.D.**
Attending Physician, Department of Emergency Medicine, Bellevue Hospital, New York, New York

**Dilip Patel, M.D.**
Director of Fellowship Training and Education, Division of Hematology/Oncology, North Shore–Long Island Jewish Health System, New Hyde Park, New York

**Nakechand Pooran, M.D.**
Assistant Professor of Medicine, Penn State University College of Medicine; Attending Physician, Division of Gastroenterology, Milton S. Hershey Medical Center, Hershey, Pennsylvania; Instructor of Medicine, Albert Einstein College of Medicine, Bronx, New York

**Leonidas Pritsiolas, M.D.**
Chief Resident, Emergency Medicine/Internal Medicine, North Shore–Long Island Jewish Health System, New Hyde Park, New York

**S. Devi Rampertab, M.D.**
Assistant Professor of Medicine, Penn State University College of Medicine; Attending Physician, Division of Gastroenterology, Milton S. Hershey Medical Center, Hershey, Pennsylvania; Instructor of Medicine, Albert Einstein College of Medicine, Bronx, New York

**Stephanie M. Reynolds, D.O.**
Assistant Professor, Mount Sinai School of Medicine; Attending Physician, Department of Emergency Medicine, Queens Hospital Center, Jamaica, New York

**Leonard J. Rossoff, M.D.**
Division Chief, Pulmonary Critical Care, North Shore–Long Island Jewish Health System, New Hyde Park, New York

### Rajasrre Roy, M.D.
Fellow, Division of Hematology/Oncology, North Shore–Long Island Jewish Health System, New Hyde Park, New York

### Angela Scicutella, M.D., Ph.D.
Attending Neuropsychiatrist, Division of Geriatric Psychiatry, The Zucker Hillside Hospital, North Shore–Long Island Jewish Health System, Glen Oaks, New York

### Hitesh Shah, M.D.
Associate Director, Division of Nephrology, North Shore–Long Island Jewish Health System, New Hyde Park, New York

### Manish Sheth, M.D.
Associate Director, Division of Hematology/Oncology, North Shore–Long Island Jewish Health System, New Hyde Park, New York

### David Shih, M.D.
Attending Physician, Department of Emergency Medicine, Huntington Hospital, Huntington, New York

### Kostas Sideridis, D.O.
Fellow, Division of Gastroenterology, North Shore–Long Island Jewish Health System, New Hyde Park, New York

### Raymond E. Suarez, M.D.
Resident Physician, Department of Psychiatry, Montefiore Medical Center and Albert Einstein College of Medicine, Bronx, New York

### Elizabeth M. Sublette, M.D., Ph.D.
Research Fellow, New York State Psychiatric Institute, New York, New York

### Sung Wu Sun, M.D.
Attending Physician, Geriatric Division, Mount Vernon Hospital, Mount Vernon, New York

### Alla M. Trubetskoy, M.D., Ph.D.
Attending Physician, Department of Emergency Medicine, Bronx Lebanon Hospital Center, Bronx, New York

**Steven A. Valassis, M.D.**
Resident, Department of Emergency Medicine, North Shore–Long Island
Jewish Health System, New Hyde Park, New York

**Catalina Vazquez, M.D.**
Attending Physician, Department of Emergency Medicine, Long Island
Jewish Hospital, New Hyde Park, New York

**Simon Vinarsky, M.D.**
Fellow, Division of Hematology and Oncology, North Shore–Long Island
Jewish Health System, New Hyde Park, New York

**Giselle P. Wolf-Klein, M.D.**
Professor of Clinical Medicine, Albert Einstein College of Medicine,
Bronx, New York; Director of Geriatric Medical Education and Research,
Parker Jewish Institute; Chief, Division of Geriatric Medicine, North
shore–Long Island Jewish Health System, New Hyde Park, New York

# Acknowledgments

This book owes its existence to the talent and dedication of a large group of residents, subspecialty fellows, and attending physicians from Long Island Jewish Medical Center, New Hyde Park, New York; North Shore University Hospital, Manhasset, New York; The Zucker Hillside Hospital, Glen Oaks, New York; Montefiore Medical Center, Bronx, New York, and Mount Sinai School of Medicine, New York City. We extend our deep appreciation to all our contributors for sharing their knowledge, insight, and discernment.

We acknowledge with gratitude and affection Steve Kamholz, Harry Steinberg, and Kumar Alagappan for invaluable help in planning the book and making it an academic priority for the faculties of the Department of Medicine and the Department of Emergency Medicine at Long Island Jewish Medical Center.

We thank John Kane, Bruce Levy, Jim Levenson, and Roger Kathol for their guidance in our effort to understand and refine the knowledge objectives of medical training in psychiatry.

We are indebted to Elisse Kramer-Ginsberg for statistical consultation during the research phase of this project.

Last, but certainly not least, we thank Bernadette Riordan for processing words, calming anxieties, and keeping it all together.

# Preface

## Medicine in Psychiatry: What Do We Need to Know?

Physical disorders are present in at least 50% of psychiatric patients, and a consensus exists that they are underrecognized, misdiagnosed, and suboptimally treated (Felker et al. 1996; Marder et al. 2004). These undesirable outcomes have been explained in terms of systemic obstacles to health care, behavioral aspects of psychiatric disorders, physical consequences of mental illnesses, and side effects of psychotropic drugs (Goldman 2000). However, psychiatrist-related reasons are clearly just as important and include inadequate history taking and premature diagnostic closure (Sternberg 1986), as well as a reluctance to perform physical assessments (Krummel and Kathol 1987).

The requirements for certification in psychiatry in the United States include 4 months of medical training but do not specify knowledge objectives (Accreditation Council for Graduate Medical Education 2000). The traditional setting for this training has been the medical ward of a teaching hospital, where psychiatry residents work alongside medical residents involved in the care of patients with acute myocardial infarction, congestive heart failure, pneumonia, respiratory failure, septicemia, phlebitis, cirrhosis, and malignancies (Thompson and Byyny 1982). We lack empirical data that show how this type of knowledge is used in psychiatric settings. What we do know is that life-threatening and terminal diseases are both infrequently encountered by and beyond the scope of care of the professional staff and support services of a self-standing psychiatric hospital. Our discussions with hundreds of psychiatry residents and attending physicians indicated their perception that the traditional training has not prepared them well for the medical problems of psychiatric patients and has not decreased their reliance on medical consultation to address symptoms of acute illnesses, side effects of psychotropic drugs, and manifestations of chronic degenerative disorders.

What do psychiatrists need to know about physical illnesses? To begin to answer this question, we performed a retrospective analysis of internal medicine evaluations requested for 1,001 patients admitted in 2002 to a 208-bed urban private psychiatric hospital.

The patients—501 men and 500 women—ranged in age from 8 to 98 years. The primary admitting diagnoses were mood disorders (57%), schizophrenia or other psychoses (33%), substance use disorders (25%), anxiety disorders (7%), dementia (6%), intermittent explosive disorder (3%), attention deficit disorders (3%), and eating disorders (2%). The average length of stay was 32 days.

A total of 2,120 medical consultations and 1,800 follow-up visits were performed for 742 patients. The highest rate of medical utilization was recorded for patients with dementia (2.3 evaluations/patient/week). Patients with schizophrenia, substance use disorders, and intermittent explosive disorder required an average of 0.9 evaluations/patient/week. Seventy-four patients (10% of the patients seen) were found to have conditions requiring immediate transfer to the nearby medical center for further evaluation or treatment.

The 2,120 initial consultations were requested to evaluate 148 specific problems. Twenty-six symptoms or abnormal laboratory test results were each the reason for evaluation of at least 3% of the psychiatric inpatients, and these problems led to the substantial majority of consultations. In the symptom category, the most common request was to evaluate patients who had just had a fall (6.4%). Other common reasons for medical evaluation were high blood pressure (6.3%), edema (5.8%), rash (5.6%), constipation (5.2%), cough (5.1%), abdominal pain (5.1%), pain in extremities (5.1%), chest pain (5%), nausea or vomiting (4.9%), soft tissue contusion (4.9%), diarrhea (3.8%), eye redness (3.7%), hypotension (3.5%), fever (3.4%), sore throat (3.4%), and back pain (3.1%). Abnormalities found through laboratory tests included hyperglycemia (8.6%), anemia (7.5%), abnormal electrocardiogram (6.3%), abnormal urinalysis (6.3%), azotemia (4.6%), abnormal potassium level (4.6%), abnormal leukocyte count (3.3%), abnormal thyroid function (3.1%), and hyponatremia (3.1%).

The reasons for the majority of medical consultations requested in the psychiatric hospital were a limited group of symptoms, signs, and abnormal laboratory test results. The three major groups of problems were potential side effects of psychotropic drugs (falls, hyperglycemia, hypotension, hyponatremia, nausea, constipation, leukopenia), pain symptoms, and respiratory and urinary tract infections. These findings made possible the elaboration of a realistic, evidence-based curriculum for enhancing the medical knowledge of psychiatrists. The curriculum is presented here as the first evidence-based overview of medicine for psychiatrists in training or practice.

This book is organized to reflect the realities confronting clinicians who work in self-standing inpatient psychiatric settings. We modified the traditional organ-system approach by grouping some of the topics according to a common feature, such as cardiac arrest, abnormal vital signs, pain, signs of common infections, and respiratory distress. The presentations are structured to discuss essential features in clinical presentation, differential diagnosis, risk stratification, and management in the psychiatric setting. We concentrated our efforts on documenting the way in which psychiatric disorders and their treatment produce pathophysiological changes and change the classic presentation of common and serious conditions.

Our work is not intended to replace well-established print and electronic resources of medical knowledge; instead, we have created a new tool for the complex practice of psychiatry in the twenty-first century.

*Peter Manu, M.D.*

*Raymond E. Suarez, M.D.*

*Barbara J. Barnett, M.D.*

## References

Accreditation Council for Graduate Medical Education: Program Requirements for Residency Training in Psychiatry. February 2000. Available at: http://www.acgme.org. Accessed May 8, 2003.

Felker B, Yazel JJ, Short D: Mortality and medical comorbidity among psychiatric patients: a review. Psychiatr Serv 47:1356–1363, 1996

Goldman LS: Comorbid medical illness in psychiatric patients. Curr Psychiatry Rep 2:256–263, 2000

Krummel S, Kathol RG: What you should know about physical evaluations in psychiatric patients. Gen Hosp Psychiatry 9:275–279, 1987

Marder SR, Essock SM, Miller AL, et al: Physical health monitoring of patients with schizophrenia. Am J Psychiatry 161:1334–1349, 2004

Sternberg D: Testing for physical illness in psychiatric patients. J Clin Psychiatry 47 (suppl 1):3–9, 1986

Thompson TL, Byyny RL: The Education of the General Internist. Denver, University of Colorado School of Medicine, 1982, pp 221–229

# PART I

# Cardiac Arrest and Airway Obstruction

Section Editors:

Jennifer Muneyyirci, M.D.

Barbara J. Barnett, M.D.

# CHAPTER 1

# Cardiac Arrest

## Catalina Vazquez, M.D.

## Clinical Presentation

Cardiac arrest encompasses a spectrum of presentations, from the patient who suddenly clutches his or her chest and collapses to the choking patient.

*Ventricular tachycardia* is defined as a rapid heart beat—usually faster than 120 beats per minute—that originates from a ventricular focus. Because the ventricles contract independently of the atria, there is no coordination between atrial emptying and ventricular filling. In ventricular tachycardia, this lack of coordination results in ineffective filling of the left ventricle and, thus, diminished cardiac output. Ventricular tachycardia is usually initiated by a series of premature ventricular contractions and is characterized on an electrocardiogram (ECG) as a tachycardia with wide QRS complexes. Ventricular tachycardia may be classified as monomorphic (a regular rhythm arising from only one focus with indistinguishable QRS complexes) or polymorphic (an irregular rhythm with QRS complexes of various morphologies). Ventricular tachycardia may be further classified by duration. Nonsustained ventricular tachycardia lasts less than 30 seconds, and sustained ventricular tachycardia has a longer duration. A variant of ventricular tachycardia is *torsades de pointes* (translated as "twisting of the points"), so named because of the appearance of the QRS complexes, which seem to undulate relative to the ECG baseline. Torsades de pointes is usually caused by drugs, such as Class IA antiarrhythmics and some antipsychotics, or by electrolyte imbalances (particularly hypomagnesemia and hypocalcemia) that prolong the ECG Q–T interval. Symptoms suggestive of ventricular tachycardia include palpitations, light-headedness, confusion, anxiety, diaphoresis, syncope, shortness of breath, seizures, and chest pain. These symptoms are the result of general hypoperfusion of the heart and brain.

| **TABLE 1-1.** Differential diagnosis of cardiac arrest |
| --- |

- Cardiac ischemia or infarction
- Occult poisoning
- Hypoxia
- Hyperkalemia
- Tension pneumothorax
- Occult blunt or penetrating trauma
- Massive internal bleeding
- Respiratory arrest due to obstructive or reactive airway disease
- Tracheal obstruction
- Opioid overdose
- Severe hypothermia
- Seizure

*Ventricular fibrillation* is defined as an abnormal heart rhythm that originates within the ventricles. If left untreated, ventricular fibrillation quickly leads to cardiac arrest. The condition is characterized by a highly disorganized and irregular pattern of ventricular contraction that results in ineffective pumping of blood to the rest of the body and thereby leads to decreased tissue perfusion and to hypoxia and complete hemodynamic collapse. This arrhythmia is usually encountered in acute myocardial ischemia, and risk factors for its development include history of coronary artery disease, severe congestive heart failure, congenital heart disease, cardiomyopathies, valvular disease, and recent cardiac surgery. Ventricular fibrillation is also found in patients who have been electrocuted or have sustained direct trauma to the heart.

## Differential Diagnosis

The clinician must assume that a patient who is unresponsive, not breathing, and without a palpable pulse is experiencing cardiac arrest. Other conditions that may be considered in this scenario include acute respiratory arrest due to tracheal obstruction, severe hypothermia, status epilepticus, and toxic overdoses (particularly of opioids) (Table 1–1).

## Risk Stratification

Patients at risk for developing sudden cardiac arrest have a history of coronary artery disease, valvular heart disease, myocarditis, cardiomyopathy, recent cardiac surgery, congenital heart disease, end-stage renal

**TABLE 1–2.**  Action algorithm/primary ABCD survey (basic cardiopulmonary resuscitation [CPR] and defibrillation) for initial treatment of a patient with cardiac arrest

- Check if the patient is responsive
- Call code team (or 911)
- Call for defibrillator and crash cart

**Airway**: Open the airway (look, listen, and feel); use jaw thrust, chin lift maneuver.

**Breathing**: Provide positive pressure ventilations; give two slow breaths; use bag-valve-mask device with tight seal around nose and mouth.

**Circulation**: Begin chest compressions for 1 minute (ratio of two ventilations for every 15 compressions); continue CPR until defibrillator becomes available.

**Defibrillation**: Attach monitor, assess for ventricular fibrillation/pulseless ventricular tachycardia. If ventricular fibrillation/pulseless ventricular tachycardia is found, shock up to three times (monophasic 200 J, 300 J, 360 J). If no response, provide CPR for 1 minute and reassess for ventricular fibrillation/pulseless ventricular tachycardia. If no electrical activity is detected, search for and treat underlying causes.

disease, chronic lung disease, pulmonary embolism, or trauma. Others at risk include patients who abuse drugs (particularly cocaine) and anyone currently taking antiarrhythmic medication.

## Assessment and Management in Psychiatric Settings

In 1991, the term "chain of survival" was created to help laypersons and healthcare workers understand the sequence of events that could lead to improved outcomes for persons with cardiac arrest (Cummins et al. 1991). The chain of survival has four links: early access (recognizing and responding to a cardiac emergency), early cardiopulmonary resuscitation (CPR), early defibrillation (for ventricular fibrillation and pulseless ventricular tachycardia), and early advanced cardiac life support maneuvers and medications (Table 1–2).

When cardiac arrest is suspected, it is necessary to first confirm that the person is unresponsive by gently shaking the person and shouting, "Are you OK?" If there is any evidence of trauma (for example, if others witnessed the person fall or if there are external signs of bleeding), the person should not be shaken but should be gently touched and spoken to. If it is determined that the patient is unresponsive, one should immediately call for help. In the community, the emergency medical service should be activated by calling 911; in the hospital, one should initiate a "code" and ask for the "crash cart" and automated external defibrillator (AED), if one is available.

Early CPR begins with proper positioning of the patient and the rescuer. If the patient is not positioned on a hard surface, every attempt should be made to gently move the patient onto his or her back with a firm support such as a backboard. If there is any question of cervical spine injury, the goal is to maintain the head, neck, and trunk in line without applying any traction while moving the patient. After the patient is properly positioned, the primary survey, including evaluation of the ABCDs (airway, breathing, circulation, defibrillation), is conducted.

## Airway

The first step should be to open the patient's mouth and inspect the airway for any foreign body. The basic head tilt and chin lift maneuver involves putting one hand on the patient's forehead and placing two fingers of the other hand under the bony part of the chin and gently lifting up. This movement lifts the tongue off the airway and allows air to pass unobstructed (Allied Mobile Health Training 2004). If there is concern about cervical spine injury, the rescuer must provide the jaw-thrust maneuver by grasping the mandible of the jaw with the fingertips while the hands are placed on the sides of the patient's face. The mandible is then lifted forward to relieve any obstruction (Cummins 1997).

## Breathing

The rescuer then looks, listens, and feels for any respirations by looking at the patient's chest to see if it is rising and falling, listening for sounds of breathing, and feeling the patient's breath on his or her cheek. All three steps should be done simultaneously (Allied Mobile Health Training 2004). If no respirations are detected or if they are agonal and sporadic, the rescuer should provide positive pressure ventilations to the patient either by using a bag-valve-mask device or by pinching the nose and delivering two slow, full breaths over a period of 2 seconds each. When a bag-valve-mask device is used, caution must be exercised to ensure a tight seal around the patient's nose and mouth to minimize gastric distention and the chance for regurgitation and aspiration of stomach contents. The adequacy of ventilations can be gauged by the symmetric rise and fall of the chest cavity.

## Circulation

Once two breaths have been successfully delivered to the patient, the rescuer should perform a pulse check. In adults, the pulse check is done by placing two fingers over the carotid artery (roughly two finger-breadths below the angle of the mandible and adjacent to the trachea). The pulse check should last at least 5–10 seconds. If no pulse is detected, 15 chest compressions should be delivered immediately to the patient. In children, after delivery of two rescue breaths, the healthcare provider checks for the following: breathing, coughing, movement, and a pulse (in an infant, brachial pulse; in a child, carotid pulse). Depth of compression varies depending on the child's age. Generally the rescuer should be positioned next to the victim's chest cavity and should place two fingers over the patient's xiphoid notch. The heel of the other hand is then placed next to the two fingers, and the other hand clasps the heel over the lower half of the sternum. Keeping elbows locked straight and using the hips as a fulcrum, the rescuer should compress roughly 1.5–2 inches deep to provide adequate chest compressions. CPR is then continued with the ratio of two ventilations for every 15 chest compressions, until a defibrillator is available at the scene.

## Defibrillation

If the patient shows signs of impaired tissue perfusion, such as chest pain, shortness of breath, low or absent blood pressure, or altered level of consciousness, it is imperative that the patient undergo synchronized cardioversion with at least 200 J of electrical energy. The defibrillator must be switched to the synchronization mode to avoid delivering the shock during the ventricular repolarization phase.

Electrical defibrillation is the definitive treatment for ventricular fibrillation and pulseless ventricular tachycardia. CPR alone cannot defibrillate the heart. If an AED is immediately available on the scene, CPR should be interrupted so that the AED can be used to assess the patient for ventricular fibrillation and pulseless ventricular tachycardia. The reason for this assessment is that ventricular fibrillation is the most frequent underlying rhythm in patients who *survive* cardiac arrest. For every minute that the heart remains in ventricular fibrillation, the chance for survival decreases by 2%–10% (Eisenberg and Mengert 2001).

The AED should first be turned on, and then the adhesive defibrillator pads should be placed on the patient (one in the right upper quadrant of the chest cavity and the other typically over the cardiac apex or adjacent to the nipple line underneath the axilla). The AED will then analyze the rhythm and announce, "Shock indicated," if ventricular fibrillation or ventricular tachycardia is detected. The rescuer must then press the shock button, stand clear of the patient, and verify that all other personnel are clear of the patient as well. The AED will then deliver the shock. These steps should be continued until the AED announces, "No shock indicated," in which case the rescuer should check for signs of spontaneous circulation and continue CPR, if indicated, until advanced cardiac life support can be initiated.

Manual or conventional defibrillators are used in a similar sequence; however, the user must initiate all steps, beginning with turning on the device, selecting 200 J of energy to start, setting the lead select switch to "paddles," placing adhesive pads on the patient, positioning the paddles over the sternum and apex of the patient, assessing the rhythm displayed on the monitor for ventricular fibrillation or pulseless ventricular tachycardia, and, if indicated, announcing to all present that the defibrillator is being charged. After pressing the charge button on the apex paddle and allowing sufficient time for the device to charge, the rescuer should announce, "I'm going to shock on three. One, I'm clear (the rescuer should check that he or she is not in contact with the patient or equipment); two, you're clear (the rescuer should check that no one else is in contact with the patient); and three, everyone's clear" (the rescuer should check again that he or she is not in contact with the patient before administering the shock). Twenty-five pounds of pressure should be applied to the paddles, and the discharge buttons should be pressed simultaneously. At this time the rescuer must look at the monitor, assess for ventricular fibrillation and pulseless ventricular tachycardia again, and immediately recharge the device and repeat all steps. This sequence should be repeated with escalating shocks at 200 J, 300 J, and 360 J. As with the AED, if no shock is indicated, the rescuer must check for spontaneous circulation and continue CPR until the final link in the chain of survival is activated (i.e., advanced cardiac life support is provided either by emergency medical service technicians or physicians trained in emergency medicine).

Table 1–3 lists clinical scenarios in which cardiac arrest may occur. If the cause can be determined with reasonable certainty, performing the maneuvers listed may indeed be lifesaving. It is important for all physicians to be familiar with and be able to recognize these potentially life-threatening conditions. Patients suspected of having hyperkalemia

**TABLE 1–3.** Causes of cardiac arrest: clinical scenarios and treatments

| Cause | Clinical scenario | Treatment |
|-------|-------------------|-----------|
| Coronary thrombosis | History of coronary artery disease | Emergent cardiac catheterization, thrombolytic therapy |
| Hypoxia | Airway obstruction, inadequate oxygenation and ventilations | Check airway positioning, check for foreign body obstruction and adequacy of ventilations |
| Pulmonary embolism | Risk factors for hypercoagulable states | Thrombolytic therapy, embolectomy |
| Toxic substance (overdose) | Toxidrome, alcohol abuse, psychiatric disease, altered mental status | Consider specific antidotes (e.g., intravenous bicarbonate for tricyclic overdose) |
| Hydrogen ion-acidosis | End-stage renal disease, diabetes, prolonged resuscitation, toxins | Check adequacy of cardiopulmonary resuscitation (CPR), consider intravenous bicarbonate |
| Hyperkalemia | End-stage renal disease, diabetes, extensive tissue injury, rhabdomyolysis | 1. 10% calcium chloride solution (10 mL slow iv) (avoid in patients taking digoxin)<br>2. Glucose (50 mL D5W) and regular insulin (10 units iv)<br>3. Bicarbonate (50 mmol iv) |
| Hypokalemia | Diabetes, poor nutrition, alcohol abuse, toxins | Intravenous potassium |
| Hypovolemia | Low blood pressure, shock, major bleeding, burns, or trauma | Volume infusion, transfusion of packed red cells if there are signs of hemorrhage |
| Tamponade | History of recent chest trauma or surgery | Emergent pericardiocentesis |

*Source.* Adapted from Marill and Williamson 2002.

should receive calcium chloride (provided that they are not taking digoxin), D50, insulin, and bicarbonate. Patients with these conditions should be transferred to the nearest emergency care facility so that further diagnosis and treatment are not delayed.

# References

Allied Mobile Health Training: Health Care Provider Study Guide. Available at: http://www.learncpr.com. Accessed January 6, 2004.

Cummins RO (ed): Advanced Cardiac Life Support. Dallas, TX, American Heart Association, 1997

Cummins RO, Ornato JP, Thies WH, et al: Improving survival from sudden cardiac arrest: the "chain of survival" concept: a statement for health professionals from the Advanced Cardiac Life Support Subcommittee and the Emergency Cardiac Care Committee, American Heart Association. Circulation 83:1832–1847, 1991

Eisenberg MS, Mengert TJ: Cardiac resuscitation. N Engl J Med 344:1304–1313, 2001

Marill KA, Williamson S: Cardiac arrest: current concepts, controversies, and evidence. Emergency Medicine Practice 4:1–24, 2002

# CHAPTER 2

# Choking and Laryngospasm

## Stephanie M. Reynolds, D.O.

## Choking

### Clinical Presentation

Choking is defined as the prevention of respiration by compression or obstruction of the airway. A recent study showed that a psychiatric patient receiving neuroleptics had a 90-times greater risk of choking and a patient receiving lithium had a 30-times greater risk of choking, compared with a healthy individual (Ruschena and Mullen 2003). The presentation of choking can be quite dramatic, and, without treatment, the patient rapidly goes from air hunger to cyanosis and, finally, death.

During normal swallowing a bolus of food or a foreign body is propelled backward by the tongue into the pharynx where the voluntary muscles constrict to move the bolus further backward toward the esophagus. While food is traveling downward, the epiglottis bends backward to cover the inlet of the larynx. This act prevents food from entering the trachea and lungs.

Certain actions by an otherwise healthy individual interfere with this process and result in choking. Taking a deep breath while swallowing or trying to speak or laugh opens the vocal cords and lifts the epiglottis simultaneously, allowing the bolus to travel into the airway. If a person who has experienced a cardiovascular accident, with the resulting paralysis of the gag reflex, attempts to swallow, the normal process of bolus propulsion does not occur, and the item can become lodged in the pharynx. When this happens, the patient begins to panic and may emit sounds such as gasps, wheezes, whistles, or stridor. Stridor is a

11

**TABLE 2–1.**   Causes of choking

| Foreign body aspiration | Trauma | Psychiatric disorders |
|---|---|---|
| **Infectious causes** | Accidental | Bradykinetic dysphagia |
| Diphtheria | Self-inflicted | Fast eating syndrome |
| Epiglottitis | **Acute edema** | **Drug-induced dysphagia** |
| Croup | Anaphylactic | Anticholinergics |
| Retropharyngeal abscess | Angioedema | Neuroleptics |
| Laryngitis | **Positioning** | |
| | Supine | |

high-pitched respiratory sound transmitted from the upper airway when it is partly obstructed and air is forced through a small opening.

## Differential Diagnosis

Airway obstruction can have various causes, including presence of a foreign body, infection, trauma, acute edema, psychiatric disorders, and patient positioning (Table 2–1).

*Foreign bodies* cause the majority of cases of choking and include a variety of objects, such as buttons, coins, balloons, chicken bones, and pieces of steak.

*Infections* can also cause airway obstruction. Croup, a viral infection also known as laryngotracheobronchitis, is an inflammation of the subglottic space caused by parainfluenza virus, respiratory syncitial virus, rhinovirus, and influenza A or B viruses. Croup manifests as a brassy, "seal barking" cough and inspiratory stridor, causing respiratory distress that can progress slowly or acutely. Signs of distress include labored breathing, subcostal retractions, and cyanosis that can be evident in a physical examination (Orenstein 2000). Croup generally occurs in children from ages 6 months to 3 years, but it has been reported in adults. Epiglottitis is a rare and often fatal viral cause of airway obstruction due to *Haemophilus influenzae* type B. Until recently, with the use of *Haemophilus influenzae* vaccine, epiglottitis was a predominately pediatric disease, but it is now more frequently encountered in the adult population. It manifests with sudden onset of high fever, severe dysphagia, and muffled voice and can rapidly progress to death. If epiglottitis is suspected, the healthcare provider should visually examine the oropharynx but not manipulate it. The oropharynx in a patient with epiglottitis can appear normal. Like croup, *laryngitis* may also be associated with influenza A and B viruses. Bacterial infections may cause airway obstruction in cases of pharyngeal or retropharyngeal abscesses. The etiology is usually group A *Streptococcus* or *Staphylococcus aureus*, and there is a prodrome of a preceding pharyngitis or otitis, fever, neck pain, and dysphagia (Melio 2002). The infection seeds itself in the space behind the pharynx in the precervical area. It may cause anterior swelling into the oropharynx, thus resulting in airway compromise and obstruction.

*Trauma* from a blow to the neck, a rope impression from a hanging attempt, or a forearm around the neck during restraint of a combative patient can collapse the trachea and obstruct the airway. A thorough history must be obtained when a patient has been involved in an altercation. Careful monitoring of the patient's respiratory status and oxygenation levels must be done if tracheal injury is suspected. The airway can swell quickly, and it may be difficult or impossible to control the airway once swelling has occurred.

*Inhalation burns*, both thermal and chemical, scorch the delicate airway tissues and cause fluid shifting into the soft spaces. Airway burns can come from hot gases released in a fire or from ingestion of corrosive substances such as gasoline or acids. These burns may not be easily visible at first, and the healthcare provider should look for clues such as singed eyebrow and nose hairs, hoarseness, a muffled voice, and oral lesions.

*Anaphylactic reactions* resulting in airway closure from laryngeal edema can be fatal. In an anaphylactic reaction, release of histamine results in an increase in vascular permeability, leading to soft tissue swelling. Triggers for allergic reactions include various foods, bee stings, exposure to latex, and medications (especially penicillin). *Angioedema* is a swelling of the face, airway, or extremities. Angioedema can be inherited or acquired (especially with use of angiotensin-converting enzyme [ACE] inhibitors), and either type can result in airway compromise. As in anaphylactic reactions, a trigger sets off a cascade of fluid shifting into the airway tissues; if the patient is not treated, this condition rapidly progresses to total occlusion of the airway and death (Schwartz 2004).

*Positional asphyxia* occurs when an individual is placed face down and restrained or when an individual under the influence of drugs or alcohol can no longer adequately protect his or her airway and may not be able to call out for help (Chicago Reporter 1999). When a patient is restrained, measures must be taken so that the person does not choke or aspirate. A restrained patient should never be placed in a prone position or left unattended where he or she can inadvertently maneuver to a dependent position and asphyxiate. Patients with altered level of consciousness should not be left supine.

*Drug-induced dysphagia* is a common cause of choking among psychiatric patients. *Bradykinetic dysphagia*, which is directly related to neuroleptic-induced extrapyramidal syndrome, predisposes patients to choking because of delayed swallowing (Bazemore et al. 1991). Many psychiatric patients, particularly those with acute psychotic episodes or mental retardation, have *fast eating syndrome*, which involves ingestion of large quantities of food in a short period of time and may increase the risk of choking.

## Risk Stratification

Certain groups of individuals are considered at risk for choking related to ingestion of a foreign body. They include especially those with impaired or immature swallowing reflexes, such as children, mentally retarded persons, persons intoxicated with drugs or alcohol, restrained patients, stroke patients, psychiatric patients, and people who wear dentures (Fioritti et al. 1997).

Psychiatric patients are at risk because medication-related side effects can suppress some of the body's natural defense systems for choking. Neuroleptics, antidepressants,and antiparkinsonian medications are often used in combination, compounding the drugs' anticholinergic effects and resulting in loss of gag and swallowing reflexes (Fioritti et al. 1997).

## Assessment and Management in Psychiatric Settings

If a patient experiences a partial airway obstruction, he or she may still be able to speak or cough forcefully. No one should physically interfere with the patient, and the patient should be verbally encouraged to expel the foreign body by forceful coughing. As long as the patient is adequately able to exchange air, the patient's efforts should be supported and he or she should not be left alone. The patient will either expel the object, or the partial obstruction will deteriorate into complete obstruction.

With complete obstruction, the patient will quickly become hypoxic and agitated, and within 1 minute the individual will become cyanotic and then unconscious. Thus, it is important to distinguish whether a choking patients needs physical intervention or verbal encouragement. The patient may become combative, but it is important to look the patient in the face and determine if he or she actually has an airway obstruction. After determining that the patient actually has an airway obstruction, the clinician should offer assistance and send someone for help. Table 2–2 and Table 2–3 list procedures for clearing a patient's airway of a foreign body.

**TABLE 2–2.**    Clearing the airway of a foreign body in an awake patient

- Determine that the patient is actually choking. The patient who is actually choking is *unable to speak or cough and does not demonstrate movement of air.*
- Look the patient in the face, and tell him or her that you are there to help.
- *Do not slap the patient on the back!*
- Stand behind the choking patient, wrap your arms around the patient's waist, and find the umbilicus and xiphoid.
- Make your left hand into a closed fist, and place it inside your right hand halfway between the umbilicus and xiphoid with the left thumb pressed against the abdomen.
- Deliver quick inward and upward thrusts, driving your fist under the ribcage and upward toward the shoulder blades.
- Continue this action until the airway is cleared or the patient collapses into unconsciousness.

**TABLE 2–3.**    Clearing the airway of a foreign body in an unconscious patient

- Lay the person on the floor on his or her back.
- Open the airway with a head tilt/chin lift. Place one hand on the forehead and two fingers from the other hand under the chin. Lift upward with the two fingers. This action moves the lower jaw forward and moves the tongue out of the airway. With the other hand pressing on the forehead, tilt the head backward.
- Look into the mouth for the obstructing object. If it is seen, remove it; if no object is seen, sweep the mouth with two fingers to clear any unseen objects from the airway.
- Straddle across the patient's hips, facing the patient's upper body.
- Clasp your hands together one on top of the other with the palmar surface toward the abdomen. Place your hands halfway between the umbilicus and xiphoid.
- Give four upward thrusts.
- Move to the head, and sweep the mouth with two fingers to see if the object can be removed.
- Attempt to ventilate the patient by pinching the nose and blowing in the mouth.
- Repeat these steps until the airway is clear or help has arrived.
- If prolonged attempts to clear the airway have been made, once the airway is clear, check for a pulse. If no pulse is found, proceed with cardiopulmonary resuscitation (refer to Chapter 1 in this volume, "Cardiac Arrest").

---

**TABLE 2–4.**    Causes of laryngospasm

---

- Hyperventilation
- Electroconvulsive therapy
- Dystonic reaction to neuroleptic medications
- Hypocalcemia
- Hypersensitivity reaction
- Anaphylaxis
- Gastroesophageal reflux disease

---

After the patient's airway is cleared, the patient should receive a medical evaluation, because there may have been considerable trauma and swelling to the airway or the thrusts may have caused intra-abdominal injury. These injuries may not be initially evident, but they can cause significant problems if left untreated.

After the crisis has been resolved, the patient may need to be evaluated to determine what caused the choking. A modified barium swallow examination with videofluoroscopy and a consultation to evaluate the patient's speech and swallowing functions must be performed without delay. In the meantime, the patient should receive a diet of pureed food with thickened fluid and should be monitored carefully at mealtimes.

## Laryngospasm

### Clinical Presentation

Laryngospasm is a spasmodic closure of the glottic aperture that can result from direct glottic or supraglottic stimulation from inhaled agents, secretions, or foreign bodies. It can be confused with choking because of the apnea that it causes.

### Differential Diagnosis

Laryngospasm can result from hyperventilation, electroconvulsive therapy (ECT), and dystonic reactions to certain neuroleptic medications (Table 2–4).

With *hyperventilation*, the patient develops tetany of the larynx muscles. The patient is able to breathe out but finds it very difficult to breathe in deeply. A hyperventilating patient who is calmed has no adverse or ill effects from the hyperventilation. A rare and dangerous side effect of ECT is posttreatment laryngospasm (National Institutes of Health 1985). Patients can develop laryngospastic *dystonia* after long-term use of certain neuroleptic medications, such as haloperidol, prochlorperazine, chlorpromazine, metoclopramide, and promethazine. Typically laryngospastic dystonia involves contractions of the involuntary muscles or clumsiness of the voluntary muscles. It may become a life-threatening side effect when it involves the larynx and vocal cords. A patient taking neuroleptics who presents with sudden onset of respiratory distress may be experiencing laryngospasm.

## Risk Stratification

Certain patients with long-term neuroleptic use are at risk for dystonias and resulting laryngospasm. Also a small group of patients who have demonstrated hypersensitivity to certain anesthetics have been known to experience laryngospasm in the recovery room after surgery. Electrolyte imbalances such as hypocalcemia can predispose patients to laryngospasm.

## Assessment and Management in Psychiatric Settings

For laryngospasm caused by hyperventilation or nonorganic causes, panting—rapid, shallow breathing performed at the onset of the laryngospasm attack—has been shown to successfully abort attacks (Pitchenik 1991).

For laryngospasm from ECT, oxygenation should be provided by means of a bag-valve-mask with a tight seal over the nose and mouth. It is important to use 100% oxygen from a wall outlet or oxygen tank. The patient should be in a controlled setting with all necessary resuscitation equipment at hand. The emergency medical service should be called for immediate assistance, if necessary.

For dystonic reactions, the common treatment is 50 mg of diphenhydramine administered immediately either intramuscularly or intravenously and discontinuation of the offending neuroleptic agent. Benztropine (1–2 mg im), as well as lorazepam (2 mg im), can also be given but not as a first-line treatment. For patients with known sensitivity to neuroleptic agents, pretreatment with diphenhydramine should be considered.

As an initial measure for dystonic laryngospasm, the patient should be admitted to the hospital and monitored for 24–48 hours. At discharge another antipsychotic should be prescribed. Delayed hypersensitivity reactions can occur 6–10 hours after the offending agent has been discontinued, so vigilance should be maintained, especially for inpatients who have recently been exposed to anesthesia.

A thorough screening program should be implemented for all inpatient facilities to identify which patients are at risk for laryngospasm. The screening should include a review of all relevant medical files, including records of any recent exposure to anesthetic agents, surgeries, and allergic reactions. Patients who undergo ECT should be in a closely monitored setting so that laryngospasm can be prevented or quickly treated.

## References

Bazemore PH, Tonkonogy J, Ananth R: Dysphagia in psychiatric patients: clinical and videofluoroscopic study. Dysphagia 6:2–5, 1991

Chicago Reporter: Chicago Police Training Bulletin on Positional Asphyxia. March 1999. Available at: http://chicagoreporter.com/1999/03–99/0399position.htm. Accessed March 2004.

Fioritti A, Giaccotto L, Melega V: Choking incidents among psychiatric patients: retrospective analysis of thirty-one cases from the west Bologna psychiatric wards. Can J Psychiatry 42:515–520, 1997

Melio FR: Upper respiratory infections, in Rosen's Emergency Medicine: Concepts and Clinical Practice, 5th Edition. Edited by Marx JA, Hockberger RS, Walls RM, et al. St. Louis, MO, Mosby, 2002, pp 978–996

National Institutes of Health: Electroconvulsive therapy. NIH Consensus Statement 5(11):1–23, 1985

Orenstein D: Bronchiolitis, in Nelson Essentials of Pediatrics, 16th Edition. Edited by Behrman RE, Kliegman RM, Jenson H. Philadelphia, PA, WB Saunders, 2000, pp 1279–1282

Pitchenik AE: Functional laryngeal obstruction relieved by panting. Chest 100:1465–1467, 1991

Ruschena D, Mullen PE: Choking deaths: the role of antipsychotic medication. Br J Psychiatry 183:446–450, 2003

Schwartz LB: Systemic anaphylaxis, in Cecil Textbook of Medicine, 22nd Edition. Edited by Goldman L, Ausiello D. Philadelphia, PA, WB Saunders, 2004, pp 1616–1618

# PART II

# Abnormal Vital Signs

Section Editor:

Pamela Arsove, M.D.

# CHAPTER 3

# Fever

## David Shih, M.D.

## Clinical Presentation

*Fever* is the elevation of core body temperature above normal. The normal temperature range depends on the time of day and is controlled by the thermoregulatory center located in the anterior hypothalamus (Blum 2002; Dale 2004; Dinarello and Gelfand 2005). Under normal circumstances, core body temperature (defined as the temperature of the blood in the right atrium) is tightly regulated to match the hypothalamic set-point temperature, traditionally 98.6°F (37°C). Fever occurs when a rise of the core temperature is secondary to the hypothalamic regulatory mechanisms, elevating the set-point. Rectal temperatures closely reflect core temperature and are generally 1°F (0.6°C) higher than oral temperatures (Blum 2002). *Hyperthermia* is the elevation of body temperature without elevation of the hypothalamic set-point. Causes of hyperthermia include insufficient heat dissipation, excessive heat production, and loss of regulation. Hyperthermia is usually associated with vigorous exercise, a hot environment, dehydration, or use of drugs (Delaney 2001; Dinarello and Gelfand 2005). *Fever of undetermined origin* (FUO) is a febrile illness of more than 3 weeks' duration in which the patient's temperature exceeds 101°F (38.3°C) on several determinations and no diagnosis is reached after 1 week of intensive evaluation (Dinarello and Gelfand 2005).The differential diagnosis of FUO includes infections (approximately 30%), neoplastic causes (30%), inflammatory disorders (15%), and miscellaneous conditions (15%–20%).

## Differential Diagnosis

### Causes of Fever

*Infections*

The most common cause of fever is an infectious process. Common infectious etiologies for fever are listed in Table 3–1. The most common causes of fever are upper respiratory illnesses, urinary tract infections, cellulitis, superficial abscesses, and pneumonia.

In general, patients with pneumonia and upper respiratory infection present with a history of fever, cough, and respiratory complaint. Treatment is dependent on the nature of the illness, comorbid factors, and suspected etiological organism.

Pathological conditions that may require surgery, such as appendicitis, cholecystitis, or diverticulitis, may be suspected in a patient with fever, abdominal pain, nausea, vomiting, diarrhea, or abnormal liver function test results. These patients may require additional tests such as a sonogram, computerized tomography (CT) scan, or hepatobiliary iminodiacetic acid (HIDA) scan, and surgical consultation in the emergency department may be needed for those patients.

Patients with altered mental status, fever, neck stiffness, photophobia, headache, and rash should be immediately suspected of having meningitis. These patients require isolation, immediate broad-spectrum intravenous antibiotics, and a lumbar puncture. Common organisms include *Streptococcus pneumoniae, Haemophilus influenzae, Neisseria meningitidis,* and viral organisms. *Listeria monocytogenes* and resistant *S. pneumoniae* must also be addressed with antibiotics.

Patients who appear ill with fever, chills, tachycardia, and symptoms of congestive heart failure (dyspnea, frothy sputum, and chest pain) may have endocarditis. A physical examiation may show new heart murmur, retinal hemorrhage (Roth's spots), nodules on fingers or toes (Osler's nodes), and plaques on the palms and feet (Janeway lesions). These patients require multiple blood cultures, appropriate intravenous antibiotics, an echocardiogram, and admission to the hospital. Common organisms are *Streptococcus viridans, Staphylococcus aureus, Enterococcus faecalis,* and various fungal organisms.

Sepsis is found in patients with suspected bacterial infection who have fever, hypotension, tachycardia, tachypnea, and complete blood count (CBC) results indicating leukocytosis. Antipyretics, intravenous antibiotics, consultations, and additional tests may be needed, depending on the nature of the illness.

**TABLE 3–1.** Causes of fever

| Infection | Drug-related fevers, effects, toxicity |
|---|---|

**Infection**

Bacterial (e.g., pneumonia, urinary tract infection/pyelonephritis, upper respiratory infection, cellulitis, meningitis, endocarditis)

Conditions that may require surgery (e.g., appendicitis, cholecystitis, diverticulitis)

Abscess (hepatic, gallbladder, splenic, perinephric, pelvic, other sites)

Granulomatous (fungal infection, tuberculosis, atypical mycobacterial infection)

Viral (e.g., common cold, HIV, cytomegalovirus, infectious mononucleosis, hepatitis)

Rickettsial (e.g., Q fever, Rocky Mountain spotted fever)

Parasitic (e.g., extraintestinal amebiasis, malaria, toxoplasmosis)

Chlamydia, Lyme disease

**Noninfectious inflammatory disorders**

Collagen vascular disease (e.g., rheumatic fever, systemic lupus erythematosus, rheumatoid arthritis, Still's disease, vasculitis)

Granulomatous (e.g., sarcoidosis, Crohn's disease, granulomatous hepatitis)

Tissue injury (e.g., pulmonary embolism, deep vein thrombosis, sickle cell disease, hemolytic anemia)

**Neoplastic disease**

Lymphoma/leukemia (e.g., Hodgkin's and non-Hodgkin's lymphoma, acute leukemia, myelodysplastic syndrome)

Carcinoma (e.g., of the kidney, pancreas, liver, gastrointestinal tract, lung, especially if metastatic)

Central nervous system tumors

**Drug-related fevers, effects, toxicity**

Antibiotics

Antiarrhythmics

Antihypertensives

Anticonvulsants

Anticholinergics, tricyclic antidepressants

Antipsychotics, lithium

Salicylate

Sympathomimetics (e.g., cocaine, phencyclidine, amphetamines)

Thyroid hormone

Ethanol

Pain medications

**Endocrine disorder**

Pheochromocytoma

Thyroid storm

Acute adrenal insufficiency

Gout

**Factitious disease**

Injection of toxic material

Manipulation of thermometer

**Hyperthermia**

Neuroleptic malignant syndrome

Malignant hyperthermia

Heatstroke

**Other causes**

Familial Mediterranean fever

Hematomas

Transfusion reactions

Transplant rejection

*Source.*   Adapted from Dinarello and Gelfand 2005 and Berkowitz 2000.

## Noninfectious Inflammatory Disease

Thromboembolic disease has been responsible for as many as 6% of FUO cases. Both deep vein thrombosis and pulmonary embolism can cause fevers.

The symptoms of collagen vascular diseases that may cause fever, such as rheumatoid arthritis and systemic lupus erythematosus, are usually well recognized by the physician in a primary care setting. However, temporal arteritis can present with fever with no clinical symptoms. In geriatric patients, temporal arteritis can manifest as little more than unexplained fever, prolonged malaise, depression, or anemia. The erythrocyte sedimentation rate is usually markedly elevated (>50 mm/hour). Because blindness is a potential complication, the diagnosis of temporal arteritis should be actively pursued with arterial biopsy. The disorder should be treated with corticosteroid therapy.

## Neoplastic Disease

Fever is a well-recognized manifestation of malignant neoplasms, especially those originating in the hematopoietic system or those with metastases to the liver. A number of mechanisms have been proposed for the cause of such fevers, including tumor necrosis, inflammation, and increased heat production from the tumor cells themselves. Current evidence points to production of pyrogenic cytokines such as interleukin (IL)-1 and tumor necrosis factor (TNF)-$\alpha$ (Dinarello and Gelfand 2005). Numerous studies have identified lymphomas as the neoplasms most commonly associated with FUO.

Patients with neutropenia and fever should be aggressively treated, and the source actively pursued. Because of the potential consequence of death in 24–48 hours, broad-coverage antibiotic therapy should be started immediately.

## Drug-Related Fever

Drug-related fever accounts for 10%–15% of unexplained fevers in hospitalized patients in the United States (Cunha 2001). It is defined as a febrile or hypersensitivity reaction to medications. Fever can occur as a result of endotoxin release in response to antibiotic therapy or the lysis of cells in chemotherapy. Table 3–2 lists drugs that are frequently implicated in drug-related fever. Drug-related fever can occur with any antibiotic but is commonly found with β-lactams and sulfonamides. Fever may also occur with antiviral, antifungal, and antiparasitic medications. Other common causes of drug-related fever include diuretics, antisei-

**TABLE 3–2.**   Drugs implicated in drug-related fevers

| Antibiotics | Antihypertensives/ antiarrhythmics | Pain medications |
|---|---|---|
| Penicillins | **antiarrhythmics** | Nonsteroidal anti- |
| Sulfonamides | β-Blockers | inflammatory drugs |
| Cephalosporins | Calcium channel | Narcotics (e.g., meperidine) |
| Nitrofurantoin | blockers | Sleep medications |
| Isoniazid and other | Diuretics | **Chemotherapy** |
| antituberculosis | Angiotensin-converting | Asparaginase |
| medications | enzyme inhibitors | Bleomycin |
| Quinidine | Nifedipine | **Others** |
| Amphotericin B | Hydralazine | Heparin |
| Azathioprine | Procainamide | Iodides |
| Aminoglycosides | Atropine | Allopurinol |
| Clindamycin | **Antiseizure/** | Thiouracil (PTU) |
| Chloramphenicol | **psychotropic** | |
| Linezolid | **medications** | |
| Macrolides | Barbiturates | |
| Tetracyclines | Methyldopa | |
| Vancomycin | Phenytoins | |

*Source.*   Adapted from Cunha 2001 and Berkowitz 2000.

zure medications, antiarrhythmics, sedatives, antihypertensives, and pain medications (Cunha 2001). The diagnosis of drug-related fever generally is a diagnosis of exclusion that is made after negative blood culture findings are obtained and other explanations for the fever are ruled out.

Drug-related fever is usually characterized by fever ≥102°F, with a usual range of 102–106°F (Cunha 2001); relative bradycardia is often present. Most patients look relatively well for the degree of fever and do not present with shaking chills unless antipyretics have been given.

Transient elevations of serum transaminase levels with eosinophils in the peripheral smears may be suggestive of drug-related fevers (Cunha 2001). Other findings include rash, hemolysis, or bone marrow suppression. Some patients may present with a serum sickness–like syndrome with rash, lymphadenopathy, arthritis, nephritis, and edema along with fever. Others may present with a systemic lupus erythematosus–like syndrome characterized by fever, arthralgias, and positive findings on the antinuclear antibody test. However, the diagnosis of drug-related fever is made when there is a decrease in temperature and transient improvement after the offending substance is withheld. In

**TABLE 3–3.** Mechanisms of drug-induced hyperthermia and drugs that cause hyperthermia

| Increased muscular activity | Impaired thermoregulation |
|---|---|
| Amphetamines | Ethanol |
| Antipsychotics, lithium (associated with neuroleptic malignant syndrome) | Phenothiazines |
| Cocaine | **Impaired heat dissipation** |
| Halothane, succinylcholine (associated with malignant hyperthermia) | Antihistamines |
| Lysergic acid diethylamide (LSD) | Phenothiazines |
| Monoamine oxidase inhibitors | Tricyclic antidepressants |
| Tricyclic antidepressants | |
| (PCP) | |
| **Increased metabolic rate** | |
| Salicylate | |
| Thyroid hormone | |

*Source.* Modified from Delaney 2001.

drug-related fever, the patient's temperature returns to near normal within 48–72 hours after discontinuing the medication.

### Drug Effects and Toxicity

Multiple medications and illicit drugs can produce hyperthermia when taken in excess (Table 3–3). Unlike drug-related fevers, these toxic effects are usually secondary to increased muscle activity, increased metabolic rate, impaired thermoregulation, and impaired heat dissipation (Delaney 2001), which can present as neuroleptic malignant syndrome (NMS), malignant hyperthermia, and febrile rhabdomyolysis.

### Factitious Fever

Factitious fever is commonly created by thermometer manipulation involving the use of external heat sources or substitute thermometers. Fraudulent fever by proxy has also been reported. In such cases, a mother manipulates the thermometer reading to create the impression of fever in her child. Others have induced fever by self-administration of pyrogenic agents, mostly consisting of bacterial suspensions. Although there may be some underlying psychiatric disorder in such cases, this practice is usually done for secondary gain.

Patients with factitious fever are generally women, approximately 50% of whom have training in health care, particularly nursing (Mackoviak and Durack 2000). Self-induced fevers are also found predominantly in women. Generally, patients with factitious fever are healthy in appearance and exhibit relative bradycardia during febrile episodes (Mackoviak and Durack 2000). They are unresponsive to antipyretics, and their laboratory test results are normal.

## Hyperthermia Syndromes

### Heatstroke

Heatstroke is a hyperthermia syndrome caused by failure of the thermoregulatory system in association with a warm environment. Heatstroke is classified as exertional or nonexertional (Dinarello and Gelfand 2005).

Exertional heatstroke is usually caused by exercise in an environment with higher than normal heat and/or humidity. It usually occurs in younger individuals during rigorous exercise without adequate hydration on hot days. Nonexertional heatstroke is more common in elderly persons, particularly during heat waves. Elderly patients at risk for nonexertional heatstroke are typically taking a medication that predisposes them to dehydration (anticholinergics, antihistamines, antiparkinsonian agents, diuretics, or phenothiazines) or a medication that may itself cause hyperthermia. These patients are at great risk of hyperthermia if they remain in a area with poor ventilation and no air conditioning (Dinarello and Gelfand 2005).

### Drug-Induced Hyperthermia

Drug-induced hyperthermia is a common side effect of psychotropic drugs such as tricyclic antidepressants and monoamine oxidase inhibitors and of stimulants, including amphetamine, cocaine, phencyclidine hydrochloride, and lysergic acid diethylamide (LSD) (see Table 3–3).

### Neuroleptic Malignant Syndrome

NMS is characterized by muscle rigidity, elevated temperature, altered mental status, and autonomic dysregulation and is associated with the use of neuroleptic medication. Signs of autonomic dysfunction in NMS include tachycardia, labile blood pressure, diaphoresis, vasoconstriction, and pallor. Motor dysfunction includes tremors, myoclonus, dystonia, dyskinesia, dysphagia, and dysarthria. Mental status changes can range from agitation to stupor to coma (Delaney 2001; Dinarello and Gelfand 2005).

*Malignant Hyperthermia*

Malignant hyperthermia is an abnormality of skeletal muscle sarcoplasmic reticulum leading to rapid increase of intracellular calcium levels in response to halothane and other inhalation anesthetics or succinylcholine. Hyperthermia and muscle rigidity are associated with malignant hyperthermia, making it difficult to distinguish from NMS.

## Risk Stratification

Greater caution is indicated for patients who are elderly, diabetic, immunocompromised, pregnant, or in postoperative recovery. Atypical symptoms with no localizing signs and symptoms are the rule in elderly and immunocompromised patients. A low threshold should be maintained for ancillary tests such as blood tests, radiograph, urinalysis, and lumbar puncture. Patients who are neutropenic, diabetic, or immunocompromised are at risk for rapid aggressive infection with a high level of morbidity and mortality. It is imperative that evaluation and empirical treatments be initiated with high priority for such patients.

## Assessment and Management in Psychiatric Settings

An algorithm that outlines the steps in assessment and management of fever is shown in Figure 3–1. In about 85% of cases of fever, the etiology may be determined by means of a history and physical examination (Blum 2002). Important historical facts are travel, social occupations, medication history, and social history. The timing and pattern of fever may offer more clues. It is also important to ascertain the risk of serious illness in a patient according to the patient's age or comorbid factors. The patient's rectal temperature, blood pressure, heart rate, respiratory rate, and pulse oximetry measurement must be obtained, and a fingerstick test and thorough physical examination must be performed. Unstable vital signs warrant transfer to an emergency department. Basic laboratory tests, including CBC with differential, urinalysis, liver function tests, blood cultures, and urine cultures, should be conducted. If the patient has headache, meningismus, or unexplained neurological deterioration, a lumbar puncture should be considered. Imaging studies such as a chest X ray are useful if pneumonia is suspected. CT scans are important if appendicitis, diverticulitis, or intra-abdominal abscess is suspected. Ultrasound or HIDA scans are the test of choice if cholecystitis is suspected. If the patient is stable, these tests can be performed in an outpatient setting.

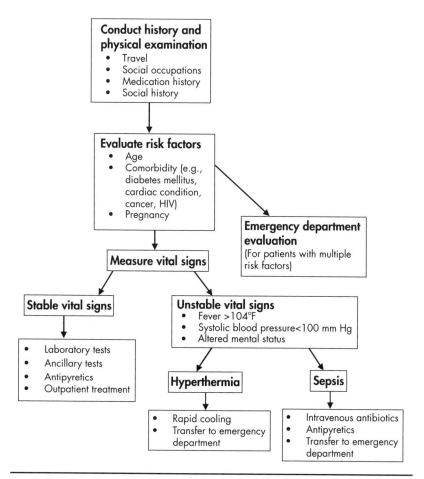

**FIGURE 3–1.** Algorithm for assessment and treatment of a patient with fever.

The need for emergency department referral and hospitalization will be dependent on the critical nature of the illness. A fever higher than 106°F in any patient or in those with hyperthermia syndrome must be treated in the emergency department. Patients who present with bacteremia or sepsis require hospitalization. In general, elderly patients, immunocompromised patients, and patients with comorbidity require hospitalization. Patients for whom outpatient therapy failed also require hospitalization. Antipyretics should be given to the patient to address the fever, and antibiotics should be given if a bacterial infection is identified or suspected in a high-risk patient. Broad-spectrum antibiotics may be necessary for immunocompromised patients and patients in whom nosocomial infection, meningitis, or sepsis is suspected.

Although in most cases antipyretics do not affect the underlying illness, the patient treated with these medications frequently feels subjectively better. For certain patients, such as those with temperatures higher than 106°F, aggressive treatment of fever is needed. Patients with myocardial ischemia, patients predisposed to seizures, and pregnant women may require treatment with antipyretics because the elevation of core temperature increases cardiac output and myocardial oxygen consumption and increases the likelihood of seizures.

The initial stabilization and treatment of hyperthermia requires rapid cooling. The goal is to reach a temperature of 101°F within the first 30 minutes of the patient's arrival in the emergency department (Blum 2002). Clothing removal, cooling with ice, ice-water immersion, or cooling with fans should be started immediately. Shivering, agitation, rigidity, and seizures from hyperthermia must be controlled with intravenous benzodiazepines (5–10 mg of diazepam every 5–10 minutes or 2–4 mg of lorazepam every 15–20 minutes). Aggressive fluid resuscitation should be started by administering a normal saline solution. Phenothiazines and butyrophenones are contraindicated in these patients because these agents interfere with thermoregulation (Delaney 2001).

For NMS, the supportive treatment described previously is essential, but specific treatment with bromocriptine (a dopamine-receptor agonist), dantrolene (a skeletal muscle relaxant), or an antiparkinsonian medication such as levodopa or amantadine may also have a role. Dantrolene can be given for malignant hyperthermia or NMS in a 1 mg/kg intravenous bolus (Delaney 2001; Dinarello and Gelfand 2005). Bromocriptine can also be given at a dose of 5 mg po bid.

## References

Berkowitz D: Fever, in Emergency Medicine: A Comprehensive Study Guide, 5th Edition. Edited by Tintinalli JE, Kelen GD, Stapczynski JS. New York, McGraw-Hill, 2000, pp 731–734

Blum F: Fever, in Rosen's Emergency Medicine: Concepts and Clinical Practice, 5th Edition. Edited by Marx JA, Hockberger RS, Walls RM, et al. St. Louis, MO, Mosby, 2002, pp 116–118

Cunha BA: Antibiotic side effects. Med Clin North Am 85:149–185, 2001

Dale D: The febrile patient, in Cecil Textbook of Medicine, 22nd Edition. Edited by Goldman L, Ausiello D. Philadelphia, PA, WB Saunders, 2004, pp 1729–1730

Delaney KA: Focused physical examination/toxidromes, in Clinical Toxicology. Edited by Ford MD, Delaney KA, Ling LJ, et al. Philadelphia, PA, WB Saunders, 2001, pp 236–243

Dinarello C, Gelfand J: Fever and hyperthermia, in Harrison's Principles of Internal Medicine, 16th Edition. Edited by Kasper D, Braunwald E, Fauci AS, et al. New York, McGraw-Hill, 2005, pp 104–108

Mackoviak PA, Durack DT: Fever of Unknown origin, in Principles and Practice of Infectious Diseases, 5th Edition. Edited by Mandell GL, Bennett JE, Dolin R. New York, Churchill Livingstone, 2000, pp 604–609

# CHAPTER 4

# Hypertension

## Alla M. Trubetskoy, M.D., Ph.D.

## Clinical Presentation

Hypertension affects approximately 50 million Americans and is a risk factor for cardiovascular disease, stroke, and renal failure. Hypertension can be divided into primary (essential) hypertension and secondary hypertension. In primary (essential) hypertension, no cause can be identified; in secondary hypertension, an underlying cause is identifiable.

The Seventh Report of the Joint National Committee on Prevention, Detection, Evaluation, and Treatment of High Blood Pressure (Chobanian et al. 2003) revised the definition of hypertension in adults ages 18 years and older who are currently not taking antihypertensive medications and are not acutely ill (Table 4–1). Hypertension is defined as a systolic reading ≥140 mm Hg or a diastolic reading ≥90 mm Hg and is identified on the basis of the mean of properly measured seated blood pressure readings determined on two or more office visits. Normal blood pressure is defined as systolic reading <120 mm Hg and a diastolic reading <80 mm Hg. Prehypertension is defined as a systolic reading of 120–139 mm Hg or a diastolic reading of 80–89 mm Hg. Patients with prehypertension have twice the risk of progressing to hypertension, compared to patients with normal blood pressure (Cushman et al. 2002).

## Differential Diagnosis

Transient elevation in blood pressure may be caused by anxiety or pain. Mild increases in blood pressure can be defined as hypertension only after an elevated reading is seen on two or more separate occasions. Most patients with hypertension have *primary* or *essential hypertension*. Al-

**TABLE 4–1.**   Systolic and diastolic blood pressure readings indicating normal blood pressure, prehypertension, and hypertension[a]

| Blood pressure category | Systolic blood pressure (mm Hg) | Diastolic blood pressure (mm Hg) |
|---|---|---|
| Normal blood pressure | <120 | <80 |
| Prehypertension | 120–139 | 80–89 |
| Hypertension | ≥140 | ≥90 |

[a]Guidelines for adults ages 18 years and older who are not taking antihypertensive medications and are not acutely ill.
*Source.*   Adapted from Chobanian et al. 2003.

though no one specific cause of essential hypertension has been identified, many factors, including genetic predisposition, age, race, and diet, may contribute to the rise in blood pressure (O'Mailia et al. 1987). Even though only 10% of hypertension is due to secondary causes, patients who are suspected of having *secondary hypertension* require further medical evaluation. The most common correctable causes of secondary hypertension include obesity, alcohol abuse, and renovascular disease.

Severe hypertension, or hypertensive crisis, can be divided into hypertensive urgency and hypertensive emergency. *Hypertensive urgency* is severely elevated blood pressure with no acute end-organ damage. In a *hypertensive emergency*, the rise in blood pressure is associated with end-organ damage.

Hypertensive emergencies include damage to various end organs and must be recognized and treated immediately. *Hypertensive encephalopathy* due to cerebral hyperperfusion can present with headache, vomiting, and altered mental status. In many of these patients, funduscopic examination shows advanced retinopathy with arteriolar changes, exudates, hemorrhages, and papilledema. Hypertensive encephalopathy is acute in onset and reversible, but if it is untreated it may rapidly lead to cerebral hemorrhage, coma, and death.

Hypertension also has a profound effect on the cardiovascular system. Left ventricular failure and coronary insufficiency may result from increased afterload that leads to decreased coronary flow and results in *myocardial ischemia* and *pulmonary edema*. Severe hypertension can cause *thoracic aortic dissection*, a true hypertensive emergency. These patients usually present with severe chest pain radiating to the back.

A marked increase in blood pressure is seen in *drug overdoses* with sympathomimetics such as amphetamines and cocaine, anticholinergics, caffeine, theophylline, nicotine, tricyclic antidepressants, phencyclidine hydrochloride, phenylpropanolamine, and methaqualone. Excessive doses of glucocorticoids are associated with hypertension. Hypertension is seen in *withdrawal from alcohol and sedative hypnotics*. Many foods containing tyramine, as well as a number of medications, can precipitate a hypertensive crisis in patients taking monoamine oxidase inhibitors (MAOIs). Hypertension is also part of *serotonin syndrome* and *neuroleptic malignant syndrome*.

*Abrupt discontinuation of antihypertensive medications* such as the $\alpha_2$-agonist clonidine may result in increased levels of catecholamines and lead to rebound hypertension 16–48 hours later. Abrupt discontinuation of β-adrenergic blockers in patients with underlying coronary disease may lead to hypertension, as well as accelerated angina, myocardial infarction, or sudden death (August 2003).

Certain *tumors*, such as pheochromocytomas, which secrete catecholamines, may also lead to a hypertensive crisis. Patients with pheochromocytoma usually present with paroxysmal episodes of hypertension, tachycardia, palpitations, sweating, malaise, and apprehension. The diagnosis can be confirmed with findings of elevated levels of catecholamines, metanephrines, and vanillylmandelic acid in the urine. Many of these patients are curable with early diagnosis. Hypertension may be a manifestation of conditions of *hormone imbalance*, including hyperthyroidism.

Hypertension is a common *complication of pregnancy*. Special consideration should be made for the pregnant patient with hypertension, because the condition is associated with increased risk of morbidity and mortality in the mother and the baby and because the pregnant woman with hypertension needs to use an antihypertensive medicine that is safe in pregnancy. Pregnancy-induced hypertension can lead to multiple obstetric complications, such as preeclampsia, eclampsia, placenta abruption, preterm birth, and low birth weight in the infant.

## Risk Stratification

The short-term risks related to uncontrolled hypertension correlate best with symptoms and physical findings suggestive of increased intracranial pressure (headache, nausea, vomiting, papilledema, and focal neurological deficits), myocardial ischemia (chest pain and arrhythmias), left ventricular failure (dyspnea, hypoxemia, jugular venous distention, S3 gallop, moist rales), aortic aneurysm dissection (pain in chest, back, or abdomen with unequal peripheral pulses), and acute renal dysfunction. Hypertensive patients with these symptoms and signs must be transferred immediately to an emergency medicine unit for evaluation and treatment.

## Assessment and Management in Psychiatric Settings

Treatment of mild hypertension generally begins with nonpharmacological therapy. These modalities include dietary sodium restriction, exercise, weight reduction, and avoidance of excess alcohol intake. If lifestyle modification techniques fail, drug therapy is instituted (August 2003). Most hypertensive patients will require two or more antihypertensive medications to achieve a goal blood pressure (Black et al. 2001). The first line of treatment in uncomplicated hypertension is usually diuretics or β-blockers. Both of these antihypertensive drugs have been shown to reduce the incidence of cardiovascular disease in patients with chronic hypertension. Diuretics should be avoided in patients with gout, and β-blockers are contraindicated in patients with asthma, chronic obstructive pulmonary disease, or heart block. Angiotensin-converting enzyme (ACE) inhibitors or angiotensin-receptor antagonists are recommended for patients with type 2 diabetes, kidney disease, or congestive heart failure (Lewington et al. 2002; Psaty et al. 1997).

Hypertensive emergency can be differentiated from hypertensive urgency with a targeted medical history and physical examination (see Figure 4–1). In the medical history, the patient should be asked about his or her history of hypertension, diabetes, cardiovascular disease, renal disease, and stroke. It is essential to obtain a complete list of medications that are being used currently or were recently discontinued. The patient should also be asked about use of nicotine, caffeine, and recreational drugs, because use of these substances may lead to a rise in blood pressure. Evidence for possible drug-drug interactions, such as the interactions of other drugs with MAOIs, should be sought.

The physical examination should include blood pressure and pulse measurement; funduscopic examination to look for papilledema and other retinal changes; auscultation for carotid, abdominal, and femoral bruits; palpation of the thyroid gland; a thorough cardiovascular and pulmonary examination; examination of the abdomen for masses or abnormal aortic pulsations; a check of the lower extremities to look for edema; and a full neurological examination. An electrocardiogram (ECG) and chest radiograph should be obtained. Laboratory tests should include measurement of cardiac enzymes, including creatine phosphokinase and troponin; a complete metabolic panel, including

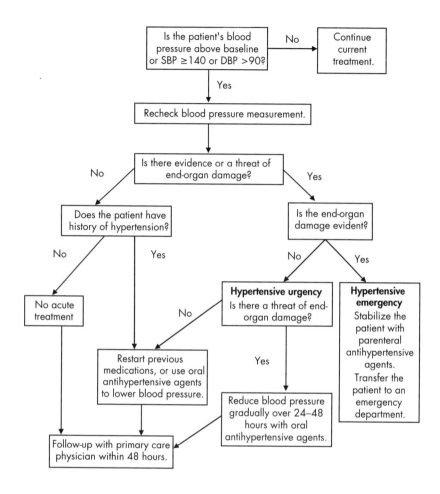

**FIGURE 4–1.**    Algorithm for assessment and treatment of a patient with hypertension.

*Note.*    SBP=systolic blood pressure; DBP=diastolic blood pressure.

measurement of sodium, potassium, blood urea nitrogen, and creatinine; and, when applicable, a pregnancy test and toxicology screen. Urine should be checked for evidence of proteinuria, red cells, and red cell casts.

Hypertensive emergency must be treated immediately. The patient must be stabilized and transferred to an emergency department as soon as possible for further management. The treatment goal for hypertensive emergency is to reduce the mean arterial pressure by 20%–25% in

**TABLE 4–2.** Medications used in the treatment of hypertensive urgency

| Drug | Dose | Onset of action (minutes) | Duration of action | Contraindication |
|------|------|---------------------------|--------------------|-----------------|
| Labetalol | 200–400 mg po every 2–3 hours | 30–120 | 6–12 hours | Asthma, chronic obstructive pulmonary disease, second-degree or third-degree heart block |
| Clonidine | 0.2 mg, then 0.1 mg every hour for a maximum of 0.8 mg | 30–60 | 3–12 hours | Drowsiness, dry mouth, sinus bradycardia, sick sinus syndrome, first-degree heart block |
| Captopril | 6.5–25 mg po | 15–30 | 4–6 hours | Renal failure, angioedema |

30–60 minutes. Lowering blood pressure too quickly can lead to cerebral hypoperfusion and stroke. The vasodilator sodium nitroprusside is considered an agent of choice for most hypertensive emergencies. Sodium nitroprusside has a very rapid onset and a short duration of action, but it may increase intracranial pressure. Good alternatives are labetalol or esmolol, respectively a short- and an ultrashort-acting β-blocker. Both are contraindicated in patients with congestive heart failure, heart block, bronchospasm, pheochromocytoma, cocaine overdose, and MAOI crisis. The α-adrenergic blocking agent phentolamine is used for management of catecholamine-induced hypertensive crisis. In acute pulmonary edema and cardiac ischemia, nitroglycerin, a venous vasodilating agent, may be used.

In hypertensive urgency the elevated blood pressure has the potential to be harmful if sustained. The goal of treatment for hypertensive urgency is to reduce the blood pressure gradually over 24–48 hours to the patient's baseline blood pressure. Patients with hypertensive urgency usually do not require hospitalization, but they should be treated with oral antihypertensive medication. There is no clear consensus on the acute management of a patient with severely elevated blood pressure (Chobanian et al. 2003). If a patient is taking a medication that has been effective in controlling blood pressure in the past, and there is no contraindication, then the same medication can be used. Otherwise, labetalol, a selective $\alpha_1$-blocker and nonselective β-blocker, can be used in most cases of hypertensive urgency. Labetalol does not cause a significant drop in cardiac output and does not affect cerebral flow or renal function. Oral labetalol is effective within 1–3 hours. In patients with pheochromocytoma, labetalol may result in paradoxical hypertension and thus should not be used. Table 4–2 shows the different medications used to treat hypertensive urgency.

# References

August P: Initial treatment of hypertension. New Engl J Med 348:610–617, 2003

Black HR, Elliott WJ, Neaton JD, et al: Baseline characteristics and elderly blood pressure control in the CONVINCE trial. Hypertension 37:12–18, 2001

Chobanian AV, Bakris GL, Black HR, et al: The Seventh Report of the Joint National Committee on Prevention, Detection, Evaluation, and Treatment of High Blood Pressure: the JNC 7 report. JAMA 289:2560–2571, 2003. Erratum in JAMA 290:197, 2003

Cushman WC, Ford CE, Cutler JA, et al: Success and predictors of blood pres-
    sure control in diverse North American settings: the Antihypertensive and
    Lipid Lowering Treatment to Prevent Heart Attack Trial (ALLHAT). J Clin
    Hypertens (Greenwich) 4:393–404, 2002
Lewington S, Clarke R, Qizilbash N, et al: Age-specific relevance of usual blood
    pressure to vascular mortality: a meta-analysis of individual data for one
    million adults in 61 prospective studies. Lancet 360:1903–1913, 2002. Erra-
    tum in Lancet 361:1060, 2003
O'Mailia JJ, Sanders GE, Giles TD: Nifedipine-associated myocardial ischemia
    or infarction in the treatment of hypertensive urgencies. Ann Intern Med
    107:185–186, 1987
Psaty BM, Smith NL, Siscovick DS, et al: Health outcomes associated with anti-
    hypertensive therapies used as first-line agents: a systematic review and
    meta-analysis. JAMA 277:739–745, 1997

# CHAPTER 5

# Hypotension and Orthostasis

### Edward Kan, M.D.

## Clinical Presentation

*Hypotension* is defined as a systolic blood pressure <90 mm Hg or a mean arterial pressure <60 mm Hg (Rivers et al. 2000). The presence of hypotension implies a physiological state in which tissue perfusion is inadequate to meet the body's needs. Blood pressure readings should always be evaluated in relation to the whole clinical picture; a young, thin woman who is noted to have a blood pressure of 85/60 mm Hg during a routine physical examination and who is otherwise asymptomatic is very much different from an 80-year-old man with history of severe hypertension who has a blood pressure of 100/50 mm Hg.

When a patient is found to have low blood pressure, the clinician should search for signs of shock. Besides hypotension, other indications of shock include altered mental status; poor urine output (0.5 mL/kg/hour); cool, pale, or mottled skin; tachycardia (heart rate >100 beats per minute [bpm]); weak peripheral pulses; and poor capillary refill. Shock is a clinical diagnosis.

*Orthostatic hypotension* is a decrease in systolic blood pressure of at least 20 mm Hg or a decrease in diastolic blood pressure of 10 mm Hg within 3 minutes of standing up.

## Differential Diagnosis

The causes of hypotension can be infectious, metabolic, endocrine, neurogenic, cardiopulmonary, traumatic or hemorrhagic, toxic, environmental, allergic, or erroneous.

Hypotension caused by *infectious etiologies* can be an indicator of very serious infection. Meningitis, urosepsis, and pneumonia are the most common infectious reasons for hypotension; endocarditis, osteomyelitis, septic arthritis, toxic shock syndrome, cellulitis, and necrotizing fasciitis are less common. *Metabolic* causes of hypotension include severe acidosis or alkalosis, as well as electrolyte abnormalities (such as hypermagnesemia, hypo- or hyperkalemia, hypo- or hyperphosphatemia, hypocalcemia, and severe hypoglycemia). *Endocrine* causes of hypotension include hypothyroidism, adrenal insufficiency, and diabetes insipidus. *Neurogenic* hypotension may present in various ways, from postural hypotension to vasovagal syncope to frank hypotension in patients with spinal shock. Autonomic nervous instability or damage may be idiopathic or be caused be spinal cord injury, long-standing diabetes mellitus, or multiple sclerosis. *Cardiopulmonary* etiologies of hypotension include cardiac tamponade, massive pulmonary embolism, myocardial infarction, tension pneumothorax, aortic stenosis or mitral stenosis, and tachycardic or bradycardic dysrhythmias. *Posttraumatic* hypotension can be the result of hemorrhage from obvious or hidden sources. Besides causing external bleeding, trauma can cause massive hemothorax and retroperitoneal or intra-abdominal bleeding, all of which may be significant enough to cause hypotension. Other sources of *hemorrhage* include massive hemoptysis, nosebleeds, gastrointestinal bleeding, hematuria, and vaginal bleeding. Hemorrhage in patients without history of trauma or any external signs of bleeding is a diagnostic challenge—one must be sure to consider the possibility of ruptured aortic aneurysms, ruptured ectopic pregnancies, occult gastrointestinal bleeding, or retroperitoneal bleeding in patients taking anticoagulant medication. *Toxic* causes of hypotension may result from drug therapy, drug side effects, and drug overdoses, as well as from environmental exposures. Drug-related hypotension may be associated with use of antihypertensive medication such as diuretics, $\alpha$- and $\beta$-blocking medications, calcium channel blockers, venodilators, and most psychotropic drugs, including sedatives, opioids, tricyclic antidepressants, monoamine oxidase inhibitors, neuroleptics, anticonvulsant medications, anticholinergic medications, and lithium (Engstrom and Aminoff 1997). *Environmental exposures*, including hypothermia and hyperthermia, envenomations, and ingestion of certain plants and herbs, may also cause hypotension. Any medication effect, side effect, or overdose that causes frank hypotension should be considered life-threatening. *Allergy*-mediated hypotension is seen in anaphylaxis. Patients with anaphylaxis present acutely with hypotension; facial, tongue, and lip swelling; hives; pruritis; skin flushing; and hoarseness, wheezing, or stridor. Finally, hypotension determined by a blood pressure cuff may be *erroneous*. One should be sure to check that patients who have low blood pressure readings are not being measured with inappropriately large cuffs.

The patient with orthostatic hypotension should first be evaluated to exclude the life-threatening causes of hypotension previously listed. After these causes of orthostatic hypotension have been excluded, causes related to medications and neurological causes should be considered. The same medications that may cause hypotension may also cause orthostatic hypotension; the benefits of medications must be weighed against the degree to which orthostatic hypotension affects the patient's life. Neurological causes of orthostatic hypotension include any disease that affects the autonomic nervous system, including diabetes mellitus, alcoholic or HIV-related polyneuropathies, Parkinson's disease, and multiple sclerosis.

## Risk Stratification

Initial evaluation of the hypotensive patient should include a full set of vital signs, including blood pressure, pulse, temperature, respiratory rate, oxygen saturation, and glucose level measured by a finger-stick test. A difference of greater than 10–20 mm Hg between blood pressures measured in the right and left arm may be suggestive of aortic dissection. Patients with early hypovolemic shock may be normotensive but tachycardic; as hypovolemia worsens, the patient will have a narrowed pulse pressure and finally will present with hypotension as compensatory mechanisms fail. Hypovolemia can often be diagnosed early through measurement of orthostatic vital signs (supine and standing vital signs). Supine vital signs should be taken after the patient has been lying down for 2 minutes; standing vital signs should then be taken after the patient has been standing for 1 minute. Findings of an increase in heart rate of >20 bpm and severe dizziness are the most predictive signs of hypovolemia (Kramer 2003). Fever suggests an infectious cause of hypotension, whereas hypothermia can suggest either severe hypovolemia or infection. A directed history and physical examination including a rectal examination should be performed to search for underlying causes of hypotension; comparisons with baseline blood pressure measurements made when the patient was healthy can be helpful. Tachypnea in a patient with hypotension can suggest lactic acidosis secondary to tissue hypoperfusion with compensatory respiratory alkalosis.

Orthostatic hypotension should be evaluated with care. Orthostatic blood pressure changes should be considered a sign of hypovolemia until proven otherwise. The patient with orthostatic hypotension may become light-headed or dizzy on standing and is at higher risk for falls. Compared with younger patients, frail, elderly patients are more likely to have orthostatic hypotension and typically experience more serious injuries from falls, including hip fractures and subdural hematomas.

## Assessment and Management in Psychiatric Settings

A physician should evaluate all patients with hypotension immediately. During the evaluation, blood pressure readings should be repeated every 5–10 minutes while one searches for signs of tissue hypoperfusion and shock, as well as for the cause of hypotension. Figure 5–1 and Figure 5–2 show action algorithms for assessment and management of, respectively, a patient with hypotension and a patient with orthostatic hypotension.

Patients who are hypotensive, show signs of shock, and are bradycardic (heart rate <50 bpm) may benefit from 0.5–1 mg of atropine administered by intravenous push; this dose may be repeated until a total of up to 3 mg has been given. Patients who are spontaneously breathing and who have a pulse but have signs of shock should be approached in the following manner: All patients should have two intravenous lines (18 gauge or larger) placed, and a fluid bolus beginning with 20 mL/kg of normal saline solution should be started (Dronen and Bobek 2000). If the appropriate equipment is available, a cardiac rhythm strip or electrocardiogram should be obtained immediately, and a full set of vital signs, including measurement of oxygen saturation and finger-stick glucose level, should be obtained. If the oxygen saturation level is low (below 93% when the patient is breathing room air), supplemental oxygen should be administered through a nasal cannula or face mask. If the oxygen level cannot be determined by pulse oximetry, supplemental oxygen should be used. Patients with hypotension and signs of shock should be transported immediately to an emergency department.

Patients with shock should be positioned in supine position to ensure adequate cerebral perfusion, and patients who have undergone trauma should have their cervical spine immobilized by using a rigid Philadelphia cervical collar. Any external hemorrhage should be stopped through direct pressure.

Anaphylactic shock should be identified and treated immediately. It is important to first stop the exposure (for example, stop any offending

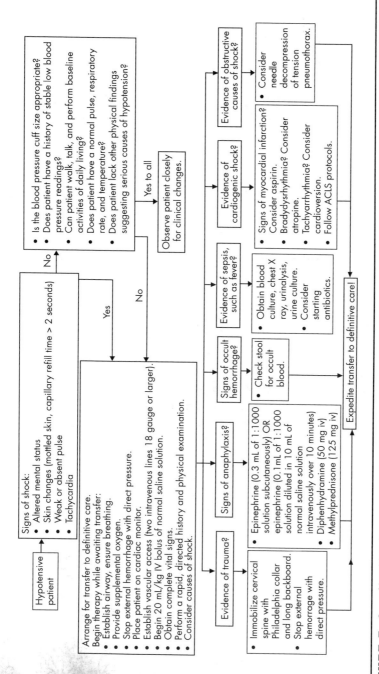

**Hypotensive patient**

Signs of shock:
- Altered mental status
- Skin changes (mottled skin, capillary refill time > 2 seconds)
- Weak or absent pulse
- Tachycardia

**No** →

- Is the blood pressure cuff size appropriate?
- Does patient have a history of stable low blood pressure readings?
- Can patient walk, talk, and perform baseline activities of daily living?
- Does patient have a normal pulse, respiratory rate, and temperature?
- Does patient lack other physical findings suggesting serious causes of hypotension?

**Yes to all** →

Observe patient closely for clinical changes.

**Yes** ↓

- Arrange for transfer to definitive care.
- Begin therapy while awaiting transfer:
- Establish airway, ensure breathing.
- Provide supplemental oxygen.
- Stop external hemorrhage with direct pressure.
- Place patient on cardiac monitor.
- Establish vascular access (two intravenous lines 18 gauge or larger).
- Begin 20 mL/kg IV bolus of normal saline solution.
- Obtain complete vital signs.
- Perform a rapid, directed history and physical examination.
- Consider causes of shock.

**No** ↓

**Evidence of trauma?**
- Immobilize cervical spine with Philadelphia collar and long backboard.
- Stop external hemorrhage with direct pressure.

**Signs of anaphylaxis?**
- Epinephrine (0.3 mL of 1:1000 solution subcutaneously) OR epinephrine (0.1 mL of 1:1000 solution diluted in 10 mL of normal saline solution intravenously over 10 minutes)
- Diphenhydramine (50 mg iv)
- Methylprednisone (125 mg iv)

**Signs of occult hemorrhage?**
- Check stool for occult blood.

**Evidence of sepsis, such as fever?**
- Obtain blood culture, chest X ray, urinalysis, urine culture.
- Consider starting antibiotics.

**Evidence of cardiogenic shock?**
- Signs of myocardial infarction? Consider aspirin.
- Bradydysrhythmia? Consider atropine.
- Tachyarrhythmia? Consider cardioversion.
- Follow ACLS protocols.

**Evidence of obstructive causes of shock?**
- Consider needle decompression of tension pneumothorax.

**Expedite transfer to definitive care!**

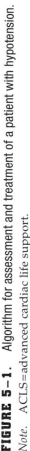

**FIGURE 5–1.** Algorithm for assessment and treatment of a patient with hypotension.

*Note.* ACLS=advanced cardiac life support.

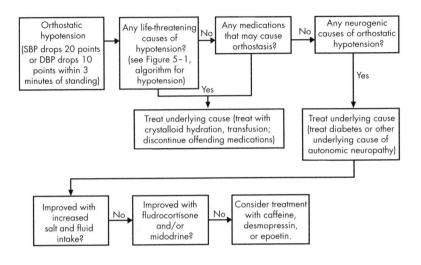

**FIGURE 5-2.**    Algorithm for assessment and treatment of a patient with orthostatic hypotension.

*Note.*    SBP=systolic blood pressure; DBP=diastolic blood pressure.

intravenous medication). If there is lip, mouth, or airway involvement, the patient should receive epinephrine. For signs of severe bronchospasm, upper airway obstruction (stridor), respiratory arrest, or shock, epinephrine should be administered intravenously (1.0 mL of a 1:10,000 epinephrine solution given over 2–5 minutes); the dose can be repeated if needed. Subcutaneous epinephrine (0.3 mL of a 1:1000 epinephrine solution administered subcutaneously) should be given for less severe signs (Koury and Herfel 2000). Patients with anaphylaxis should also receive oxygen, fluid resuscitation, antihistamines (50 mg iv of diphenhydramine hydrochloride), and steroids (125 mg iv of methylprednisolone) (Trunkey et al. 1992). Both treated and untreated patients should be transported to an emergency department immediately.

Patients who have hypotension but have no signs of shock or hypoperfusion may be approached differently. Initial steps in evaluating the stable patient with hypotension include a review of medications, a review of current medical problems, and a careful history and physical examination to assess for the possible causes listed earlier. If the etiology of hypotension cannot be determined or if the hypotension is caused by a disease process that may progress rapidly (such as gastrointestinal bleeding), the patient should be transferred to an emergency department for further care.

Patients with orthostatic hypotension should be treated for the underlying cause. Medications that may cause orthostatic hypotension should be adjusted or stopped. If neurological causes of orthostatic hypotension are suspected and nonneurological causes have been ruled out, a number of interventions may be used to combat orthostatic hypotension. First, the patient should be encouraged to increase sodium and fluid intake in order to increase intravascular volume. The patient should be encouraged to exercise and continue physical activity. Certain physical positions, such as leg crossing and squatting, may temporarily alleviate symptoms of orthostatic hypotension. Medications that can combat orthostasis include fludrocortisone (a synthetic mineralocorticoid) at a starting dose of 0.1 mg po once daily up to 1 mg po daily, and midodrine (an $\alpha_1$ receptor agonist) at a dose of 10 mg po three times a day. Other medications that may be of benefit include epoetin in the anemic patient, caffeine, and the vasopressin analogue desmopressin.

In certain populations additional tests may be conducted. In a patient with gastrointestinal bleeding, insertion of a nasogastric tube and gastric lavage may be indicated. A patient with an upper gastrointestinal hemorrhage may need emergent endoscopy to control bleeding. Patients with lower gastrointestinal bleeding require surgical consultation and may need to be evaluated with colonoscopy or bleeding scans.

A pelvic examination and pelvic ultrasound should be included in the evaluation of the pregnant patient with hypotension. The patient should be placed in the left lateral decubitus position, and a gynecological consultation should be obtained.

Patients with suspected intra-abdominal bleeding might benefit from abdominal ultrasound to search for free peritoneal fluid and aortic aneurysms. An abdominal computed tomography (CT) scan may also be indicated to search for retroperitoneal bleeding, intra-abdominal infections, or a leaking abdominal aortic aneurysm.

The septic patient will be evaluated with a chest X ray, urinalysis, and urine culture, in addition to blood cultures. A patient with a suspected overdose that is causing hypotension should be assessed with blood and urine toxicology screens and should receive activated charcoal for gut decontamination.

Patients with suspected pulmonary embolism will need evaluation with a ventilation perfusion scan or a spiral CT scan; they will likely need systemic anticoagulation therapy or may even need thrombolytic therapy for pulmonary embolism that is causing persistent hypotension. Patients with pneumothorax should receive a chest X ray to confirm the diagnosis; however, patients with tension pneumothorax with shifting of the trachea and hypotension must be treated immediately with needle thoracostomy followed by chest tube placement. Patients with suspected cardiac tamponade should receive bedside echocardiography; subxiphoid needle pericardiocentesis may be lifesaving in a patient with hemodynamic failure secondary to cardiac tamponade.

## References

Dronen SC, Bobek EM: Fluid and blood resuscitation, in Medicine: A Comprehensive Study Guide, 5th Edition. Edited by Tintinalli JE, Kelen GD, Stapczynski JS. New York, McGraw-Hill, 2000, pp 222–228

Engstrom JW, Aminoff MJ: Evaluation and treatment of orthostatic hypotension. Am Fam Physician 56:1378–1384, 1997

Koury SI, Herfel LU: Anaphylaxis and acute allergic reactions, in Medicine: A Comprehensive Study Guide, 5th Edition. Edited by Tintinalli JE, Kelen GD, Stapczynski JS. New York, McGraw-Hill, 2000, pp 242–247

Kramer GC: Hypertonic resuscitation: physiologic mechanisms and recommendations for trauma care. J Trauma 54 (suppl 5):S89–S99, 2003

Trunkey DD, Salber PR, Mills J: Shock, in Current Emergency Diagnosis and Treatment, 4th Edition. Edited by Saunders CE, Ho MT. Norwalk, CT, Appleton and Lange, 1992, pp 51–67

Rivers EP, Rady MY, Bilkovski R: Approach to the patient in shock, in Medicine: A Comprehensive Study Guide, 5th Edition. Edited by Tintinalli JE, Kelen GD, Stapczynski JS. New York, McGraw-Hill, 2000, pp 215–222

# CHAPTER 6

# Tachycardia

## Bon S. Ku, M.D.

## Clinical Presentation

Tachyarrhythmia is defined as a heart rate exceeding 100 beats per minute (bpm). Tachyarrhythmias include supraventricular tachycardia (SVT), which originates above the ventricle, and ventricular arrhythmia, which arises within the ventricle. Patients may or may not experience clinical symptoms. Some patients may complain of dizziness, palpatations, shortness of breath, or chest pain, whereas others are relatively assymptomatic. On an electrocardiogram (ECG), SVT generally presents as a narrow complex tachycardia, and ventricular arrhythmia has a QRS complex that is greater than 0.12 seconds or 120 milliseconds.

This chapter focuses on SVTs. SVT is defined as a rhythm with a rate greater than 100 bpm and a QRS complex that is less than 0.12 seconds. The range of SVTs includes sinus tachycardia, atrial fibrillation, atrial flutter, multifocal atrial tachycardia, and Wolff-Parkinson-White syndrome. Digoxin and tricyclic antidepressant toxicities can present as a variety of tachyarrhythmias.

Sinus tachycardia results from an increase in the firing of the sinoatrial node. On an ECG, there is a P wave preceding each QRS complex, the rhythm is regular, and the QRS complex is less than 0.12 seconds. The heart rate in sinus tachycardia usually does not exceed 160 bpm. The maximum heart rate normally achieved can be roughly estimated for a given patient by using the following formula: 220–the patient's age.

Atrial fibrillation, one of the most common arrhythmias, appears to be caused by multiple microreentrant circuits within the atria (Yealy and Delbridge 2002). On an ECG, the rhythm appears chaotic or irregular and without distinct P waves. Atrial fibrillation is associated with a plethora of underlying diseases, including valvular heart disease, hyperthyroidism, ischemic heart disease, pericarditis, acute ethanol ingestion, cardiomyopathy, pulmonary embolism, and congestive heart failure (Krimm and Minczak 2004).

Atrial flutter is often associated with atrial fibrillation, and it is not uncommon to see a cardiac rhythm oscillate between the two. Atrial flutter is generated by a high number of atrial impulses reaching the atrioventricular (AV) node. On an ECG, atrial flutter classically presents in a "sawtooth" pattern, which represents flutter waves. It is easy to mistake these flutter waves (which are best seen in leads II, III, and aVF) for P waves (Krimm and Minczak 2004). Atrial flutter typically presents with a ventricular rate of 150 bpm, representing a 2:1 AV conduction ratio. Like atrial fibrillation, atrial flutter is associated with valvular disease, congestive heart failure, and metabolic disturbances.

Multifocal atrial tachycardia is caused by the firing of several ectopic foci within the atria. On an ECG, the rhythm is irregular with at least three different P wave morphologies. The rate is typically 100–180 bpm. Multifocal atrial tachycardia is usually seen in patients with chronic pulmonary disease and hypoxemia. Multifocal atrial tachycardia is typically not seen acutely but usually reflects chronic underlying pulmonary disease.

Wolff-Parkinson-White syndrome, the most common accessory pathway syndrome, is caused by atrial impulses conducting not only through the AV node but also through an accessory bypass tract such as Kent's bundle. On an ECG there is a wide QRS complex (>0.12 seconds), a shortened P–R interval (<0.12 seconds), and a delta wave that is an "upslurring" at the beginning of the QRS complex. Wolff-Parkinson-White syndrome is most commonly idiopathic, but it is also associated with cardiomyopathy and mitral valve prolapse (Krimm and Minczak 2004).

The term paroxysmal supraventricular tachycardia (PSVT) can be applied to any intermittent SVT other than atrial fibrillation, atrial flutter, or multifocal atrial tachycardia (Arnsdorf and Ganz 2003).

## Differential Diagnosis

The causes of SVTs include but are not limited to fever, hypoxemia (secondary to a pulmonary embolism), hyperthyroidism, electrolyte disturbance, pain, anxiety, agitation, hypovolemia, sepsis, myocardial infarction, ingestion of stimulants such as caffeine, and drug toxicities and overdoses.

Certain psychotropic medications such as fluoxetine, clozapine, and tricyclic antidepressants have been associated with tachyarrhythmias. A multicenter study showed that tachycardia was a major presenting symptom in patients who acutely ingested fluoxetine (Borys et al. 1992). A case report described SVT in a patient who was taking fluoxetine during an inpatient psychiatric stay (Allhoff et al. 2001). Clozapine has been shown to caus a persistent sinus tachycardia by inducing a dilated cardiomyopathy. Patients with tricyclic antidepressant overdoses often present with sinus tachycardia, which may progress to a lethal rhythm and therefore requires immediate referral to an emergency department. Other common drugs that in overdose cause sinus tachycardia include sympathomimetics (such as cocaine and amphetamines), anticholinergics (scopolamine, atropine), salicylates, and hypoglycemic agents (sulfonylureas, insulin).

Although patients with digoxin toxicity commonly do not present with tachyarrhythmia, it is important to include this toxicity in the differential diagnosis of tachyarrhythmias because the management of potentially life-threatening digitalis toxicity is considerably different from that of other tachyarrhythmias.

Sinus tachycardia may also be a common underlying rhythm in some psychiatric conditions. One investigator found that a significant proportion of patients with schizophrenia had an underlying sinus tachycardia when their resting heart rates were monitored (Lovett Doust 1980).

## Risk Stratification

In general, sinus tachycardia does not represent an unstable rhythm and does not need to be treated with cardioversion. On the other hand, atrial fibrillation, atrial flutter, and PSVT can potentially be unstable rhythms for which cardioversion is required. Signs and symptoms of unstable rhythms include hypotension, chest pain suggestive of myocardial ischemia, dyspnea, and altered sensorium (Krimm and Minczak 2004). A patient who gives a history of chest pain, syncope, dizziness, or palpitations may have an unstable rhythm and should be transferred immediately to the nearest emergency department.

## Assessment and Management in Psychiatric Settings

Expedient and accurate interpretation of an ECG is vital in the treatment of the patient with tachyarrhythmia. It is necessary to answer three questions regarding ECG interpretation: 1) What is the rate? 2) Is the rhythm regular or irregular? 3) Is the QRS complex narrow or wide? If there is an irregular rhythm, then the tachycardia is likely to be atrial fibrillation or multifocal atrial tachycardia. Multifocal atrial tachycardia rarely requires electrical cardioversion, because it is most often a manifestation of chronic cardiopulmonary disease. If the rhythm occurs at a regular rate, the rhythm is likely to be a sinus tachycardia, atrial flutter, or PSVT. A wide QRS complex points to Wolff-Parkinson-White syndrome, ventricular tachycardia, ventricular fibrillation, or tachycardia associated with an underlying bundle branch block.

A complete set of vital signs measurements, including temperature, heart rate, blood pressure, respiratory rate, and oxygen saturation, must be obtained for all patients with tachycardia. An increased respiratory rate and low pulse oximetry measurement may signify pulmonary embolism or chronic obstructive pulmonary disease.

Immediate transfer to the nearest emergency department for cardioversion is mandatory if a patient is found to have an SVT other than sinus tachycardia and has signs and symptoms of instability, including hypotension. Cardioversion for SVTs should always be performed under the synchronized mode because an unsynchronized cardioversion may convert a rhythm into ventricular fibrillation (Cummins 2001). Until cardioversion is performed, the patient should be connected to a cardiac monitor, provided with supplemental oxygen, and prepared for intravenous administration of the cardioversion agent. Chemical cardioversion requires intravenous administration of adenosine, rapidly acting β-blockers, or calcium channel blockers and should be attempted only at the instruction of an emergency medicine physician.

# References

Allhoff T, Bender S, Banger M, et al: Atrial arrhythmia in a woman treated with fluoxetine: is there a causal relationship? (letter) Ann Emerg Med 37:116–117, 2001

Arnsdorf M, Ganz L: Approach to narrow QRS complex tachycardias [UpToDate Web site]. May 6, 2003. Available at: http://uptodate.com. Accessed January 15, 2004.

Borys DJ, Setzer SC, Ling LJ, et al: Acute fluoxetine overdose: a report of 234 cases. Am J Emerg Med 10:115–120, 1992

Cummins RO: ACLS Provider Manual. Dallas, TX, American Health Association, 2001, pp 157–166

Krimm MJ, Minczak B: Defibrillation and cardioversion, in Clinical Procedures in Emergency Medicine, 4th Edition. Edited by Roberts J, Hedges J. Philadelphia, PA, WB Saunders, 2004, pp 213–225

Lovett Doust JW: Sinus tachycardia and abnormal cardiac rate variation in schizophrenia. Neuropsychobiology 6:305–312, 1980

Yealy D, Delbridge T: Dysrhythmias, in Rosen's Emergency Medicine: Concepts and Clinical Practice, 5th Edition. Edited by Marx JA, Hockberger RS, Walls RM, et al. St. Louis, MO, Mosby, 2002, pp 1053–1088

# CHAPTER 7

# Bradycardia

## Leonidas Pritsiolas, M.D.

## Clinical Presentation

Bradycardia is defined as a heart rate less than 50 beats per minute (bpm). Most sources report that the normal heart rate is 60–100 bpm. However, studies conducted with outpatients showed that the normal heart rate, within two standard deviations, is 46–93 bpm for men and 51–95 bpm for women (Spodick 1995). These data were presented to members of the American College of Cardiology, most of whom were in favor of a definition of a normal heart rate as 50–90 bpm, compared to <50 bpm for bradycardia.

Bradycardia can be the result of sinus node dysfunction, atrioventricular (AV) node dysfunction, or a block at a level lower in the conduction system, such as the His-Purkinje system or bundle branches. These disturbances may be the result of an intrinsic malfunction of the conduction system or may be caused by outside influences, such as medicines or alterations in neural tone.

The symptoms associated with bradycardia include light-headedness, dizziness, near-syncope or syncope, confusion, fatigue, increasing angina, or symptoms of congestive heart failure, although some patients with bradycardia are asymptomatic. A patient with symptomatic bradycardia may present for evaluation after a fall.

## Differential Diagnosis

*Natural pacemaker failure* is the result of abnormal firing of the sinoatrial (SA) node and usually leads to sinus bradycardia. However, if SA nodal disease is severe enough and impulse formation does not occur, then pacemaker function is usually picked up by one of the latent pacemaker areas, such as the AV node. In this case, the rhythm may be regular but would not be sinus in origin and would most definitely occur at a lower rate, as latent pacemakers have a slower intrinsic rate of firing than the SA node. Examples of pacemaker malfunction include sinus pauses, sinus block, sick sinus syndrome, and sinus bradycardia.

Sinus bradycardia can occur secondary to increased vagal activity, acute coronary syndrome (explained later in this chapter), obstructive sleep apnea, hypothyroidism, hypothermia, hypoxia, infiltrative diseases (e.g., sarcoidosis, amyloidosis, hemachromatosis), and drug effects. Medications that can cause sinus bradycardia include β-blockers, digitalis, nondihydropyridine calcium channel blockers (verapamil and diltiazem), amiodarone, sotalol, cimetidine, and lithium. In addition, parasympathomimetic agents such as pyridostigmine, opioids, and pesticides can cause bradycardia. Withdrawal of sympathomimetic agents such as amphetamines and cocaine can cause sinus bradycardia, but this effect is usually transient and rarely symptomatic.

Bradycardia caused by psychiatric medicines is less pronounced than that caused by β-blockers and calcium channel blockers. The selective serotonin reuptake inhibitors, especially fluoxetine, have been implicated in symptomatic bradycardia. This effect is thought to be caused by the direct action of the increased serotonin on the medulla (Ellison et al. 1990). Antipsychotics such as clozapine have also been found to cause bradycardia, particularly in elderly patients (Pitner et al. 1995). Medications that have cholinergic effects should also, in theory, cause bradycardia. Cholinergic stimulation enhances vagal activity and thus slows the rate of sinus firing and AV conduction. However, studies of donepezil, a cholinesterase inhibitor used to treat Alzheimer's dementia, failed to show a significant difference in heart rates between subjects taking donepezil and control subjects (Relkin et al. 2003; Tariot et al. 2001). The studies also showed that even patients taking AV nodal blockers in conjunction with donepezil had no significant difference in heart rate, compared with control subjects. In contrast, medications with anticholinergic effects, such as the tricyclic antidepressants, can indirectly cause bradycardia. These drugs can also cause urinary retention. Finally, electroconvulsive therapy (ECT) causes excessive vagal stimulation that can lead to severe bradycardia and even asystole. These effects occur immediately after ECT and are responsive to high doses of atropine (Robinson and Lighthall 2004).

Heightened vagal activity deserves special mention as it is considered to be the most likely cause of syncope (termed *vasovagal syncope*). Unless the patient is examined immediately after the event, the patient will likely not be found to have bradycardia.

Bradycardia can also be caused by a block at the level of the AV node, which leads to a *conduction abnormality* in which the sinus rhythm is normal but does not propagate normally. These conduction abnormalities are classified as first-degree, second-degree, and third-degree heart blocks. They may be caused by medicines such as β-blockers and calcium channel blockers, or they may be caused by intrinsic disease of the conduction system. Withdrawal of possibly offending agents will cause the conduction abnormality to disappear within days if there is no intrinsic disease. Intrinsic disease of the conduction system can be caused by fibrosis or scarring. Prior myocardial infarction, chronic ischemia, and infiltrative diseases are but a few of the causes of an intrinsic conduction block.

In first-degree AV block, there is a conduction delay at the level of the AV node, which is manifested on an electrocardiogram (ECG) as a prolongation of the P–R interval to greater than 200 milliseconds. Each P wave is conducted, and generally these patients have a good prognosis. The QRS complex is usually narrow, indicating that the block is at the AV node and not at the His-Purkinje system. Conduction blocks at the AV node are considered more stable than blocks further down the conduction system; even if the block at the AV node becomes complete, the latent pacemaker of the AV node has an intrinsic firing rate that is fast enough to avoid a decrease in cardiac output and the subsequent onset of symptoms (Mymin et al. 1986). A block below the AV node characteristically produces bradycardia with a wide QRS complex, as this block originates within the ventricles and disrupts normal ventricular depolarization. These blocks are inherently more unstable; they are more likely than AV nodal blocks to progress to complete heart block and, because the pacemaker function would then be picked up by slower pacemaker cells in the ventricle, are more likely to cause symptoms.

Second-degree heart blocks are divided into two categories: type I (Wenckebach) and type II. Type I second-degree heart blocks occur at the level of the AV node and lead to a progressive lengthening of the P–R interval until one P wave fails to propagate and does not cause a QRS complex to follow. This conduction abnormality does not involve the bundle branches, and so the QRS complexes tend to be narrow. This type of block rarely progresses to complete heart block. In the situations where it does progress to complete heart block, the patient tolerates the block fairly well because the escape pacemaker at this level in the conduction system is sufficiently fast for the patient to avoid symptomatic bradycardia. Type II second-degree heart block is more ominous, as the block is usually below the AV node and often lies within the bundle branches. This type of block typically has wide QRS complexes. In addition, some of the P waves fail to initiate a QRS complex and ventricular contraction, similar to the characteristics of a type I block. In a type II block, however, the failure to propagate is unpredictable, as the P–R interval is often normal and there are sudden nonconducted P waves. A type II block can usually be distinguished from a type I block because the P–R interval in the type II block is constant.

It is important to be able to differentiate between the two types of blocks, because type II blocks have a higher probability of progressing to complete heart block. The following rule can be used to differentiate between the two types of second-degree heart block: generally, if the P–R interval is prolonged and the QRS complexes are narrow, it is a type I block. Conversely, if the P–R interval is normal and the QRS complexes are wide, it is a type II block.

Third-degree blocks are complete heart blocks and result in AV dissociation. The P waves are regular and have no relation to the QRS complexes, which are also regular and tend to occur at a slower rate. The QRS complexes can be either wide or narrow, depending on the level of the block. Often the ventricular rate will be markedly slow.

*Artificial pacemaker failure* can present with complete or intermittent heart block, brady-tachy syndrome, atrial fibrillation with slow ventricular response, or symptomatic bradycardia. Any patient with a pacemaker who is found to be bradycardic should have an ECG. If the ECG shows a pacer spike preceding every QRS complex and the rhythm is regular, then the pacer is functioning at that time. The pacemaker may still be intermittently malfunctioning, and further evaluation is warranted if the patient has any symptoms that may be related to bradycardia or a low cardiac output.

## Risk Stratification

The morbidity and mortality secondary to bradycardia are related to the patient's symptoms and the presence of myocardial injury. Symptomatic bradycardia can present as light-headedness, dizziness, near-syncope or syncope, confusion, fatigue, increasing angina, or congestive heart failure. These symptoms are caused by decreased cardiac output, and all patients with symptomatic bradycardia need to be treated as soon as possible on site or in the nearest emergency department.

Poisoning, whether accidental or with intent to harm, can impair conduction and may need to be managed aggressively to prevent the symptoms from worsening. Also, ischemia to the nodal artery during myocardial infarction or unstable angina can cause significant brady-cardia; in fact, bradycardia may be one of the only clues in the ECG that the patient is having an acute coronary syndrome. This pattern may be especially likely in elderly, diabetic, or otherwise incapacitated patients who may not present with typical chest pain. However, bradycardia secondary to cardiac ischemia or infarction is almost always associated with involvement of the right coronary artery and inferior wall (Serrano et al. 1999). On an ECG, this condition usually manifests as either ST segment elevation or depression in limb leads II, III, and aVF.

For patients who are not symptomatic and are found to be brady-cardic in a routine examination, risk stratification becomes more com-plicated. An ECG should be obtained for these patients, and the results will guide management. If the ECG shows sinus bradycardia but is oth-erwise normal, the asymptomatic patient usually does not need acute treatment and can often be followed expectantly. If the ECG is abnormal and shows a high-degree block (type II second-degree heart block or complete heart block), then the patient is at risk, even though he or she is asymptomatic, and should be placed in a monitored setting.

## Assessment and Management in Psychiatric Settings

The algorithm shown in Figure 7–1 outlines the steps that should be fol-lowed when a patient is found to have bradycardia.

All symptomatic patients need to be stabilized with advanced car-diac life support protocols. Intravenous access must be established, as the patient is likely to need intravenous fluid support and specific ther-apy based on the cause of the bradycardia. If an overdose or toxidrome is suspected, the patient should receive activated charcoal if the inges-tion has occurred within the last several hours, and an antidote should be administered (see Table 7–1). In addition, all symptomatic patients should be monitored with a cardiac monitor, and atropine and transcu-taneous pacing should be available (Hayden et al. 2004).

Laboratory investigations must include a basic metabolic panel with measurement of electrolytes, urine and serum toxicological screens, and measurement of serum drug levels if applicable (for patients taking digoxin or lithium).

Patients with complete heart block or high-degree heart block with slow ventricular rates and evidence of brain or heart hypoperfusion (such as confusion, dizziness, chest pain, and hypotension) should be given atropine sulfate and have pacemaker pads placed in an anterior-posterior position on the chest wall. The amount of current needed to

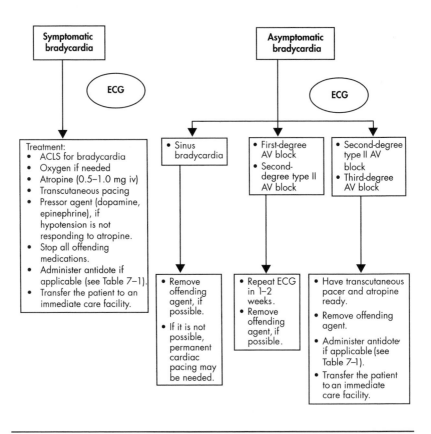

**FIGURE 7–1.**    Algorithm for assessment and treatment of a patient with bradycardia.

*Note.*   ACLS=advanced cardiac life support; AV=atrioventricular; ECG=electrocardiogram.

pace the heart externally is more than 30 mA, which is uncomfortable for the patient and causes muscle twitching. Transvenous pacing offers the advantage of more reliable capturing and less patient discomfort. Permanent pacing may be required for complete heart block, second-degree type II heart block, and other forms of heart block that are symptomatic and in which the symptoms are clearly related to the bradycardia (Gregoratos et al. 2002).

Patients with bradycardia require close follow-up. Those who have sinus bradycardia with no secondary cause and who continue to be asymptomatic need no further assessment. If no bradycardia is documented at the time of the physician's examination, but the patient has

**TABLE 7-1.**   Antidotes for medications and toxins known to cause bradycardia

| Medication/toxin | Antidote |
|---|---|
| β-Blockers | Glucagon (50–100 μg/kg bolus followed by infusion) |
| | Pressor agent (dopamine preferred), if no increase in blood pressure after treatment with glucagon |
| Calcium channel blockers | Calcium chloride (1 g bolus followed by infusion) |
| Digoxin | Glucagon (100 μg/kg bolus followed by infusion) |
| | Pressor agent (dopamine preferred) if needed |
| | Digoxin immune Fab (Digibind) (dose based on either amount ingested or serum digoxin level) |
| Clonidine | Atropine (0.5–1.0 mg iv) |
| Opiates | Atropine (0.5–1.0 mg iv), multiple doses likely to be needed |

symptoms that may be related to bradycardia, or if a first-degree or type I second-degree heart block is present, the patient should be further evaluated with either a Holter monitor or event recorder. Some patients may need to continue the very medicines that may have contributed to the bradycardia. Patients who have congestive heart failure or previous myocardial infarction clearly benefit from taking β-blockers, and these patients need to be followed up closely to make sure their heart rate stays in an acceptable range (Rapaport and Gheorghiade 1996). Psychiatrists must be aware that certain drugs can cause bradycardia and should monitor their patients' resting heart rates regularly. When treating a patient with agents known to decrease conduction through the AV node, such as β-blockers and the nondihydropyridine calcium channel blockers, the clinician must be careful to avoid prescribing more than one such agent for the patient. It is important to titrate the dosage of these agents to avoid precipitating symptomatic bradycardia and possibly heart block.

Once bradycardia is diagnosed, it is important to consider whether referral to a cardiologist and use of a pacemaker may be indicated to prevent some of the more disabling effects of symptomatic bradycardia, such as falls and syncope. If a patient presents after a fall and with a history of dizziness or syncope, it is important to evaluate possible cardiac causes of these events before the next episode occurs. In these situations, a baseline ECG and use of a Holter monitor (or event recording) can aid in ruling out bradycardia or other cardiac precipitants of the symptoms (Linzer et al. 1992).

## References

Ellison JM, Milofsky JE, Ely E: Fluoxetine-induced bradycardia and syncope in two patients. J Clin Psychiatry 51:385–386, 1990

Gregoratos G, Abrams J, Epstein AE, et al: ACC/AHA/NASPE 2002 guideline update for implantation of cardiac pacemakers and antiarrhythmia devices: summary article. A report of the American College of Cardiology/American Heart Association Task Force on Practice Guidelines (ACC/AHA/NASPE Committee to Update the 1998 Pacemaker Guidelines). J Cardiovasc Electrophysiol 13:1183–1199, 2002

Hayden GE, Brady WJ, Pollack M, et al: Electrocardiographic manifestations: diagnosis of atrioventricular block in the emergency department. J Emerg Med 26:95–106, 2004

Linzer M, Varia I, Pontinen M, et al: Medically unexplained syncope: relationship to psychiatric illness. Am J Med 92:18S–25S, 1992

Mymin D, Mathewson FA, Tate RB: The natural history of primary first-degree atrioventricular heart block. N Engl J Med 315:1183–1187, 1986

Pitner JK, Mintzer JE, Pennypacker LC, et al: Efficacy and adverse effects of clozapine in four elderly psychotic patients. J Clin Psychiatry 56:180–185, 1995

Rapaport E, Gheorghiade M: Pharmacologic therapies after myocardial infarction. Am J Med 101:4A61S–4A69S, 1996; discussion in Am J Med 101:4A69S–4A70S, 1996

Relkin NR, Reichman WE, Orazem J, et al: A large, community-based, open-label trial of donepezil in the treatment of Alzheimer's disease. Dement Geriatr Cogn Disord 16:15–24, 2003

Robinson M, Lighthall G: Asystole during successive electroconvulsive therapy sessions: a report of two cases. J Clin Anesth 16:210–213, 2004

Serrano CV Jr, Bortolotto LA, Cesar LA, et al: Sinus bradycardia as a predictor of right coronary artery occlusion in patients with inferior myocardial infarction. Int J Cardiol 68:75–82, 1999.

Spodick DH: Operational definition of sinus tachycardia and sinus bradycardia. Cardiovasc Rev Rep 16:12,20,47, 1995

Tariot PN, Cummings JL, Katz IR, et al: A randomized, double-blind, placebo-controlled study of the efficacy and safety of donepezil in patients with Alzheimer's disease in the nursing home setting. J Am Geriatr Soc 49:1590–1599, 2001

# PART III

# Respiratory Distress

Section Editors:

Jill Karpel, M.D.

Peter Manu, M.D.

# CHAPTER 8

# Dyspnea

Boris I. Medarov, M.D.

Leonard J. Rossoff, M.D.

## Clinical Presentation

Dyspnea is a term used to characterize a subjective experience of breathing discomfort that derives from interactions among multiple physiological, psychological, social, and environmental factors and may induce secondary physiological and behavioral responses (American Thoracic Society 1999).

Dyspnea or breathlessness may or may not be associated with objective findings (tachypnea, hyperpnea) of respiratory distress and respiratory failure. Dyspnea is similar, even perhaps identical, to the sensation of shortness of breath experienced by healthy individuals during significant exertion.

The mechanism of dyspnea remains unclear despite decades of research. The relation between abnormal levels of oxygen and carbon dioxide in the blood and the perception of dyspnea is not straightforward. A classic example is the patient with emphysema who frequently complains of severe dyspnea despite normal oxygen and carbon dioxide levels in the blood.

## Differential Diagnosis

### Organic Disorders

Organic disorders causing dyspnea generally belong to one of the following subgroups: ventilation and gas exchange–related diseases, hemodynamic disorders, metabolic conditions, and oxygen-transport–related conditions.

The initial step of effective gas exchange is delivering oxygen to the blood in the alveolar capillaries. This ventilatory system comprises the oral and nasopharynx airways and the thoracic cage, including the respiratory muscles and the lung parenchyma. A pathological condition affecting any of these components may lead to dyspnea.

*Upper airway obstruction* is perhaps the most acute form of ventilatory failure and, therefore, produces one of the most distressing forms of dyspnea. In some cases, a brief history may reveal the diagnosis (e.g., history of upper airway edema after a bee sting). In others, a more detailed history and examination are necessary (e.g., in cases of foreign body aspiration). Stridor, a high-pitched inspiratory sound audible over the trachea, is a classic sign of extrathoracic airway obstruction. Stridor is caused by an incomplete obstruction that becomes more prominent on inspiration as the airway collapses. Significant obstruction or stenosis may cause stridor during both inspiration and expiration.

*Chronic obstructive pulmonary disease* (COPD) is a common lung disorder that leads to chronic and disabling shortness of breath. Classically, dyspnea is more prominent in the emphysematous form of COPD and less so in chronic bronchitis. An exacerbation of COPD typically manifests with dyspnea, cough, wheezing, and excessive sputum production.

*Pneumonia* typically presents with high fever, productive cough, and malaise. Chest pain or discomfort that worsens with deep inspiration (pleurisy) is a sign of pleural inflammation. Significant dyspnea is unusual in a young and otherwise healthy patient. The physical examination typically reveals crackles, signs of consolidation such as dullness, increased fremitus, and egophony.

*Congestive heart failure* is commonly associated with dyspnea. Generally, the dyspnea associated with congestive heart failure is worse when the patient is in a recumbent position (orthopnea), and the patient may have nocturnal awakenings (paroxysmal nocturnal dyspnea). However, orthopnea has been reported in virtually every type of respiratory failure. Measurement of serum B-type natriuretic peptide (BNP) is a fairly sensitive and specific test for congestive heart failure. The causes of congestive heart failure include coronary artery disease, hypertensive or diabetic heart disease, cardiomyopathy, valvulopathies, myocarditis, thyroid disorders, and drug effects (e.g., clozapine-induced myocarditis). A precipitating factor, such as fluid/salt overload, nonadherence to medical treatment, hypertensive emergency, or acute coronary syndrome, must be sought in a patient with a long history of well-compensated congestive heart failure who develops shortness of breath. In all cases of new or worsening congestive heart failure, acute coronary syndrome must be ruled out by using serial electrocardiograms (ECGs) and myocardial necrosis markers. Echocardiography is usually necessary to assess left ventricular function and any wall motion abnormalities.

*Pulmonary embolism* is a significant, difficult-to-detect, source of in-hospital morbidity and mortality. As a life-threatening condition, pulmonary embolism always needs to be considered in the differential diagnosis of dyspnea, especially in patients at risk. Risk factors include previous history of deep vein thrombosis, neoplasm, immobility (in restrained or bed-bound patients), smoking, obesity, congestive heart failure, and hereditable factors. For patients at risk for deep vein thrombosis, the importance of prophylaxis with unfractionated or low-molecular-weight heparin or with intermittent compression devices cannot be overemphasized. Pulmonary embolism classically presents with sudden-onset shortness of breath, pleuritic chest pain, and, often, hemoptysis. In severe cases, the presenting symptoms can be hypotension, syncope, or sudden death. ECG findings can be normal, or they can reveal tachycardia, complete or incomplete right bundle branch block, atrial fibrillation/atrial flutter, right atrium enlargement, or the S1Q3T3 pattern. Tachycardia is common, but its specificity for pulmonary embolism is very low. Findings from the physical examination range from normal to severe respiratory distress and shock. Lung auscultation is generally unrevealing. A ventilation/perfusion (V/Q) scan or computer tomograpic angiography can confirm suspected pulmonary embolism. An elevated level of serum D-dimer—a fibrin degradation product—is a sensitive but not specific sign of pulmonary embolism and deep venous thrombosis.

*Pneumothorax* must be considered in all patients presenting with shortness of breath and chest pain. The spontaneous form generally affects young asthenic male smokers and people with underlying lung disease, such as COPD. There is also an increased frequency of pneumothorax in patients with HIV. Findings in the physical examination include decreased breath sounds and increased resonance to percussion on the side of the pneumothorax. A chest radiograph is generally necessary to confirm the diagnosis. Increasing intrapleural pressure (tension pneumothorax) can rapidly cause hemodynamic collapse and death and thus requires emergent intervention.

*Deconditioning* is a very common contributing factor to dyspnea. Deconditioning never causes shortness of breath at rest, but it restricts the patient's ability to exercise, which leads to a sedentary lifestyle and further deconditioning.

*Obesity-hypoventilation syndrome* may manifest with dyspnea and chronic hypercapnic respiratory failure, usually in morbidly obese patients. The mechanism appears to be a combination of restriction, obstruction, and central hypoventilation. Most patients experience dyspnea on exertion or at rest, which is likely related to the increased work of breathing, cor pulmonale, and deconditioning.

Any *neuromuscular disease* affecting the respiratory muscles can cause respiratory failure and dyspnea. Acute inflammatory demyelinating polyneuropathy (Guillain-Barré syndrome) is a classic example. Idiopathic or secondary unilateral phrenic nerve paralysis should be considered in the case of exertional dyspnea and a finding of unilateral hemidiaphragm elevation on the chest radiograph. The effects of various poisons (curare, strychnine) and tetanus are other dramatic examples of neuromuscular respiratory failure. A careful physical examination and a detailed history may uncover the etiology of this dyspnea.

*Metabolic acidosis* causes increased respiratory drive that leads to higher tidal volume and higher respiratory rate. The most prominent example is Kussmaul breathing in diabetic ketoacidosis. The higher ventilation requirements may result in shortness of breath, particularly in patients with low cardiopulmonary reserve. Similarly, anemia imposes an increased burden on the cardiovascular system. To maintain oxygen delivery to the peripheral tissues, the cardiac output may increase significantly, which can lead to a high-output cardiac failure with resulting dyspnea on exertion or at rest.

A large number of *pulmonary conditions* may also result in dyspnea. They include pleural effusions, acute respiratory distress syndrome, pulmonary hypertension, and lung fibrosis of any etiology. Evaluation usually starts with a chest radiograph and lung function testing.

## Drug Adverse Effects

Neuroleptic-related side effects deserve special attention in the psychiatric population. Tardive dystonia and dyskinesia are late complications of long-term use of neuroleptic drugs. Among other muscle groups, the laryngeal muscles can be affected, and dysphonia and stridor may result.

As opposed to tardive dyskinesia, *neuroleptic-induced acute laryngeal dystonia* (NALD) is an acute complication of antipsychotic therapy. NALD is an extrapyramidal adverse reaction to neuroleptics, including antiemetic phenothiazines and metoclopramide. The symptoms usually develop within 7 days of initiation of the neuroleptic medication and include dysphonia, respiratory distress, and stridor. Laryngoscopy may show no evidence of physical abnormality. NALD may be associated with other neuroleptic-induced acute dystonic reactions, such as torticollis, oculogyric crisis, and trismus. Risk factors for NALD include young age, male gender, previous episodes of acute dystonia, recent cocaine use, hypocalcemia, and dehydration. Medications used to treat NALD include diphenhydramine, benztropine, benzodiazepines, and barbiturates. Although NALD is a rare disorder, it should be included in the differential diagnosis of acute respiratory distress in patients who recently starting taking a neuroleptic or recently had an increase in their neuroleptic dosage.

*Opioids and most sedatives* have a respiratory depressant effect and need to be used with caution in patients with chronic lung disease. Occasionally, they are administered in small doses to relieve dyspnea, particularly in patients with malignancy. The effect of antidepressants on breathing is controversial. Some studies have suggested that tricyclic antidepressants may decrease the responsiveness of the ventilatory center. Paradoxically, this phenomenon may be associated with improved exercise tolerance and alleviated dyspnea (Greenberg et al. 1993).

## Psychiatric Disorders

Dyspnea is a common complaint in the general psychiatric population. The complex nature of the process of breathing and its regulation makes it vulnerable to interference at various levels.

During a *panic attack*, there is an increase in sympathetic discharge. Chest pain, a feeling of impending doom, hyperventilation, and dyspnea are among the most common symptoms of a panic attack. Hyperventilation and respiratory alkalosis may be the intrinsic elements of the vicious cycle that leads to a panic attack. The physical examination reveals significant distress, tachycardia, hyperventilation, and excessive sweating without evidence of respiratory failure, heart failure, or hypoxemia.

The *co-occurrence of panic disorder and anxiety* in patients with chronic dyspnea deserves particular attention. The psychological model of anxiety implicates noncritical sensations misinterpreted as dangerous ones. Thus, it is not surprising that chronic dyspnea frequently lays the groundwork for the development of anxiety. This phenomenon has been studied mostly in COPD (Brenes 2003). The prevalence of generalized anxiety disorder and panic disorder was found to be three to five times higher in patients with COPD than in the general public. The rate of anxiety symptoms may be as high as 50% in patients with COPD and appears to be higher than in other chronic conditions, such as congestive heart failure and cancer. Antidepressants and buspirone may be helpful in treating patients with COPD and anxiety. Cognitive and behavioral techniques, as well as pulmonary rehabilitation, are useful.

*Hyperventilation syndrome* is psychogenic hyperventilation associated with anxiety states. The increased minute ventilation leads to respiratory alkalosis and a decreased level of ionized calcium. The symptoms include shortness of breath, chest discomfort, paresthesias, dizziness, faintness, palpitations, muscle spasms, diaphoresis, and cold extremities. As many as one-half of cases of hyperventilation syndrome may be diagnosed in association with the symptoms of panic disorder or other psychiatric conditions.

*Vocal cord dysfunction* ("functional" asthma, psychogenic stridor) is an increasingly recognized disorder that usually manifests as refractory asthma. It is clearly more prevalent among psychiatric patients and women ages 30–50 years, but the prevalence appears to be increasing in adolescents. Vocal cord dysfunction is characterized by abnormal adduction of the vocal cords during inspiration and, less commonly, during expiration as well. The symptoms include wheezing, stridor, and shortness of breath. The condition frequently seems refractory to traditional asthma treatments, and the patient may have a history of multiple intubations. More than 50% of patients who have vocal cord dysfunction also have coexisting mild asthma. Vocal cord dysfunction is also associated with a variety of psychiatric disorders and underlying neurological diseases (e.g., spasmodic dysphonia or vocal cord paralysis), and it may be idiopathic as well. The mechanism of vocal cord dysfunction is unclear and may represent a learned unconscious, involuntary reaction that results in secondary gain. It may be suspected in cases of asthma attacks that do not respond to appropriate therapy, have a rapid onset and an abrupt resolution, and include wheezing that is alleviated by simple distraction, panting, or phonation. The diagnosis can be established by direct laryngoscopy.

*Psychogenic dyspnea* is a poorly defined concept that has been used to describe the functional complaint of shortness of breath without an organic cause. This term has been applied to dyspnea in vocal cord dysfunction and panic attacks as well. Patients with psychogenic dyspnea are generally female and ages 20–40 years. The attacks usually occur at rest. They are characterized by deep respirations without tachypnea and are often associated with chest discomfort or pressure. The symptoms are usually produced by stressful situations and may be alleviated by distraction. Organic causes of dyspnea need to be excluded.

**TABLE 8-1.** Initial evaluation of dyspnea

| Assessment | Findings | Differential diagnosis |
|---|---|---|
| Physical examination | Stridor | Upper airway obstruction (laryngeal edema, vocal chord dysfunction, neuroleptic-induced acute laryngeal dystonia) |
| | Wheezing | Asthma<br>Bronchiectasis<br>COPD |
| | Diffuse basilar crackles | Congestive heart failure<br>Pulmonary fibrosis |
| | Dullness on percussion | Pleural effusion |
| | Localized crackles, egophony | Pneumonia |
| | Clubbing | Lung cancer<br>Fibrosis<br>Bronchiectasis |
| | Peripheral edema, gallop rhythms, heart murmur | Congestive heart failure |
| | Unilateral leg edema, Homans' sign | Deep venous thrombosis, possible pulmonary emobolism |
| Chest X ray | Pneumothorax | Pneumothorax |
| | Infiltrate | Pneumonia |
| | Triangular peripheral infiltrate | Pulmonary embolism with lung infarction |
| | Cephalization, "batwing" edema, cardiomegaly | Congestive heart failure |
| | Hyperinflation | Asthma<br>COPD |
| | Pleural effusion | Congestive heart failure<br>Pneumonia<br>Pulmonary embolism<br>Malignancy |
| Electrocardiogram | Ischemic changes, new LBBB | Acute coronary syndrome |

**TABLE 8−1.**   Initial evaluation of dyspnea *(continued)*

| Assessment | Findings | Differential diagnosis |
|---|---|---|
| | Tachycardia, right bundle branch block, atrial fibrillation/ atrial flutter, S1Q3T3 pattern | Pulmonary embolism |
| | Left ventricular hypertrophy, atrial fibrillation, left atrium enlargement | Congestive heart failure |
| Arterial blood gas analysis | Hypercarbic respiratory failure | CNS disorder (e.g., drug effects, hypothyroidism, alkalosis) Airway obstruction (e.g., COPD, asthma) Neuropathy (e.g., Guillain-Barré syndrome) Restrictive chest wall disease (e.g., kyphoscoliosis) Neuromuscular disorder (myasthenia gravis, neuromuscular blockers) |
| | Hypoxemic respiratory failure | Pneumonia Pulmonary fibrosis Congestive heart failure COPD (e.g., emphysema) Adult respiratory distress syndrome Pulmonary embolism |

*Note.*   CNS=central nervous system; COPD=chronic obstructive pulmonary disease.

## Risk Stratification

The risk of death in the dyspneic patient is predicted by the presence of airway obstruction, severe or rapidly worsening hypoxemia (with oxygen saturation less than 86%), change in mental status (lethargy or coma), and the presence of symptoms and signs of acute coronary syndrome or pulmonary embolism.

## Assessment and Management in Psychiatric Settings

The approach to the dyspneic patient starts with checking the upper airways for a critical obstruction. If there is an obstruction, advanced cardiac life support protocols should be initiated. Patients in severe respiratory distress, especially if they are also hypoxemic, require intubation and mechanical ventilation, regardless of the etiology. A quick physical examination should include checking for tension pneumothorax, which may require immediate needle decompression. Table 8–1 summarizes procedures for initial evaluation of dyspnea.

## References

American Thoracic Society: Dyspnea: mechanisms, assessment and management—a consensus statement. Am J Respir Crit Care Med 159:321–340, 1999

Brenes GA: Anxiety and chronic obstructive pulmonary disease: prevalence, impact, and treatment. Psychosom Med 65:963–970, 2003

Greenberg HE, Scharf SM, Green H: Nortriptyline-induced depression of ventilatory control in a patient with chronic obstructive pulmonary disease. Am Rev Respir Dis 147:1303–1305, 1993

# CHAPTER 9

# Wheezing

Jacob K. Goertz, M.D.

## Clinical Presentation

Wheezing is a multifaceted complaint that can causes distress to patients. Wheezes are high-pitched breath sounds with a musical quality caused by a disruption in the normal laminar flow of air through the airways that results in turbulence. In the physical examination, wheezes can be generalized or localized to one segment or lobe of the lung. Any process that causes airway narrowing or any foreign body can cause airflow disruption and wheezing (Table 9–1). Wheezing must be differentiated from stridor, which is inspiratory in nature, located over the neck and upper airway, and caused by turbulent flow of air through the larynx and upper airway.

## Differential Diagnosis

### Asthma

*Definition*

Asthma is a a complex disease marked by a variable degree of airway obstruction, bronchial hyperreactivity, and airway inflammation (Busse and Lemanski 2001). Clinically, patients present with bouts of wheezing, chest tightness, and cough that resolve spontaneously or with treatment.

*Risk Stratification*

The history and physical examination of a patient with asthma should be directed toward determining the adequacy of oxygenation and venti-

| **TABLE 9–1.**    Causes of wheezing |
| --- |

**Respiratory**
Asthma
Chronic obstructive pulmonary disease
Foreign body
Pneumonia, aspiration
Bronchitis, bronchiolitis

**Cardiovascular**
Congestive heart failure
Pulmonary embolism

**Allergic reaction**

lation, signs of impending respiratory failure, high-risk elements of the history, and examination of the chest and upper airway. Wheezing may not necessarily be present; the patient may complain only of a nonproductive cough. The severity of the patient's symptoms should be assessed, including symptom frequency, triggers, exercise tolerance, nocturnal awakenings, and need for use of rescue medication. Exacerbations are typically triggered by viral infections, weather changes (e.g., cold or humid weather), allergen or irritant exposure (e.g., tobacco smoke or odors), or exercise. Patients with symptoms requiring use of short-acting $\beta_2$-agonist medications more than two times per week or two nights per month are considered to have poorly controlled asthma and are at risk for frequent exacerbations. Risk factors for death from asthma include a past history of sudden severe exacerbations, prior intubation or intensive care unit admission for asthma, two or more hospitalizations or three or more emergency department visits for asthma in the past year, a hospitalization or emergency department visit for asthma within the past month, use of more than two canisters per month of short-acting $\beta_2$-agonists, current or recent use of systemic steroids, comorbid medical or psychiatric disease, and severe psychosocial problems, including low socioeconomic status and illicit drug use (Nunn and Gregg 1989). The patient's baseline asthma medications and use of rescue medication during the current episode should be ascertained.

## Assessment and Management in Psychiatric Settings

The physical examination should be focused on determining the severity of the airway obstruction and identifying impending respiratory failure. A preliminary assessment can be made by observing the patient's respiratory rate and effort, level of alertness, and ability to talk during the examination. As airway constriction progresses, the patient's respiratory rate will increase in an attempt to maintain minute ventilation. The patient may become increasingly anxious or agitated, have difficulty speaking, and feel unable to breathe. Use of accessory muscles (suprasternal, intercostal, and subcostal muscles) becomes apparent as the work of breathing increases. Finally, as the patient tires, the normal pattern of ventilation cannot be maintained, and paradoxical abdominal and thoracic breathing occurs. Respiratory failure then develops with resulting carbon dioxide retention and hypoxemia. *If a patient is unable to talk, is drowsy or confused, or exhibits paradoxical thoracic or abdominal breathing, respiratory failure is imminent, and the patient requires immediate respiratory support.*

As the patient's ability to move air diminishes, the loudness of the wheezing decreases. A patient with asthma who is dyspnic and not wheezing may have impending respiratory failure and requires emergent treatment, including respiratory support.

Two rapid bedside tests that can aid in determining the severity of an asthma exacerbation are measurement of oxygen saturation and peak expiratory flow rate (PEFR). Hypoxia develops at an oxygen saturation of less than 90%, corresponding to an arterial oxygen partial pressure of about 60 mm Hg. PEFR is inversely proportional to the degree of obstruction of the large airways. Normal PEFR is predicted by the patient's age, height, and sex (Schmaling and Bell 1997). PEFR during an asthma exacerbation should be compared to the patient's predicted normal PEFR or "best" PEFR. Serial measurements during treatment can also be used to determine responsiveness to therapy.

In the majority of asthma exacerbations, arterial blood gas analysis is unnecessary; the decision to provide ventilatory support for respiratory failure is clinically based. However, if the patient's PEFR remains less than 150 L/minute or the patient's forced expiratory volume in 1 second (FEV1) is less than 1 L after intensive therapy with bronchodilators, an arterial blood gas analysis should be performed to assess for impending respiratory failure. Patients initially develop respiratory alkalosis, which is a decrease in alveolar partial pressure of carbon dioxide ($PaCO_2$) secondary to the increased respiratory rate. In these patients, an increase in $PaCO_2$ to a normal or above-normal level is an indicator of impending respiratory failure.

The goal of therapy is to preserve oxygenation. Supplemental 100% oxygen should be used to keep the oxygen saturation greater than 90%–92%. The mainstays of therapy are inhaled bronchodilators ($\beta_2$-

agonists and anticholinergics) and inhaled and systemic corticosteroids. Ultimately, respiratory support with intubation and mechanical ventilation may be required. The National Asthma Education and Prevention Program asthma treatment guidelines (National Asthma Education and Prevention Program 1997) are presented in Figure 9–1.

**Bronchodilators.**    Inhaled $\beta_2$-agonists are the primary therapy for asthma exacerbations. They stimulate the $\beta_2$ receptors on the smooth muscle of the bronchioles, causing direct muscle relaxation and bronchial dilation. Albuterol, the most commonly used medication, is administered as two puffs from a metered dose inhaler used with a spacer or 2.5 mg of the nebulized form every 4–6 hours as needed. For an acute exacerbation, nebulized albuterol or four to eight puffs from a metered dose inhaler is given every 15–20 minutes during the first hour and continued as needed. Inhaled anticholinergic agents, such as ipratropium bromide, have been used to promote bronchodilation; they have a synergistic effect with inhaled $\beta_2$-agonists in patients with severe asthma exacerbations (Adams and Cydulka 2003; Nunn and Gregg 1989).

**Steroids.**    Corticosteroids treat the inflammatory component of asthma, and early treatment with steroids decreases hospitalization and relapse rates (Adams and Cydulka 2003). Systemic steroids, given either orally or parenterally, are used during exacerabations, and inhaled steroids are used for chronic control. Precise dosing is not known, but generally burst therapy with either oral prednisone or intravenous methylprednisolone is given at a dose of 2 mg/kg/day divided once or twice daily (maximum of 60 mg/day) for a total of 5–10 days. A taper is not needed after short-burst therapy but should be considered in patients treated with chronic or recurrent systemic steroid therapy or in whom symptoms persist or the PEFR remains less than 80% after completion of the steroid burst. Inhaled corticosteroids should be started as well to maintain chronic control (Adams and Cydulka 2003; Nunn and Gregg 1989).

**Magnesium.**    Magnesium at a dose of 2 g (40 mg/kg in children) given intravenously over 15–20 minutes in patients with severe asthma improved pulmonary mechanics and decreased the admission rate (Adams and Cydulka 2003; Bloch et al. 1995). Patients should be monitored for cardiac arrhythmias and hypotension during infusion.

**Intubation and mechanical ventilation.**    Intubation and ventilatory support are lifesaving in patients with impending respiratory failure. The

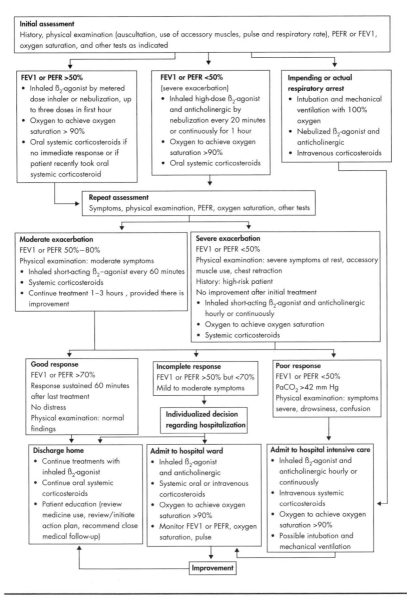

**FIGURE 9–1.** Asthma treatment guidelines.

*Note.* FEV1=forced expiratory volume in 1 second; PaCO₂=alveolar partial pressure of carbon dioxide; PEFR=peak expiratory flow rate.

*Source.* Modified from National Asthma Education and Prevention Program 1997.

parameters of ventilatory support in the asthmatic patient should reflect the patient's underlying bronchoconstriction, which necessitates low respiratory rates, high flow rates, and prolonged expiratory times (Adams and Cydulka 2003).

### Asthma and the Psychiatric Patient

The difficulty of treating the asthmatic psychiatric patient is well documented. Sonin and Patterson (1984) reported on a case series of schizophrenic patients with asthma and found that these patients missed medical appointments and were nonadherent to their medication regimens. These characteristics may place schizophrenic patients with asthma at increased risk for death (Stoppe et al. 1992).

Determining the cause of wheezing in the psychiatric patient may be difficult. Confounding factors include medication side effects, allergic reactions to medications, and manifestations of the patient's underlying psychiatric disease. At least one case of a bronchospastic allergic reaction to clozapine has been reported (Stoppe et al. 1992). Furthermore, the signs and symptoms of psychiatric conditions such as anxiety and panic disorder and the signs and symptoms of asthma frequently overlap, and differentiating the underlying etiology can be difficult. However, the presence of wheezing, mucous congestion, and coughing is clearly predictive of asthmatic airway obstruction (Snow et al. 2001).

## Chronic Obstructive Pulmonary Disease

### Definition

Chronic obstructive pulmonary disease (COPD) is "a disease state characterized by the presence of airflow obstruction due to chronic bronchitis or emphysema" (American Thoracic Society 1995). Chronic bronchitis is a clinical diagnosis of chronic productive cough, while emphysema is an "abnormal permanent enlargement of the airspaces...accompanied by destruction of their walls" (American Thoracic Society 1995).

### Risk Stratification

The evaluation of a patient with an exacerbation of COPD is similar to that of a patient with an asthma exacerbation. Specific attention should be directed toward determining the adequacy of oxygenation and ventilation and signs of impending respiratory failure. Compared with asthma patients, patients with COPD have a later onset, are more likely to smoke tobacco, and are more likely to have their symptoms begin with exertional dyspnea. During an acute episode, COPD patients complain of increasing shortness of breath that is often accompanied by a productive cough. Frequently the patient may report that a viral upper respiratory tract infection preceded the exacerbation. Fever suggests pneumonia.

The physical examintaion should be focused on determining the severity of the airway obstruction and on identifying impending respiratory failure. Because the lungs of a patient with COPD have lost their elasticity as a result of alveolar destruction, the patient may attempt to keep the airway open at the end of expiration by breathing against pursed lips to produce positive end expiratory pressure.

All patients with COPD exacerbation should be evaluated with pulse oximetry. Unlike patients with asthma, patients with COPD may have varying degrees of hypoventilation and carbon dioxide retention at baseline. Therefore, arterial blood gas analysis can be helpful in determining the patient's oxygenation and ventilatory status. A chest radiograph should be obtained to rule out pulmonary infections or other potential complications.

### Management in Psychiatric Settings

The objectives in the treatment of the patient with COPD are to reverse hypoxia, to treat any reversible bronchoconstriction and airway inflammation, and to treat underlying pulmonary infections. The mainstays of therapy are oxygen, inhaled bronchodilators, systemic steroids, antibiotics, and noninvasive positive pressure ventilation. Smoking cessation is the only measure that will prevent the continued progression of COPD.

**Oxygen.**    In patients with an arterial oxygen partial pressure of 55 mm Hg or oxygen saturation of 85% or less, survival is prolonged with supplemental low-flow oxygen to keep oxygen saturation greater than 90%. During an acute exacerbation, *never withhold supplemental oxygen from a hypoxic patient!*

**Bronchodilators.**    In stable symptomatic patients, a combination inhaler containing both albuterol and ipratropium (Combivent) or a long-acting $\beta_2$-agonist can be prescribed. In acute exacerbation, both albuterol and ipratropium can be given by nebulizer or metered dose inhaler. Up to three albuterol (2.5 mg) and ipratropium (0.5 mg) nebulizers can be given in the first hour and should be given continuously to patients in severe respiratory distress.

**Steroids.**    During acute exacerbations, either oral or parenteral systemic corticosteroids have been shown to decrease symptoms and should be given to treat the bronchial inflammation. The initial dose is 60 mg of prednisone orally or 125 mg of methylprednisolone intravenously. A steroid taper should be given for a total of 2 weeks. Inhaled corticosteroids are also recommended for patients with severe COPD who require systemic steroids or antibiotics to treat exacerbations.

**Antibiotics.**    COPD exacerbations are often triggered by pulmonary infections. For the patient with a COPD exacerbation, it is reasonable to initiate systemic broad-spectrum antibiotics covering both typical pathogens (including *Streptococcus pneumoniae* and *Haemophilus influenzae*) and atypical pathogens (including *Mycoplasma* and *Moraxella*) for 7–14 days.

**Noninvasive positive pressure ventilation.**    Noninvasive positive pressure ventilation is frequently used in the management of patients with COPD exacerbations. It has been shown to improve ventilation, improve oxygenation, and decrease the need for intubation in patients with impending hypercarbic respiratory failure (Sonin and Patterson 1984).

## Congestive Heart Failure

### Definition

Left ventricular failure results in increased pulmonary vascular pressures that cause alveolar flooding (causing rales) and bronchiolar wall edema (causing wheezing, or "cardiac asthma"). Right ventricular failure results in increased venous pressures and systemic fluid overload.

### Risk Stratification

Patients with congestive heart failure complain of exertional dyspnea, worsening shortness of breath, particularly at night and when lying supine (orthopnea), and increasing lower extremity edema. There may also be complaints of chest pain or of palpitations. In the physical examination, left ventricular failure is evident as rales or wheezing, and right ventricular failure leads to jugular venous distention and edema in the extremities. The cardiac examination may demonstrate an abnormal rate or rhythm or abnormal cardiac gallops (S3 and S4). Evaluation should include an electrocardiogram (ECG), chest radiograph, and echocardiogram.

### Management in Psychiatric Settings

The goal of treatment for acute decompensated heart failure is to maintain adequate oxygenation and rapidly reverse fluid overload. Supplemental 100% oxygen should be given to maintain an oxygen saturation of greater than 90%–92%. If underlying ischemia is suspected, the patient should be given 162 mg of aspirin, which should be chewed, assuming no contraindications for aspirin exist. Nitroglycerin (0.4 mg sl every 5 minutes for a total of three doses, provided the patient has a systolic blood pressure above 100 mm Hg) works as a vasodilator, resulting in preload reduction. Parenteral loop diuretics, such as furosemide (at a dose of 40–80 mg iv, which may be repeated after 15 minutes), may be given to promote diuresis of excess fluid. Chronic management includes the use of nitrates, diuretics, digoxin, β-blockers, and angiotensin-converting enzyme (ACE) inhibitors.

## General Approach to the Wheezing Patient

The general approach to the wheezing patient should follow the ABCs of basic and advanced life support. The goals of the rapid primary and secondary surveys are to determine the degree of respiratory distress, identify respiratory failure, and provide information to guide treatment (Figure 9–2).

The goals of the secondary survey are to obtain a history and perform a directed physical examination, as detailed in the following paragraph. The results provide the basis for elucidating the etiology of the patient's wheezing, determining risk stratification, and selecting appropriate therapy. A brief summary of the features that differentiate asthma, COPD, and congestive heart failure is presented in Table 9–2.

Pulse oximetry measurements should be obtained, and, if the patient is in severe respiratory distress, an arterial blood gas analysis should be considered to determine if the patient has adequate oxygenation (by measurement of alveolar partial pressure of oxygen [$PaO_2$]) and ventilation (measurement of $PaCO_2$). Bedside pulmonary function tests (PEFR or FEV1) provide a rapid objective measurement of bronchoconstriction and the degree of airflow obstruction. A chest radiograph should be obtained if the patient has a history of COPD or congestive heart failure, is febrile, has focal lung findings, is suspected of having a bronchial foreign body, or has unexplained wheezing. An ECG and echocardiogram should be obtained for any patient in whom congestive heart failure is suspected and for any patient complaining of shortness of breath or chest pain in whom cardiac ischemia is suspected. If pulmonary embolism is suspected, a ventilation/perfusion nuclear scan or a computed tomography pulmonary angiogram should be performed, and anticoagulation with heparin should be considered.

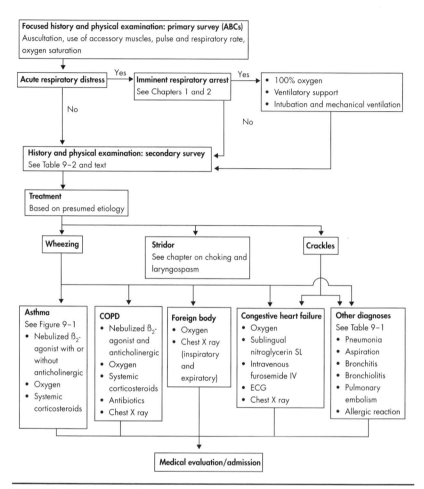

**FIGURE 9–2.**     Algorithm for the assessment and treatment of a wheezing patient.

*Note.*     ABC=airway, breathing, circulation; COPD=chronic obstructive pulmonary disease; ECG=electrocardiogram.

## Treatment

The results of the history and physical examination should be used to determine the underlying etiology of the patient's wheezing, and the patient should be treated accordingly. If the patient is hypoxic, supplemental 100% oxygen should be provided to keep the oxygen saturation above 90%–92%. The patient's respiratory status should be continually observed, especially if the patient has a history of COPD. If the etiology

**TABLE 9-2.** Characteristics of asthma, chronic obstructive pulmonary disease, and congestive heart failure

| Disorder | Symptoms | History | Physical examination findings |
|---|---|---|---|
| Asthma | Episodic dyspnea Episodic wheezing Nocturnal cough | Asthma | Wheezing Prolonged expiratory phase |
| Chronic obstructive pulmonary disease | Progressive dyspnea Wheezing Cough/sputum | Chronic obstructive pulmonary disease Chronic bronchitis Emphysema Smoking | Wheezing Pursed-lip breathing Hyperinflation of lungs |
| Congestive heart failure | Dyspnea Orthopnea Chest pain | Heart attack Heart failure Hypertension | Crackles/rales Jugular venous distention Lower extremity edema Abnormal cardiac gallops (S3, S4) |

of the patient's wheezing is uncertain, the patient should be treated for both bronchoconstriction (asthma and COPD) and congestive heart failure. Initial treatment consists of giving the patient oxygen, 2.5 mg of albuterol and 0.5 mg of ipratropium by nebulizer, and 40 mg iv of furosemide.

## References

Adams BK, Cydulka RK: Asthma evaluation and management. Emerg Med Clin North Am 21:315–330, 2003

American Thoracic Society: Standards for the diagnosis and care of patients with chronic obstructive pulmonary disease. Am J Respir Crit Care Med 152:S77–S120, 1995

Bloch H, Silverman R, Mancherje N, et al: Intravenous magnesium sulfate as an adjunct in the treatment of acute asthma. Chest 107:1576–1581, 1995

Busse WW, Lemanski RF: Advances in immunology: asthma. N Engl J Med 344:350–362, 2001

National Asthma Education and Prevention Program: Expert Panel Report 2: Guideline for the Diagnosis and Management of Asthma (NIH Publ No 97–4051). Bethesda, MD, National Institutes of Health, 1997

Nunn AJ, Gregg I: New regression equations for predicting peak expiratory flow in adults. BMJ 298:4068–4070, 1989

Schmaling KB, Bell J: Asthma and panic disorder. Arch Fam Med 6:20–23, 1997

Snow V, Lascher S, Mottur-Pilson C: Evidence base for management of acute exacerbations of chronic obstructive pulmonary disease. Ann Intern Med 134:595–599, 2001

Sonin L, Patterson R: Corticosteroid-dependent asthma and schizophrenia. Arch Intern Med 144:554–556, 1984

Stoppe G, Müller P, Fuchs T, et al: Life-threatening allergic reaction to clozapine. Br J Psychiatry 161:259–261, 1992

# CHAPTER 10

# Sleep Apnea

Harly E. Greenberg, M.D.

Aung Htoo, M.D.

## Clinical Presentation

Obstructive sleep apnea (OSA) is characterized by repetitive episodes of obstruction of the upper airway during sleep that are usually associated with decreases in arterial oxygen saturation and brief arousals from sleep. Common symptomatic manifestations of OSA include heavy snoring with intermittent pauses during apneas, complaints of nocturnal gasping, apneas witnessed by the bed partner, restless sleep, and awakening with a dry mouth or headache. Apnea-induced arousals fragment sleep, reduce sleep continuity, and disrupt the normal progression of sleep stages across the night. These sleep disturbances lead to excessive daytime somnolence (EDS), a major clinical manifestation of OSA, which can range in severity from a sensation of fatigue to inability to maintain wakefulness during daily activities. It is worth noting that in some cases EDS may be obvious but not reported by the patient, and in other cases it may be more subtle. Symptoms of EDS can often be elicited by querying patients about unintentional sleep episodes, either while inactive or while active and especially while driving, and about decreased vigilance and concentration during monotonous tasks. Often, the spouse or other family members can provide valuable insight into the severity of functional impairment and daytime somnolence that may not be fully recognized by the patient. Deficits in vigilance and concentration, as well as in short- and long-term memory, have been documented in this disorder and appear to have the strongest associations with measures of sleep disturbance. Decreased global intellectual and executive functions have been most closely associated with nocturnal hypoxemia (Camacho and Morin 1995; Hoffstein and Szalai 1993).

## Differential Diagnosis

Although the clinical signs and symptoms mentioned earlier are characteristic of OSA, clinical impression alone is insufficient to identify this syndrome. In a study of 594 patients, subjective clinical impression had a sensitivity and specificity of only 60% and 63%, respectively (Hoffstein and Szalai 1993). Surprisingly, the positive predictive value of a report of snoring and of witnessed apneas was only 49% and 56%, respectively. Thus, polysomnographic confirmation is required for diagnosis.

In the evaluation of patients with complaints suggestive of OSA, other sleep disorders should be considered. Within the category of sleep-related upper airway obstruction, a spectrum of disorders has been identified, ranging from primary snoring, in which respiration and sleep quality are not compromised, to overt obstructive apnea, in which airflow completely ceases during the apnea, resulting in oxygen desaturation and arousal from sleep. Between these extremes are disorders of partial airway obstruction, including hypopneas, which induce at least a 50% reduction in airflow and may be associated with arousals and oxygen desaturation, and inspiratory flow limitation, which results from less severe upper airway obstruction but may also be associated with arousals and decreased oxygenation.

Other forms of disordered breathing during sleep that are not related to upper airway obstruction include central sleep apnea and Cheyne-Stokes respiration, which may occur in the setting of cardiovascular or cerebrovascular disease. These disorders can impair sleep continuity and nocturnal oxygenation and may result in complaints of insomnia and daytime somnolence. In addition to being at risk for OSA, morbidly obese patients may have concomitant obesity-hypoventilation syndrome, which results in hypercapnia and hypoxemia that persists even when obstructive apneas are treated. Nocturnal hypoventilation, which may be particularly severe during rapid eye movement (REM) sleep, may also occur in neuromuscular or chest wall diseases, such as myasthenia gravis and kyphoscoliosis. The associated sleep disruption may cause EDS. Compromised respiration during sleep, with associated sleep complaints, may also occur in the setting of underlying pulmonary disorders such as asthma or chronic obstructive pulmonary disease. It is also worth noting that hypothyroidism predisposes the patient to development of OSA, possibly because of effects associated with hypothyroidism, including macroglossia and effects on upper airway muscles and ventilatory control.

Many disorders that cause anatomical abnormalities of the upper airway or abnormalities in the upper airway musculature or its neural control have been associated with snoring and OSA. These disorders are listed in Table 10–1. In addition, many other sleep disorders, listed in Table 10–2, can cause excessive daytime somnolence and should be considered in the evaluation of sleep complaints. Furthermore, many of these sleep disorders can coexist with OSA and may be responsible for persistent symptoms after treatment of sleep apnea.

## Risk Stratification

Obesity is a major risk factor for OSA, and strong associations between body mass index and apnea severity have been observed in most studies. The association of OSA with obesity may reflect obesity-related changes in upper airway size and conformation that predispose the airway to collapse during sleep. In addition to body mass index, neck circumference has been shown to correlate with the presence and severity of OSA (>17 inches in males and >16 inches in females) (Hoffstein and Szalai 1993). Because of the strong positive association of OSA with body mass index and the increasing prevalence of obesity in the United States, the burden of OSA is expected to increase in the future.

Epidemiological studies of the general population have shown a male-to-female ratio of 2–4:1 for OSA. Among females, menopausal status has been conclusively shown to play an important role in the development of sleep apnea (Jordan and McEvoy 2003).

Aging also appears to have a strong impact on OSA. Most patients with clinically apparent OSA are in the 30–60-year age range. However, studies of subjects ages 65 years and older have revealed prevalence rates for OSA that are two to four times greater than those in middle-aged adults (Partinen and Telakivi 1992).

Although OSA is more common among elderly persons, its strong associations with obesity, hypertension, EDS, and decreased functional capacity, which have been clearly documented in middle-aged subjects, are not as apparent in elderly subjects.

Crowding of the upper airway due to anatomical features such as enlargement of the tonsils, soft palate, uvula, and base of the tongue, as well as retrognathia or micrognathia, may lead to obstruction of the upper airway during sleep. Rarely, tumors and other masses can contribute to upper airway obstruction. Enlargement of these upper airway

---

**TABLE 10−1.**    Causes of snoring

---

**Conditions that compromise the nasopharyngeal area**
Congenital
    Achondroplasia
    Down syndrome
    Enlarged uvula
    Klippel-Feil syndrome
    Low-hanging soft palate
    Macroglossia
    Micrognathia
    Midface hypoplasia
    Pierre Robin syndrome
    Prader-Willi syndrome
    Retrognathia
    Storage diseases
Traumatic
    Deformity of upper airway
Systemic disease
    Acromegaly
    Amyloidosis
    Hypothyroidism
    Obesity
Other
    Nasal septal deviation
    Rhinitis/sinusitis
    Tonsillar/adenoid hypertrophy

**Conditions that affect collapsibility of the upper airway**
Congenital
    Hypotonia
    Muscular dystrophies
    Myopathies
Neurological
    Cranial nerve palsy
    Guillain-Barré syndrome (Miller-Fisher variant)
    Myasthenia gravis
    Parkinson's disease
Medications
    Alcohol
    Narcotics
    Sedative/hypnotics

**TABLE 10–2.**  Disorders other than obstructive sleep apnea that cause excessive daytime somnolence and sleep disturbances

**Hypersomnia due to sleep disorders**
Insufficient sleep time
Inadequate sleep hygiene
Restless legs syndrome/periodic limb movement disorder
Central sleep apnea
Cheyne-Stokes respiration
Obesity-hypoventilation syndrome
Parasomnias
   Sleep terrors
   Somnambulism
   Rapid eye movement sleep behavior disorder
Narcolepsy
Idiopathic hypersomnia
Circadian rhythm disorders
   Jet lag
   Shift work sleep disorder
   Delayed sleep phase syndrome
   Advanced sleep phase syndrome
   Irregular sleep-wake pattern
Kleine-Levin syndrome

**Hypersomnia due to psychiatric disorders**
Major depressive disorder
Bipolar disorder
Schizophrenia and schizoaffective disorder
Personality disorder

**Hypersomnia due to medications/substances**
Sedatives and hypnotics
Narcotics
Antidepressants (some)
Antipsychotics
Antiepileptic drugs
Antihistamines
Withdrawal of central nervous system stimulants
Alcohol

structures compromises the airway lumen. The retropalatal airway is the most severely narrowed region and is the most common site of upper airway collapse in OSA.

## Assessment and Management in Psychiatric Settings

After historical and physical features suggest the potential presence of OSA, laboratory confirmation of the diagnosis and assessment of its severity are required. Polysomnography, performed in a sleep laboratory, is the standard means of evaluating sleep and is useful in the assessment of complaints of EDS as well as difficulty initiating and maintaining sleep.

OSA patients should be advised to avoid alcohol consumption, particularly shortly before bedtime. Alcohol depresses one of the major compensatory mechanisms opposing upper airway collapse during sleep. As a result, the severity of OSA can be considerably worsened after alcohol consumption (Partinen and Telakivi 1992).

Although studies of the effects of sedative/hypnotic agents on respiratory control are limited and have yielded somewhat conflicting results, several studies have shown that benzodiazepines decrease ventilatory drive, inspiratory ventilatory load compensation, and upper airway muscle tone (Rapoport et al. 1991; Stepanski 2002). The combination of these effects may promote upper airway collapse and worsen OSA. However, other studies have failed to confirm worsening of sleep-disordered breathing after benzodiazepine administration in hypnotic doses in patients with mild to moderate OSA (Lim et al. 2003). Nevertheless, given the potential adverse effects of benzodiazepines on ventilatory control and upper airway muscle tone, prudence would dictate minimizing use of such agents in untreated OSA patients. When administration of these medications is necessary for other medical or psychiatric purposes, use of therapeutic continuous positive airway pressure (CPAP) with close respiratory monitoring is advised. Similar precautions would apply to the use of narcotics, which have more pronounced respiratory depressant effects. The limited data available on the effects of the newer nonbenzodiazepine hypnotics zolpidem, zaleplon, and zopiclone suggest that these agents do not have significant respiratory depressant effects (George 2000).

Most antidepressants can be safely administered in OSA. In fact, protriptyline and fluoxetine have been shown to have either no adverse effect or a minimally beneficial effect on sleep-disordered breathing (Hanzel et al. 1991).

Otolaryngology consultation with fiber-optic nasopharyngoscopy may identify upper airway abnormalities that are not evident in routine physical examination and may be particularly useful if a surgical intervention is being considered. The vibratory trauma of snoring may also be reflected by edema and erythema of these structures. Tonsillar hypertrophy along with enlargement of the tonsillar pillars, as well as redundant posterior pharyngeal tissue, is also commonly observed. In addition, relative enlargement of the base of the tongue, as well as retrognathia, may contribute to crowding in the retroglossal region. Nasal obstruction caused by nasal septal deviation, turbinate hypertrophy, or prior nasal fracture or trauma may lead to increased nasopharyngeal resistance that contributes to downstream airway obstruction.

Nasal continuous positive airway pressure (nCPAP) is first-line medical therapy for OSA. It functions as a "pressure splint" to maintain upper airway patency during sleep. When it is administered to patients with OSA, dramatic improvements in sleep quality are often observed in association with elimination of apneas and snoring. Prescription of nCPAP is best accomplished by nocturnal CPAP titration polysomnography that accurately determines CPAP pressure requirements during all stages of sleep. Many types and styles of CPAP masks are available. Selection of a comfortable, properly fitting mask is essential to maximize adherence to therapy. Once CPAP is prescribed, follow-up is required to assure continued adherence. Common interventions to improve comfort include heated humidification of the CPAP system to alleviate upper airway dryness, use of an oronasal mask or chin straps for mouth breathing, and provision of alternative mask sizes and styles to optimize fit and comfort.

Oral appliance therapy, another noninvasive modality, utilizes a custom-fit dental appliance to advance the mandible and increase upper airway patency. The devices are most effective in mild to moderate OSA and provide a useful alternative for treatment of patients who are intolerant of CPAP. Efficacy studies have shown improvements in the apnea hypopnea index with oral appliances, although improvement may not be as complete as with CPAP (Remmers et al. 1978).

In patients intolerant of CPAP or oral appliances, surgical therapy can be considered. Surgical treatments include uvulopalatopharyngoplasty, which may be combined with nasal septoplasty and tonsillectomy if appropriate. Reported success rates range from 40% to 70% (Pepin 1996). Other less invasive procedures such as radiofrequency ablation surgery of the upper airway can be performed on an ambulatory basis in patients with snoring and mild OSA.

# References

Camacho ME, Morin CM: The effect of temazepam on respiration in elderly insomniacs with mild sleep apnea. Sleep 18:644–645, 1995

George CF: Perspectives on the management of insomnia in patients with chronic respiratory disorders. Sleep 23 (suppl 1):S31–S35, 2000

Hanzel DA, Proia NG, Hudgel DW: Response of obstructive sleep apnea to fluoxetine and protriptylline. Chest 100:416–421, 1991s

Hoffstein V, Szalai JP: Predictive value of clinical features in diagnosing obstructive sleep apnea. Sleep 16:118–122, 1993

Leiter JC, Knuth SL, Krol RC, et al: The effect of diazepam on genioglossal muscle activity in normal human subjects. Am Rev Respir Dis 132:216–219, 1985

Lim J, Lasserson TJ, Fleetham J, et al: Oral appliances for obstructive sleep apnea. Cochrane Database Syst Rev 4:CD004435, 2003

Jordan AS, McEvoy RD: Gender differences in sleep apnea: epidemiology, clinical presentation, and pathogenic mechanisms. Sleep Med Rev 7:377–389, 2003

Partinen M, Telakivi T: Epidemiology of obstructive sleep apnea syndrome. Sleep 15 (suppl 6):S1–S4, 1992

Pepin JL, Veale D, Mayer P, et al: Critical analysis of the results of surgery in the treatment of snoring, upper airway resistance syndrome (UARS), and obstructive sleep apnea (OSA). Sleep 19 (suppl 9):S90–S100, 1996

Rapoport DM, Greenberg HE, Goldring RM: Differing effects of the anxiolytic agents buspirone and diazepam on control of breathing. Clin Pharmacol Ther 49:394–401, 1991

Remmers JE, deGroot WJ, Sauerland EK, et al: Pathogenesis of upper airway occlusion during sleep. J Appl Physiol 44:931–938, 1978

Stepanski EJ: The effect of sleep fragmentation on daytime function. Sleep 25:268–276, 2002

# PART IV

# Pain Symptoms

Section Editor:

Kumar Alagappan, M.D.

# CHAPTER 11

# Chest Pain

Lorna Breen, M.D.

Barbara J. Barnett, M.D.

## Clinical Presentation

Chest pain is a common complaint that may indicate life-threatening disorders. Aortic dissection, pulmonary embolism, and pneumothorax usually cause sudden onset of pain, whereas musculoskeletal etiologies are more likely to have an insidious onset. Cardiac ischemia classically causes a pressure-like pain, but there are many different presentations of ischemia. Gupta et al. (2002) showed that of 721 patients with acute myocardial infarction at a large, urban public hospital emergency department, only 53% had a chief complaint of chest pain.

Aortic dissection pain is usually described as excruciating, tearing, and maximal at onset and may be described as migrating. Pleuritic pain may be due to pulmonary embolism, pneumothorax, pleurisy, or pneumonia. Pneumothorax causes sharp pain that may be well localized. Chest pain with a gastrointestinal cause may be described as burning.

Cardiac pain often radiates to one arm, both arms, or the neck/jaw. Pain that radiates to the back may indicate aortic dissection, posterior ulcer, or pancreatitis. Aortic dissection may also cause pain that is localized primarily in the back (especially in the interscapular region). Pericarditis pain may radiate to the trapezius area. Herniated thoracic disc may cause band-like chest pain.

Associated symptoms may help to differentiate among the different types of chest pain. Cardiac pain is often associated with diaphoresis and dyspnea. Hemoptysis may indicate pulmonary embolism. Nausea and vomiting can come from cardiac or gastrointestinal causes of pain. Syncope suggests aortic dissection, large pulmonary embolism, acute myocardial infarction, or critical aortic stenosis. Myocarditis may be seen with systemic symptoms of fever, myalgias, and muscle tenderness. Aortic dissection may be seen with symptoms of cardiac tamponade caused by a rupture of aorta into the pericardial space. Patients with gastroesophageal reflux disease often experience dyspepsia, regurgitation of food, and acid taste in the mouth.

Angina may last less than 2–10 minutes, and unstable angina usually lasts less than 20 minutes. Pain from myocardial infarction usually lasts longer than 15–30 minutes. Aortic dissection pain is usually unrelenting.

Cardiac ischemia is often precipitated by activity and emotional stress and is relieved by rest or nitroglycerin (although a myocardial infarction will *not* be relieved by rest and nitroglycerin). Improvement with a "GI cocktail," such as viscous lidocaine plus antacid, does *not* distinguish gastrointestinal versus cardiac chest pain. Esophageal reflux may be aggravated by a large meal and postprandial recumbence and relieved with an antacid, but biliary colic may be worse with fatty food intake. Pain from pulmonary and musculoskeletal causes is often worse with breathing. Pericarditis pain often worsens when the patient is in the supine position and with swallowing and inspiration and improves when the patient sits up.

## Differential Diagnosis

Although physicians often focus on the cardiovascular system while evaluating a patient with chest pain, several other organ systems can cause identical symptoms that require a different focus in evaluation and treatment. The major systems that should be considered while evaluating a patient with chest pain are the cardiovascular, pulmonary, gastrointestinal, musculoskeletal, neurological, and psychiatric systems. Although ischemic cardiac events can cause a range of acute coronary syndromes, inflammatory conditions such as pericarditis and myocarditis should also be considered. Another life-threatening condition that should always be considered is aortic dissection, which classically presents with tearing chest pain that radiates to the back in a patient with history of hypertension. In the pulmonary system, the history and physical examination should help separate infectious sources (e.g., pneumonia, pneumomediastinum) from structural diseases such as pneumothorax or pulmonary embolism. Another fairly common cause of chest pain that may be discovered incidentally on a chest X ray is malignancy. Multiple gastrointestinal abnormalities can cause epigastric pain that is difficult to differentiate from cardiac pain. Herpes zoster can cause severe neuropathic pain in a dermatomal distribution that is present days before the vesicular lesions appear.

Chest pain may be a presenting symptom of several psychiatric disorders, including anxiety disorders, depression, hypochondriasis, and factitious disorder with predominantly physical signs and symptoms (Munchausen syndrome). In one study, two groups of patients—one with and one without significant coronary artery disease at cardiac catheterization—underwent psychiatric testing; major depressive disorder and panic disorder were found in 42% and 19%, respectively (Carney et al. 1990). It was also noted that of the patients with no significant coronary artery disease but with major depressive disorder or panic disorder, 80% had mitral valve prolapse. In a review of the literature, Carter et al. (1997) found that 30%–50% of patients with recurrent chest pain and normal coronary arteries met the criteria for panic disorder. Corruble and Guelfi (2000) evaluated pain complaints in 150 depressed patients on the day of admission and after 10 and 28 days of treatment. They found that headache and chest pain were more common complaints in women than in men and that pain complaints decreased between the evaluation on the day of admission and the evaluation after 10 days of treatment. Another study found that of 441 consecutive emergency department patients with complaints of chest pain, 25% ($n=108$) had panic disorder (Fleet et al. 1996). The interplay between psychiatric conditions and physical symptoms should not be overlooked in patients with a known psychiatric history.

## Risk Stratification

Multiple factors can increase a patient's risk for having coronary artery disease. The major risk factors are a high level of low-density lipoprotein (LDL) cholesterol and a low level of high-density lipoprotein (HDL) cholesterol (various cutoff points for high and low values, depending on the patient's other medical problems), age (men: 45 years; women: 55 years or premature menopause without estrogen replacement therapy), family history of premature coronary heart disease (definite myocardial infarction or sudden death before age 55 years in the father or first-degree male relative or sudden death before age 65 years in the mother or first-degree female relative), cigarette smoking, hypertension, and diabetes mellitus. Cocaine is the major toxic substance that needs to be considered as a cause of chest pain in any patient presenting with that complaint. One study showed that 17% of patients evaluated for myocardial infarction in an urban/suburban setting had cocaine metabolites in their urine (Hollander et al. 1995). Use of cocaine can lead to vasospastic ischemic events that must be treated differently from occlusive coronary artery disease. It is critical that all patients experiencing chest pain be questioned about their possible use of cocaine.

## Assessment and Management in Psychiatric Settings

The initial evaluation begins with a complete history of the patient. Inquiry about the patient's past medical history should include questions about cardiac risk factors and history of alcohol use, smoking, and illicit drug use. The clinician should ascertain the qualities of the chest pain, including time of onset, nature of the pain, severity, duration, palliative or provocative features, and associated symptoms.

The physical examination must include evaluation of vital signs, the neck, heart sounds, breath sounds, the chest wall, abdomen, musculoskeletal system, skin, and neurological structures. Irregular vital signs can help point to the etiology of the discomfort. Inferior wall myocardial infarction may cause bradycardia or heart block. Right ventricular myocardial infarction often causes hypotension, and nitroglycerin and morphine should be used sparingly or not at all in these patients. Pulsus paradoxus—an accentuation of the normal decrease in the systolic blood pressure during inspiration of greater than 20 mm Hg—is seen with pericardial tamponade. A marked difference in blood pressure measurements between the two arms suggests aortic dissection. Pulse oximetry is likely to indicate hypoxemia in patients with pulmonary embolism, pneumothorax, pneumonia, and acute mycoadial infarction with left ventricular dysfunction. Tachypnea is the most common physical finding with pulmonary embolism, although tachypnea may be present in other disorders as well. Elevated temperature should lead the clinician to consider pneumonia or mediastinitis, although a low-grade temperature elevation is possible in pulmonary embolism and acute myocardial infarction.

While examining the neck, it is important to look for jugular venous distention, which may indicate congestive heart failure. Kussmaul's sign, a paradoxical increase in jugular venous distention with inspiration, may be seen in pericardial tamponade, right heart failure, pulmonary embolism, or tension pneumothorax. The presence of carotid bruits increases the likelihood of coronary artery disease, and Beck's triad of hypotension, distended neck veins, and muffled heart sounds may be seen with pericardial tamponade. With tension pneumothorax, the trachea is seen to be deviating away from the injured side.

Careful examination of the heart sounds can also help elucidate the cause of the patient's chest pain. Acute myocardial infarction may cause an S3 sound secondary to congestive heart failure. Pericarditis may cause a pericardial friction rub that may be heard only intermittently. Aortic dissection may cause an aortic insufficiency murmur that is diastolic and heard at the upper left sternal border. Hamman's sign, an audible systolic "crunch" heard on cardiac examination, may be found with esophageal rupture or mediastinitis.

The chest wall examination is very important in cases of chest pain that are thought less likely to be caused by cardiac disease. Costochondritis may lead to tenderness with palpation in the area of the costal cartilage, especially in the upper costochondral junctions. Pain due to compression of ventral nerve roots is usually worse with neck movement, coughing, sneezing, or axial loading by applying pressure to the top of the head (Spurling's maneuver). Pneumothorax, esophageal rupture, and mediastinitis can all cause subcutaneous emphysema, but only pneumothorax causes hyperresonance to percussion and decreased breath sounds.

The abdominal examination must include a search for an enlarged or tender aorta. The musculoskeletal examination should include a search for enlarged lower extremity or extremity with cord, especially in a patient suspected of having pulmonary embolism. The skin examination should reveal any evidence of vesicular rash in dermatomal pattern. A rapid neurological examination should uncover any focal neurological deficit that may be the result of an aortic dissection, which would be suspected in any patient with chest pain and associated stroke symptoms.

The electrocardiogram (ECG) should be read in a systematic fashion, by considering rate, rhythm, axis, intervals, hypertrophy, and ischemia. Cardiac ischemia is indicated by hyperacute T waves (the first ECG change of cardiac ischemia), left bundle branch block, Q waves, flipped T waves, and ST elevation or depression in anatomic distribution. Ischemic ECG findings may be present with aortic dissection. The S1Q3T3 pattern is suggestive of pulmonary embolism. Incomplete right bundle branch block and sinus tachycardia are commonly found in patients with pulmonary embolism. The earliest ECG change with pulmonary embolism is T wave inversion in the anterior precordial leads. Diffuse ST elevation and P–R segment depression suggest pericarditis. Electrical alternans on the ECG may be seen with pericardial tamponade. Whenever possible, one should compare the patient's current ECG to the most recent available ECG to check for changes.

For any patient with a complaint of chest pain, a chest X ray should be obtained to rule out skeletal, pleuropulmonary, or mediastinal pathology. The X ray should be examined closely for pneumothorax, which may be more visible on an expiratory film. A combination of pneumothorax, pneumomediastinum, and pleural effusion is suggestive of esophageal rupture. A finding of a widened mediastinum on a nonrotated X ray may be a sign of aortic dissection. Infiltrate should be seen with pneumonia or acute chest syndrome. Pleural effusion can be caused by multiple underlying processes, such as pulmonary embolism, pneumonia, malignancy, or congestive heart failure. A finding of a "water bottle"–shaped heart on a chest X ray suggests cardiac tamponade.

Laboratory investigations for patients with chest pain should include measurement of creatine phosphokinase and troponin for suspected myocardial infarction. Troponin may be elevated with renal failure, pulmonary embolism, myocarditis, and pericarditis. The test for D-dimer should be considered for patients with suspected pulmonary embolism. The test is very sensitive but not very specific; thus a negative D-dimer test may rule out pulmonary embolism in patients with a low pretest probability of this condition (Kruip et al. 2003). Arterial blood gas analysis may reveal a widened alveolar-arterial gradient or respiratory alkalosis in patients with pulmonary embolism.

Figure 11–1 shows an algorithm for evaluation of chest pain. Serious pathology should be considered first. If there is any suspicion of a cardiac event, the patient should be treated with aspirin (81 or 325 mg chewed), oxygen, cardiac monitoring, and sublingual nitroglycerin. A 0.4-mg tablet of nitroglycerin may be given up to three times 5 minutes apart, but an intravenous line should be established first in case the patient's blood pressure drops after nitroglycerin administration. Use of nitroglycerin should be avoided in any patient with hypotension or right ventricle infarction and in patients who have used sildenafil (Viagra) within the last 24 hours. The patient should be transferred to the nearest emergency department.

If aortic dissection is diagnosed, the patient should be treated with a β-blocker as soon as possible. If there is evidence of tension pneumothorax (respiratory distress, shock, decreased breath sounds), the patient needs immediate intervention with a needle/tube thoracostomy.

If pneumonia is suspected, antibiotics should be started as soon as possible, ideally within 4 hours. If there is evidence of pericardial tamponade (diffuse ST elevation on an ECG, cardiomegaly seen on a chest X ray, shock), pericardiocentesis should be performed as soon as possible.

The vital signs of patients with acute coronary syndromes should be monitored closely, and these patients should be watched for recurrence of chest pain. Because the goal "door-to-drug time" for thrombolytic

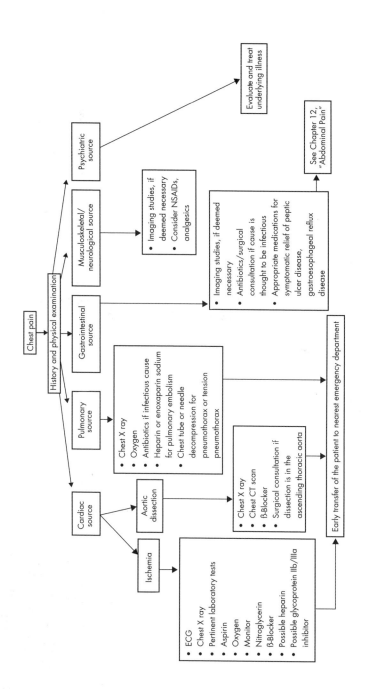

**FIGURE 11–1.** Algorithm for the assessment and treatment of a patient with chest pain.

*Note.* CT=computed tomography; ECG=electrocardiogram; NSAIDs=nonsteroidal anti-inflammatory drugs.

therapy for acute myocardial infarction is 30 minutes, the patient should be transferred to the nearest emergency department as soon as possible.

## References

Carney RM, Freedland KE, Ludbrook PA, et al: Major depression, panic disorder, and mitral valve prolapse in patients who complain of chest pain. Am J Med 89:757–760, 1990

Carter CS, Servan-Schreiber D, Perlstein WM: Anxiety disorders and the syndrome of chest pain with normal coronary arteries: prevalence and pathophysiology. J Clin Psychiatry 58 (suppl 3):70–73, 1997

Corruble E, Guelfi JD: Pain complaints in depressed inpatients. Psychopathology 33:307–309, 2000

Fleet RP, Dupuis G, Marchand A, et al: Panic disorder in emergency department chest pain patients: prevalence, comorbidity, suicidal ideation, and physician recognition. Am J Med 101:371–380, 1996

Gupta M, Tabas JA, Kohn MA: Presenting complaint among patients with myocardial infarction who present to an urban, public hospital emergency department. Ann Emerg Med 40:180–186, 2002

Hollander JE, Todd KH, Green G, et al: Chest pain associated with cocaine: an assessment of prevalence in suburban and urban emergency departments. Ann Emerg Med 26:671–676, 1995

Kruip MJ, Leclercq MG, van der Heul C, et al: Diagnostic strategies for excluding pulmonary embolism in clinical outcome studies: a systematic review. Ann Intern Med 138:941–951, 2003

# CHAPTER 12

# Abdominal Pain

Douglas A. Isaacs, M.D.

Barbara J. Barnett, M.D.

## Clinical Presentation

Causes of abdominal pain can be divided into intra-abdominal and extra-abdominal causes. Intra-abdominal causes are further characterized by organ systems, which include gastrointestinal, genitourinary, gynecological, and vascular systems (King and Wightman 2002). The evaluation of abdominal pain is approached by dividing the abdomen into four quadrants. A variant of this approach includes four additional regions that are a blend of two of these quadrants (Gallagher 2000) (Table 12–1). Extra-abdominal pain can also be divided into broad divisions (Table 12–2) (Cheskin and Lacy 2003; Gallagher 2000). Pain can be referred to the abdomen from the chest, spine, or pelvis, further complicating the clinical picture.

The pain should be characterized according to location, time course, quality, intensity, and associated symptoms. Being able to define and localize the pain may help determine the etiology. For example, appendicitis initially causes periumbilical pain, but as the inflammation worsens and involves the overlying peritoneum, the pain relocates to the right lower quadrant. Radiation of pain can be an important clue. It is important to determine whether the pain is acute or chronic. Sudden onset of severe pain may suggest a serious disorder, such as aortic dissection or a perforated viscus. However, patients with kidney stones may also present with severe abrupt onset of pain. Insidious onset of pain does not rule out serious pathology.

Constant pain suggests an inflammatory process, while cramping may be from obstruction or an increase in intraluminal pressure from

**TABLE 12-1.**   Causes of abdominal pain, by location

| Location of pain | Causes |
|---|---|
| Right upper quadrant | Acute cholecystitis, biliary colic, acute hepatitis, peptic ulcer, hepatomegaly secondary to congestive heart failure, acute pancreatitis, hepatic abscess, retrocecal appendicitis, herpes zoster, myocardial ischemia, right lower lobe pneumonia, empyema, pericarditis, renal colic |
| Right lower quadrant | Appendicitis, regional enteritis, diverticulitis, leaking aneurysm, abdominal wall hematoma, ectopic pregnancy, ovarian cyst, ovarian torsion, pelvic inflammatory disease, mittelschmerz, endometriosis, renal colic, seminal vesiculitis, psoas abscess, intestinal obstruction, inguinal hernia, inflammatory bowel disease, testicular torsion |
| Left upper quadrant | Gastritis, gastric ulcer, acute appendicitis, splenic pathology (enlargement, infarction, rupture, or aneurysm), myocardial ischemia, left lower lobe pneumonia, renal colic |
| Left lower quadrant | Diverticulitis, intestinal obstruction, appendicitis, ectopic pregnancy, mittelschmerz, ovarian cyst, ovarian torsion, pelvic inflammatory disease, endometriosis, renal colic, seminal vesciulitis, psoas abscess, leaking aneurysm, inguinal hernia, testicular torsion |
| Epigastric | Peptic ulcer disease, gastroesophageal reflux disease, gastritis, acute pancreatitis, myocardial ischemia/ infarction, pericarditis, abdominal aortic aneurysm |
| Periumbilical | Early appendicitis, gastroenteritis, intestinal obstruction, abdominal aortic aneurysm |
| Suprapubic | Ectopic pregnancy, mittelschmerz, ovarian cyst, pelvic inflammatory disease, endometriosis, urinary tract infection, acute urinary retention |
| Flank | Abdominal aortic aneurysm, pyelonephritis, renal colic, acute cholecystitis |
| Diffuse | Peritonitis, acute pancreatitis, mesenteric thrombosis/ ischemia, intestinal obstruction, sickle cell crisis, gastroenteritis, metabolic disorder (diabetic ketoacidosis, porphyria), irritable bowel syndrome |
| Front to back | Ruptured abdominal aortic aneurysm, acute pancreatitis, posterior duodenal ulcer, acute cholecystitis |

**TABLE 12–2.** Extra-abdominal causes of abdominal pain

| | |
|---|---|
| **Cardiopulmonary** | **Toxic** |
| Congestive heart failure | Drugs |
| Empyema | Lead poisoning |
| Myocardial ischemia/infarction | Methanol poisoning |
| Myocarditis | Venoms |
| Pneumonia | **Genitourinary** |
| Pulmonary embolism | Epididymitis |
| **Vascular** | Pyelonephritis |
| Aortic aneurysm rupture, | Renal colic |
| dissection, or expansion | Testicular torsion |
| Periarteritis | **Psychogenic** |
| **Hematological** | Irritable bowel syndrome |
| Leukemia | |
| Sickle cell crisis | |
| **Metabolic** | |
| Addisonian crisis | |
| Diabetic ketoacidosis | |
| Hypercalcemia | |
| Hyperlipidemia | |
| Porphyria | |
| Uremia | |

distention. Dysuria, urinary urgency, and increased urinary frequency suggest involvement of the bladder. Nausea, vomiting, obstipation (inability to pass flatus or stool), and diarrhea suggest involvement of the gastrointestinal tract. Jaundice and pruritis suggest liver or gallbladder disease.

## Differential Diagnosis

Table 12–1 lists possible causes of abdominal pain by location in the abdomen. Table 12–2 lists extra-abdominal causes of abdominal pain.

## Risk Stratification

The temporal development of pain helps dictate the urgency of the clinical situation, directs the evaluation of the patient, and may be an important prognostic factor. An abrupt onset of pain may be an ominous sign. Some causes of pain in relation to time of onset are noted in Table 12–3 (Bullard and Rothenberger 1994; White and Counselman 2002).

**TABLE 12–3.**   Timing of onset and causes of abdominal pain

| Timing of onset | Causes | |
|---|---|---|
| Abrupt onset (seconds) | • Acute myocardial infarction <br> • Perforated ulcer <br> • Ruptured abdominal aortic aneurysm or aortic dissection | • Mesenteric infarction <br> • Pulmonary embolism <br> • Ruptured ectopic pregnancy |
| Rapid onset (minutes) | • Acute pancreatitis <br> • Diverticulitis <br> • Strangulated hernia | • Biliary colic <br> • Renal colic <br> • Volvulus |
| Gradual onset (hours) | • Appendicitis <br> • Chronic pancreatitis <br> • Inflammatory bowel disease <br> • Mesenteric lymphadenitis <br> • Prostatitis | • Cystitis <br> • Diverticulitis <br> • Intestinal obstruction <br> • Peptic ulcer disease <br> • Salpingitis <br> • Urinary retention <br> • Strangulated hernia |

Two groups of patients requiring special attention are elderly patients and women of reproductive age. Their differential diagnoses can be more extensive and complicated. Elderly patients often have more atypical presentations than their younger counterparts. They may delay seeking help, their pain may be less severe, and their fever may be less pronounced. Often, in elderly patients, peritoneal signs are either minimal or not present, and laboratory values are less sensitive (Cheskin and Lacy 2003). Gynecological diseases are of primary consideration in women of childbearing age. These diseases include ectopic pregnancy, pelvic inflammatory disease, tubo-ovarian abscess, torsion, hemorrhage, cysts, and mittelschmerz.

## Assessment and Management in Psychiatric Settings

The assessment begins with an evaluation of the patient's appearance. Is the patient lying still, as would be seen in diffuse peritonitis, or writhing in pain, as might be seen in an obstructive state (e.g., renal or biliary colic)? An abnormal vital sign should never be disregarded. In addition to an assessment of the four basic vital signs, pulse oximetry and a finger-stick test should be performed. The patient should by inspected for scars indicating prior surgeries and any asymmetry. In the auscultation for bowel sounds, a complete lack of bowel sounds is suggestive of peritonitis or an ileus. High-pitched or hyperactive bowel sounds associated with cramping abdominal pain are highly suggestive of an obstruction. Bruits may indicate an aortic aneurysm or stenosis of a blood vessel. The clinician should gently percuss the patient's abdomen and note any dullness or tympany. Dullness may be caused by an abdominal mass, fluid (ascites), or fluid-filled loops of bowel. Tympany indicates free-air or fluid-filled loops of bowel. Next, the abdomen is palpated, starting from an area away from where the patient has pain and slowly working toward the painful region. Any rigidity or guarding should be noted. Voluntary guarding is the conscious contraction of the abdominal musculature, whereas involuntary guarding is a reflex contraction of the abdominal musculature from the underlying inflammation. Involuntary guarding signifies that serious pathology is present (White and Counselman 2002). The clinician should check if any hernias are present and whether they are reducible, tender, or warm or are associated with a change in color of the overlying skin. The patient should also be assessed for urinary bladder distention.

The main utility of a rectal examination is to identify intraluminal hemorrhage, in which case the stool may be black or bright red. The presence of any fecal impaction or perirectal disease should be noted. A prostate examination should be performed in male patients, and any tenderness, nodularity, or enlargement of the prostate should be noted. In male patients, the genital area should be examined for signs for testicular torsion, epididymitis, tumor, penile discharge, and inguinal or femoral hernias. A pelvic examination should be performed in all female patients who complain of lower abdominal pain.

An elevated white blood cell count (WBC) can be a sign that an infectious process is occurring. A low hemoglobin level can indicate gastrointestinal bleeding. A pregnancy test should be performed in women of childbearing age. A urinalysis should also be performed. If nephrolithiasis is being considered, the urine test may be positive for hematuria, although it has been noted that 10% of patients with nephrolithiasis have urine tests that are negative for hematuria (White and Counselman 2002). An increase in the ratio of blood urea nitrogen to creatinine may suggest gastrointestinal bleeding or dehydration (Overton 2000). An increase in the creatinine level can also indicate renal dysfunction. Elevated blood glucose and serum ketones levels are indicative of diabetic ketoacidosis. Abnomal liver function test results can give clues for the direction for further evaluation. An elevation of the alkaline phosphatase level is suggestive of a cholestatic or infiltrative process; in these cases, an abdominal ultrasound examination should be obtained for further evaluation. The most likely causes of high transaminase levels are either viral or related to alcohol or drugs. Transaminase levels >5,000 U/L may indicate acetaminophen overdose. If pancreatitis is present, elevated amylase and lipase levels should be found. As opposed to an elevation of the lipase level, a high amylase level is not specific for pancreatitis, nor does the absolute level correlate with the severity of the pancreatitis.

Plain radiographs have limited utility in assessing abdominal pain, but they may be useful if bowel obstruction, perforated viscus, foreign object ingestion, or lower lobe pneumonia is suspected. An electrocardiogram should be done if a cardiac etiology is suspected.

Initial management is dictated by the severity of the abdominal pain and other variables, as mentioned previously. If the patient appears well and is hemodynamically stable, an attempt could be made to treat the pain in the psychiatric setting and the patient's response could be observed. Referral to an emergency department is needed in some cases (Figure 12–1).

## Peptic Ulcer Disease

Duodenal ulcer symptoms present 1–3 hours after a meal, give nocturnal discomfort, and are immediately relieved with either food, antacids, or vomiting. Gastric ulcers have a more variable presentation but tend to be immediately relieved by food and antacids. Symptoms are mid-epigastric discomfort with a feeling of gnawing hunger and an aching or burning sensation. Ulcers may be caused by *Helicobacter pylori*, nonsteroidal anti-inflammatory drugs (NSAIDs), or a hypersecretory acid state.

Treatment includes both nonpharmacological and pharmacological approaches. The patient should be encouraged to quit cigarette smoking and stop all NSAID, aspirin, and alcohol use. These substances are risk factors for development of ulcers and prevent healing of ulcers (Dempsey 2005). Pharmacological treatment includes the use of antisecretory agents, such as histamine type 2 ($H_2$) antagonists or proton pump inhibitors (PPIs).

Patients who have peptic ulcer disease should be tested for *H. pylori*. Although a large percentage of the healthy population test positive for *H. pylori*, failure to treat patients with symptoms who test positive will result in recurrent disease. The most practical test is to check the patient's serum for the IgG antibody against *H. pylori*. The most effective treatment regimen currently used is PPI-based triple therapy (Bullard and

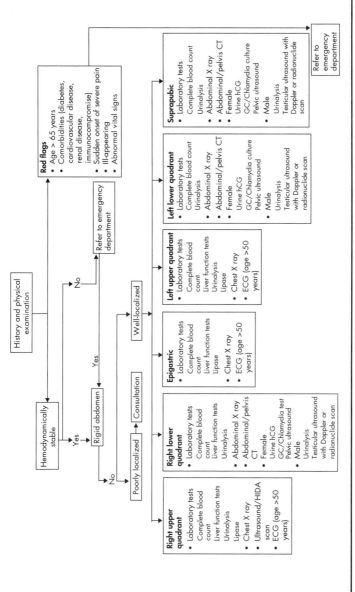

**FIGURE 12–1.** Algorithm for the assessment and treatment of a patient with abdominal pain.

*Note.* CT=computed tomography; ECG=electrocardiogram; GC=*Neisseria gonoroohoae* test; hCG=human chorionic gonadotropin; HIDA=hepatobiliary iminodiacetic acid.

Rothenberger 2005), which includes the use of a PPI twice a day, amoxicillin (1 g twice a day), and clarithromycin (500 mg twice a day). If there is a contraindication to amoxicillin, metronidazole (500 mg twice a day) can be substituted. Treatment should continue for 10–14 days. Specialty consultation must be obtained to rule out a gastrointestinal malignancy.

## Irritable Bowel Syndrome

Most clinicians consider irritable bowel syndrome (IBS) when a patient has chronic intermittent mild abdominal pain with a change in frequency or character of bowel movements (Bullard and Rothenberger 2005). Often there is a temporal relationship between relief of the abdominal pain and defecation or change in the consistency of the stool. The abdominal pain is described as cramping, sharp, or burning. The patient may also have complaints of gaseous symptoms, such as bloating and belching. Many IBS patients experience symptoms similar to those of gastroesophageal reflux disease (GERD). The most important identifier of IBS is completely normal findings in the physical examination.

Treatment is focused on alleviating the symptoms. It is important to elucidate if there are any psychological factors that may be contributing to the onset of the symptoms. Patients with such factors may require psychological management for anxiety, depression, or other psychological disorders. Also, it may be helpful to determine if there is an association between the patient's diet and IBS symptoms (e.g., lactose intolerance). However, no specific correlation has been demonstrated between specific foods and IBS symptoms. For patients who complain of constipation, symptoms should be ameliorated by increasing the amount of dietary fiber by adding supplementary fiber, increasing fluid intake, and following the same bowel regimen each day. For patients with diarrhea as the predominant symptom, a low-dose fiber supplement should be started. Pharmacological agents such as analgesics should be avoided for the abdominal pain, especially narcotics, because IBS tends to be a chronic disorder. Dietary restrictions and avoidance of caffeine, alcohol, and tobacco may help alleviate symptoms (Bullard and Rothenberger 2005).

## Gastroesophageal Reflux Disease

The cause of GERD is the abnormal reflux of acid from the stomach into the esophagus. The underlying mechanisms are the abnormal relaxation of the lower esophageal sphincter, abnormal clearing of the gastric acid, and abnormal esophageal mucosa that is susceptible to the gastric acid. Patients may experience substernal chest pain, described as burning, that radiates up, a sour taste in the mouth, and worsening pain with large meals and when lying down or bending over. Symptoms improve when the patient is sitting up or with the use of antacids. Other serious pathology such as cardiac disease should be considered before making a diagnosis of GERD.

For mild cases, patients can make changes in both their diet and lifestyle. They should avoid such foods as caffeine (coffee, chocolate), citrus juices, alcohol, fatty meals, and spices. Some lifestyle changes include keeping the head of the bed elevated, eating smaller meals, avoiding tight fitting clothing, not lying down for at least 3 hours after eating, and losing weight. For more moderate or severe cases, antisecretory medications, such as $H_2$ antagonists, and PPI are indicated. Initially antacids should be prescribed, and the patient's response should be observed. This step can be both diagnostic and therapeutic. The patient should subsequently be referred to a gastroenterologist as an outpatient.

## Urinary Tract Infection

Patients with urinary tract infection (UTI) frequently complain of dysuria, increase in urinary frequency and urgency, nocturia, and hematuria. A physical examination may show that the patient has a low-grade fever and mild suprapubic tenderness or costovertebral angle tenderness. A urine sample should be sent for both urinalysis and urine culture.

Treatment with antibiotics (trimethoprim-sulfamethoxazole or ciprofloxacin) for 3 days is often effective. If there are comorbidities, the dosage and length of treatment may have to be adjusted. The patient's failure to respond to treatment could suggest other possibilities (e.g., a sexually transmitted disease, prostatitis or epididymitis in a male patient, vaginitis in a female patient, or bacterial resistance) and would warrant a referral for further treatment. It is unusual for male patients to have a UTI, and a urology consultation should be requested for such patients.

Pyelonephritis shoul be suspected if the patient appears sicker and has an elevated temperature, costovertebral angle tenderness, and an elevated white blood cell count. A medical consultation should be requested. The patient will require a longer course of antibiotics and possible hospitalization. It is highly unusual for a male patient younger than age 35 years to have a UTI, and a sexually transmitted disease should be suspected in such cases. A culture taken from the patient's urethra should be sent for testing for both *Chlamydia trachomatis* and *Neisseria gonorrhoeae*, and therapy should be empirically started with 125 mg/day intramuscularly of ceftriaxone (or 400 mg po of ofloxacin in patients who are allergic to penicillin) plus 1 g po of azithromycin (or alternatively 100 mg po bid of doxycycline for 10 days). The patient's partner should also be tested or be treated empirically.

## Urinary Retention

Urinary retention is more common in men. The patient reports a history of inability to void or decreased voiding with a sensation of postvoid incomplete bladder emptying. A physical examination should include examination of the meatus for any obvious strictures, a rectal examination to note any masses, and assessment of the size and consistency of the prostate. If there is an obstruction, the bladder should be easily palpated.

A Foley catheter should be placed. Initial urine output greater than 200 cc is suggestive of retention, and the patient generally feels immediate relief after catheterization. The patient's electrolytes may need to be monitored, and the patient should be checked to ensure that he is receiving adequate fluids by mouth. The Foley catheter should be left in place until a urology consultation can be obtained.

## References

Bullard K, Rothenberger D: Colon, rectum, and anus, in Schwartz's Principles of Surgery, 8th Edition. Edited by Brunicardi FC, Anderson D, Billiar TR, et al. New York, McGraw-Hill, 2005, pp 1055–1066

Cheskin L, Lacy B: Abdominal pain, in Principles of Ambulatory Medicine, 6th Edition. Edited by Barker LR, Burton JR, Zieve PD, et al. Philadelphia, PA, Lippincott Williams & Wilkins, 2003, pp 623–631

Dempsey D: Esophagus and diaphragmatic hernia, in Schwartz's Principles of Surgery, 8th Edition. Edited by Brunicardi FC, Anderson D, Billiar TR, et al. New York, McGraw-Hill, 2005, pp 933–960

Gallagher EJ: Abnominal pain, in Emergency Medicine: A Comprehensive Study Guide, 5th Edition. Edited by Tintinalli JE, Kelen GD, Stapczynski JS. New York, McGraw-Hill, 2000, pp 497–515

King K, Wightman J: Abdominal pain, in Rosen's Emergency Medicine: Concepts and Clinical Practice, 5th Edition. Edited by Marx JA, Hockberger RS, Walls RM, et al. St. Louis, MO, Mosby, 2002, pp 185–194

Overton D: Gastrointestinal bleeding, in Emergency Medicine: A Comprehensive Study Guide, 5th Edition. Edited by Tintinalli JE, Kelen GD, Stapczynski JS. New York, McGraw-Hill, 2000, pp 520–521

White MJ, Counselman FL: Troubleshooting acute abdominal pain (part 1). Emerg Med 20:34–42, 2002

# CHAPTER 13

# Low Back Pain

## Tom Kuo, M.D.

## Clinical Presentation

*Low back pain* (LBP) is classified by duration of symptoms. Acute LBP is defined as pain for less than 6 weeks. Subacute LBP is pain with a duration between 6 and 12 weeks. Chronic LBP is pain that lasts longer than 12 weeks. *Sciatica* is an S1 nerve root injury classically described as numbness or shooting pain from the back through the buttock and down the posterior thigh to the foot. *Spinal stenosis* is an often diffuse, bilateral neurological deficit (pain, numbness, and tingling) in which pain is worse with activity such as walking, prolonged standing, and back extension. *Cauda equina syndrome* is injury to the spinal cord that presents with bowel or bladder dysfunction, urinary retention, saddle anesthesia with decreased sphincter tone, and bilateral leg weakness and/or numbness.

## Differential Diagnosis

The differential diagnosis (Table 13–1) is broad. Ninety percent of cases of LBP are benign, but in the remaining cases, LBP signifies a life-threatening disorder. One end of the spectrum consists of musculoligamentous injuries with localized pain and no neurological deficit. On the other end of the spectrum, cancer, compression fracture, and infection can produce pain with neurological deficits. Other less common but still important considerations in LBP include connective tissue disease (systemic lupus erythematosus), abdominal aortic aneurysm, ankylosing spondylitis, and cauda equina syndrome. Furthermore, one must consider drug-seeking behavior in chronic LBP patients who consistently require narcotics for relief. Alternatively, chronic LBP patients may have

**TABLE 13–1.**    Differential diagnosis of low back pain

| | |
|---|---|
| **Primary structural or mechanical** | **Metabolic disease** |
| Ligamentous strain | Osteoporosis |
| Facet joint disruption or degeneration | Osteomalacia |
| Intervertebral disc degeneration or | Hemochromatosis |
|   herniation | Ochronosis |
| Vertebral compression fracture | **Inflammatory rheumatologic disorders** |
| Vertebral end-plate microfractures | Ankylosing spondylitis |
| Spondylolisthesis | Reactive spondyloarthropathies |
| Spinal stenosis |   (Reiter's syndrome) |
| Diffuse idiopathic skeletal | Psoriatic arthropathy |
|   hyperostosis | Polymyalgia rheumatica |
| Scheuermann's disease (vertebral | Paget's disease of the bone |
|   epiphyseal aseptic necrosis) | **Referred pain** |
| **Infection** | Abdominal or retroperitoneal visceral |
| Epidural abscess |   process |
| Vertebral osteomyelitis | Retroperitoneal vascular process |
| Septic diskitis | Retroperitoneal malignancy |
| Pott's disease (tuberculosis) | Herpes zoster |
| **Nonspecific manifestation of** | **Other** |
| **systemic illness** | Somatization disorder |
| Bacterial endocarditis | Fibromyalgia |
| Influenza | Malingering |
| **Neoplasia** | |
| Epidural or vertebral carcinomatous | |
|   metastases | |
| Multiple myeloma, lymphoma | |
| Primary epidural or intradural tumors | |

somatoform pain disorder, depression, and malingering if there are issues of secondary financial or emotional gain. More than 85% of patients with isolated LBP cannot be given a precise pathoanatomical diagnosis (Deyo and Weinstein 2001).

## Risk Stratification

The challenge for the physician is to identify LBP patients with symptoms that require further investigation and possibly aggressive intervention. A clinical guideline published by the Agency for Health Care Policy and Research includes a list of "red-flag" characteristics to help identify LBP patients who require further evaluation (Table 13–2) (Bigos

**TABLE 13–2.** "Red flag" characteristics of patients with low back pain who require additional evaluation

| History | Physical examination findings |
| --- | --- |
| Age <18, >50 years | Saddle anesthesia |
| Unexplained weight loss | Loss of anal sphincter tone |
| Cancer | Major motor weakness in lower |
| Immunosuppression | extremities |
| Prolonged use of steroids | Fever |
| Intravenous drug use | Vertebral tenderness |
| Urinary tract infection | Limited spinal range of motion |
| Increased pain or pain unrelieved by rest | Neurological findings with a duration of more than 6 weeks |
| Fever | |
| Trauma | |
| Bladder or bowel incontinence | |
| Urinary retention | |

*Source.* Modified from Bigos et al. 1994.

et al. 1994). Elderly patients (age >65 years) have higher incidences of cancer, compression fracture, spinal stenosis, and aortic aneurysms and should be more carefully evaluated. Patients with a history of intravenous drug use, HIV-positive patients, and immunocompromised patients have higher incidences of spinal abscess and osteomyelitis. Patients with history of trauma, disc herniation, or cancer can present with spinal cord compression or cauda equina syndrome and require immediate attention.

## Assessment and Management in Psychiatric Settings

A detailed history, an assessment of risk factors, and a careful neurological evaluation are vital to proper diagnosis. Most acute LBP can be treated without further studies. However, if more severe disorder is suspected, additional evaluation includes laboratory tests, radiographic studies, and consultation.

### Medical History

Common presentations of acute LBP range from localized pain over the lumbosacral area to nonspecific back pain and neurological symptoms. A careful history is key to the diagnosis of LBP. The history should include the patient's age, the location and distribution of the pain, and the characteristics, temporal sequence, and severity of the pain, as well as any exacerbating and remitting factors and predisposing factors. The review of systems should include the symptoms of claudication and pseudoclaudication, as well as neurological symptoms such as numbness, weakness, radiating pain, and bowel and bladder dysfunction. If the patient reports pain that radiates down to the foot, the patient should be asked whether the pain travels behind the thigh (indicating S1 radiculopathy) or the lateral side (L5 radiculopathy). Furthermore, it is important to inquire about a history of trauma, previous therapy, efficacy of previous therapy, and the functional impact of the pain on the patient's work and activities of daily living. A duration of LBP greater than 6 weeks should raise the suspicion of a more serious etiology and suggests the need for additional diagnostic studies.

LBP with sciatica symptoms occurs in only 2%–3% of all LBP patients but in 95% of patients with a herniated disc or a herniated nucleus pulposus. The most common sites of disc herniations are at the L4–L5 or L5–S1 level, producing L5 or S1 radiculopathies. In patients with a herniated disc, pain occurs during flexion and prolonged sitting, and relief occurs with extension. Common etiologies include central disc herniation, spinal canal hematoma, abscess, tumor, and traumatic compression. On the other hand, in patients with spinal stenosis, relief from pain occurs with forward flexion and rest, and pain in worsened by extension (Hall et al. 1985).

## Physical Examination

The physical examination should begin with an assessment of vital signs to look for fever, tachycardia, and hyper- or hypotension. In the abdominal examination, the clinician should check for a pulsatile mass (a sign of abdominal aortic aneurysm), epigastric tenderness (pancreatitis), and flank pain (renal stones, pyelonephritis). A detailed neurological evaluation, including assessment of tendon reflex, tactile senses, and motor strength, should be performed. The examination should include assessment of gait and posture (to check for scoliosis) and assessment of range of motion, including forward flexion, extension, lateral flexion, and lateral rotation. Spinal stenosis is a possible diagnosis if pain occurs with back extension. Point tenderness over the spine suggests fracture or infection. The clinician may ask the patient to walk heel to toe and then to squat and rise; a patient's inability to do so may suggest severe cauda equina syndrome. In the straight leg raising test, the patient lies in a supine position, and each leg is raised until pain occurs. If pain is reproduced when the leg is at an angle between 30° and 60°, nerve root irritation is suggested. Bending the knee while maintaining hip flexion will relieve the pain, and pressure in the popliteal region (popliteal compression test) will worsen the pain (Kirkpatrick 1996). If pain is increased when the knee is placed in full extension during straight leg raising and if pain is increased with dorsiflexion of the ankle (Lasègue's sign), nerve root and sciatic nerve irritation is likely. The straight leg test is positive in 95% of cases of herniated disc at surgery, but it is also positive in 80%–90% of patients without disc disease.

Recovery from nonspecific acute LBP is usually short and requires only conservative therapy. A gradual return to normal daily function with minimal bed rest is recommended (Deyo et al. 1986). Nonsteroidal anti-inflammatory drugs (NSAIDs) and acetaminophen are effective for pain relief. Opioid analgesic drugs may be given during the first few days, but no studies have proved that they are more effective than NSAIDs. Controversy remains in regard to the effectiveness of muscle relaxants. Muscle relaxants plus NSAIDs have been found to be no more effective than NSAIDs alone (Turturro et al. 2003). In general, medication should be used in a regular and timely manner and not on an as-needed basis. One dosing regiment consists of 800 mg of ibuprofen orally every 8 hours with food for a maximum of 2,400 mg/day if the patient is younger than age 60 years. Ketorolac (60 mg im for patients younger than age 60 years or 30 mg im for patients ages 60 years and older) is commonly given for immediate pain relief, but it has the potential for misuse by opioid-dependent patients, and it lowers the seizure threshold. A superficial heat or cold pack can be applied for 20–30 minutes every 2 hours for analgesia and reduction of muscle spasms. Studies have shown that 60% of patients with new-onset LBP improve within 7 days, and 90% improve within 2–4 weeks (Connelly 1996; Coste et al. 1994).

If the patient does not improve after 6 weeks of medical management with NSAIDs, the patient should be reevaluated, and imaging of the spine should be performed at the recommendation of a neurologist or orthopedic surgeon (Figure 13–1). The association between symptoms and imaging results is weak (White and Gordon 1982). A plain X ray is not routinely done during the initial evaluation of acute LBP. Several large retrospective studies showed low sensitivity and specificity of lumbar spine films. In one study, plain-film X ray done for assessment of acute LBP had either normal findings or showed changes of equivocal clinical significance in more than 75% of the study group (Scavone et al. 1981). However, plain films maybe useful if the patient's

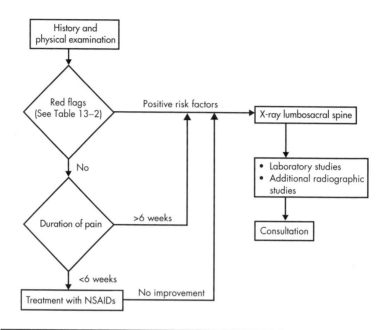

**FIGURE 13-1.**    Algorithm for assessment and treatment of a patient with low back pain.

*Note.*   NSAIDs=nonsteroidal anti-inflammatory drugs.

symptoms are suggestive of systemic disease or trauma (Table 13–3) (Deyo and Diehl 1986).

Alternative radiographic studies include computed tomography (CT), magnetic resonance imaging (MRI), combined myelography and CT, and bone scintigraphy (bone scan). CT or MRI should be considered emergently if the patient has worsening motor/sensory deficits or if a neurological emergency such as cauda equina syndrome or a systemic etiology such as infection or cancer is suspected. CT provides better images of cortical bone, and MRI is better for imaging of a soft tissue phenomenon such as a herniated disc or tumor. MRI is currently a popular tool in the study of LBP, but one study showed herniated discs in approximately 25% of asymptomatic patients younger than age 60 years and in 33% of those ages 60 years and older (Jensen et al. 1994). A bone scan may be useful if the results of spine films are normal. Exercise programs that facilitate weight loss, trunk strengthening (strengthening of the oblique and rectus abdominis muscles), and stretching of the musculotendinous structure of the spine are most beneficial for alleviating

| **TABLE 13-3.** | Indications for radiography in a patient with low back pain |
|---|---|

Age >50
Significant trauma
Neurological deficits
Unexplained weight loss (10 lb in 6 months)
Suspicion of ankylosing spondylitis
Drug or alcohol abuse
History of cancer
Use of corticosteroids
Temperature >38°C (100.4°F)
No improvement after 1 month
Patient is seeking compensation for back pain

*Source.* Modified from Deyo and Diehl 1986.

LBP and should be included as part of the prevention and treatment for chronic back pain.

Patients with cauda equina syndrome present with bowel and bladder dysfunction (i.e., urinary retention), numbness in saddle distribution around the anus and perineum, and bilateral leg pain, weakness, and numbness. Cauda equina syndrome is considered a surgical emergency that requires immediate steroid treatment, emergent MRI, and neurology and neurosurgery consultation. Emergent corticosteroid treatment is initiated with 10–100 mg iv of dexamethasone or with methylprednisolone (30 mg/kg bolus over 15 minutes).

Most sciatica symptoms resolve in 6 weeks, but some patients with sciatica need further imaging and advanced treatments. Initially, sciatica should be treated as acute LBP with pain control and minimal bed rest. Epidural steroid injection may improve symptoms in 10%–15% of patients. Surgical intervention may also be considered if pain is not improved after 6–8 weeks.

Some patients with chronic back pain have no radiculopathy or anatomical abnormalities that clearly correlate with their symptoms. Psychosocial factors must be considered in such cases; these factors may encompass economic (financial compensation), social (job dissatisfaction), and legal (pending litigation) issues.

Signs indicating the presence of a functional component of back pain have been proposed by Weddell et al. (1980). A patient with three of the five signs is likely to have a somatoform pain disorder (Table 13–4).

**TABLE 13-4.**  Signs suggesting a functional component of low back pain[a]

Superficial, nonanatomic tenderness

Pain with simulated tests (e.g., axial load or pelvic rotation)

Inconsistent responses with distraction (e.g., straight leg raises while the patient is sitting)

Nonorganic regional disturbances (e.g., sensory loss inconsistent with dermatome)

Overreaction

[a]A patient with three of the five signs is likely to have a somatoform pain disorder.
*Source.*  Modified from Weddell et al. 1980.

In a study of 200 patients with chronic LBP who were assessed with a structured psychiatric interview, a significantly higher proportion of the patients (98%) met the criteria for a DSM-III-R Axis I diagnosis, compared with the base rate in the general population (Polatin et al. 1993). When patients with somatoform pain disorder (97%) were excluded, 77% of the patients still had one or more Axis I disorders, with depression (64%), substance abuse (36%), and anxiety disorder (19%) the most common diagnoses. It is interesting to note that among the chronic LBP patients in this study, substance abuse and anxiety disorder commonly preceded the onset of LBP. Furthermore, although major depression was common, the patients were nearly equally divided into groups with onset of depression before and after the onset of LBP (54% and 46%, respectively).

# References

Bigos S, Bowyer O, Braen G, et al: Acute Low Back Problems in Adults. Clinical Practice Guideline, Quick Reference Guide Number 14 (AHCPR Publ No 95-0643). Rockville, MD, US Department of Health and Human Services, Public Health Service, Agency for Health Care Policy and Research, 1994

Connelly C: Patients with low back pain: how to identify the few who need extra attention. Postgrad Med 100:143–156, 1996

Coste J, Delecoeuillerie G, Cohen de Lara A, et al: Clinical course and prognostic factors in acute low back pain: an inception cohort study in primary care practice. BMJ 308:577–580, 1994

Deyo RA, Diehl AK: Lumbar spine films in primary care: current use and effects of selective ordering criteria. J Gen Intern Med 1:20–25, 1986

Deyo RA, Weinstein JN: Low back pain. N Engl J Med 344:363–370, 2001

Deyo RA, Diehl AK, Rosenthal M: How many days of bedrest for acute low back pain? A randomized clinical trial. N Engl J Med 315:1064–1070, 1986

Hall S, Bartleson JD, Onofrio BM, et al: Lumbar spinal stenosis: clinical features, diagnostic procedures, and results of surgical treatment in 68 patients. Ann Intern Med 103:271–275, 1985

Jensen MC, Brant-Zawadzki MN, Obuchowski N, et al: Magnetic resonance imaging of the lumbar spine in people without back pain. N Engl J Med 331:69–73, 1994

Kirkpatrick JS: Oh my aching back: evaluation and surgical treatment of lumbar spine disorders. South Med J 89:935–939, 1996

Polatin PB, Kinney RK, Gatchel RJ, et al: Psychiatric illness and chronic low-back pain. Spine 18:66–71, 1993

Scavone JG, Latshaw RF, Rohrer GV: Use of lumbar spine films: statistical evaluation at a university teaching hospital. JAMA 246:1105–1108, 1981

Turturro M, Frater CR, D'Amico FJ:. Cyclobenzaprine with ibuprofen versus ibuprofen alone in acute myofascial strain: a randomized, double-blind clinical trial. Ann Emerg Med 41:818–826, 2003

Weddell G, McCulloch JA, Kummel E, et al: Nonorganic physical signs in low-back pain. Spine 5:117–125, 1980

White AA III, Gordon SL: Synopsis: workshop on idiopathic low-back pain. Spine 7:141–145, 1982

# CHAPTER 14

# Pain in Extremities

Michael Bennett, M.D.

Peter Manu, M.D.

## Clinical Presentation

Pain in extremities is a very common complaint. In community studies, widespread chronic pain is reported by 10%–15% of people at any one time (Elliott et al. 1999) and intermittent regional joint pain, primarily of the knees or back, is present in 25% of the population (Linaker et al. 1999). The anatomical classification of pain in extremities differentiates conditions that produce generalized pain, such as myofascial pain syndromes and fibromyalgia, and those involving only one region, such as the neck, shoulder, elbow, wrist/hand, hip, knee, and ankle/foot (Linaker et al. 1999). Most cases of regional pain occur in the elderly and are related to the degenerative joint changes of osteoarthritis (Dieppe and Lohmander 2005). The pathogenesis of pain in extremities is mainly related to structural injury or inflammatory changes in the subchondral bone, periosteum, synovium, ligaments, and muscles (Kidd et al. 2004). Patients with fibromyalgia have no evidence of muscle pathology, and their pain syndrome is considered to be related to an alteration in sleep physiology (i.e., alpha intrusion during delta sleep)(Abeles 1998).

## Differential Diagnosis

The challenge in the evaluation of the psychiatric patient with pain in extremities focuses on the identification of the structure most likely to be responsible for the chief complaint. The examiner must systematically evaluate the skin and soft tissue, individual muscles and muscle compartments, and joints and bones for posttraumatic, degenerative, inflammatory, infectious, and drug-induced abnormalities.

## Risk Stratification

At the highest risk are the patients with acute pain in extremities associated with fever, swelling, and erythema, because they may have necrotizing fasciitis and require immediate surgical intervention (Valeriano-Marcet et al. 2003). Psychiatric patients with recent history of trauma may have nondisplaced fractures that are difficult to diagnose clinically and should be sent for radiological examinations. Diffuse muscle pain in an elderly patient should be investigated for the presence of polymyalgia rheumatica, a condition that may be associated with temporal arteritis and visual loss. Finally, patients with suspected septic arthritis and septic bursitis must have joint and bursa fluid examined for definitive diagnosis (Valeriano-Marcet et al. 2003).

## Assessment and Treatment in Psychiatric Settings

### Neck Pain

The evaluation of the patient with neck pain begins with observation of range of motion and of any limitations because of pain. A complete neurological examination of the upper and lower extremities is necessary, including observation of any deficits with respect to dermatomes and myotomes, altered reflex arcs, decreased anal tone, and any changes in bowel, bladder, or sexual function. If there is any evidence of cervical myelopathy or radiculopathy with motor or sensory deficits, the patient must be urgently referred for magnetic resonance imaging of the spine and for neurosurgical evaluation. For neck pain without neurological findings, treatment consists of nonsteroidal anti-inflammatory drugs (NSAIDs) with the possible addition of muscle relaxants.

### Shoulder Pain

The shoulder has many structures that may become inflamed. All movements must be evaluated through observation of both passive and active range of motion. The patient should be evaluated for possible tendonitis and partial or complete tendon tear. For evaluation of a suspected large or complete tendon tear, orthopedic consultation is required. If the examination is unrevealing, the patient may be experiencing referred pain, and an evaluation for other sources of pain, such as the neck or chest, is required.

Pain with palpation of the anterior shoulder joint and increased pain with flexion of the biceps against resistance suggest biceps tendonitis.

Treatment consists of rest and an NSAID. The rotator cuff consists of the supraspinatus, infraspinatus, teres minor, and subscapularis. Rotator cuff injuries are the most common shoulder injury and usually present with weakness or increased pain with resistance in the mid-range or middle third of external rotation or abduction. Pain is decreased with passive movement and is increased with resisted active movement. Treatment consists of limiting movement with a sling, use of range-of-motion exercises as tolerated, and NSAIDs. Steroid injections into the subacromial bursa may be helpful. Pain with minimal passive motion may indicate a fracture or shoulder dislocation, and an X ray would be indicated.

## Elbow Pain

Tennis elbow usually presents with pain with palpation at the lateral epicondyle or where the extensor tendons attach to the epicondyle, especially with wrist extension against resistance. Treatment consists of NSAIDs and limiting the extension of the wrist with a splint. Golfer's elbow presents with tenderness of the medial epicondyle or where the flexor tendons attach to the epicondyle, especially with flexion of the wrist against resistance. The treatment is the same as that for tennis elbow.

## Wrist and Hand Pain

Carpal tunnel syndrome, which usually results from repetitive movement, is caused by a narrowing of the channel at the wrist through which the median nerve travels. Patients may develop a neuropathy in the median distribution; decreased sensation of the thumb, second, third, or half of the fourth finger; and eventually atrophy of the thenar muscle. Phalen's test (sustained wrist flexion) or Tinel's test (tapping on the carpel tunnel) both can reproduce the symptom. Electromyograph studies may confirm the diagnosis. Wrist splints are used in initial treatment, but treatment may eventually include surgery to relieve the median nerve compression.

## Knee Pain

The knees should be evaluated for an effusion, pain with palpation, and range of motion. The painful knee should be compared with the opposite knee, and the ipsilateral hip and ankle should be examined. Minor sprains may be treated with rest and an NSAID. Severe sprains are treated by immobilization and orthopedic referral. Suspected meniscus injuries are treated by knee immobilization, NSAIDs, and orthopedic referral.

In the knee, a bursa in prepatellar (in front of and below the patella), suprapatellar (above the patella), infrapatellar (between the patella and the tibia), or anserine (medial knee below the joint line) area may become inflamed and painful. After infection is excluded, treatment begins with limiting activity and use of NSAIDs, such as ibuprofen. (See the following section, "Bursitis.")

Baker's cyst, which develops near a bursa located behind the knee, may cause discomfort in the knee, calf, or popliteal space and may cause more intense pain if it ruptures. Frequently this process has a presentation similar to that of deep vein thrombosis, and an ultrasound must be obtained to distinguish between the two. Treatment is rest and NSAIDs, such as ibuprofen.

## Bursitis

A bursa is a small, synovial sac that provides lubrication between moving surfaces. Common locations of *bursitis,* which is inflammation of a bursa from minor trauma or overuse, include the prepatellar, olecranon, supraspinatus, subacromial, trochanteric, and anserine bursa (Hellman 2003). Treatment includes NSAIDs and limiting motion that irritates the bursa. Additional treatment may include steroid injections of the bursa. If infection of the bursa is suspected (i.e., if the patient has fever, chills, erythema, and warmth of the bursa), the synovial fluid should be aspirated and sent for laboratory studies.

## Claudication/Pseudoclaudication Pain

Claudication pain is pain in the buttocks, thighs, or calves that occurs after walking some distance. The pain is caused by limited oxygen supply to the muscles because of narrowing of the arteries leading to the muscles. Risk factors associated with claudication are diabetes, high blood pressure, smoking, and age. The physical examination of a patient with claudication pain includes checking the lower extremity pulses, including the dorsal pedis and posterior tibial pulses. If the pulses are significantly reduced, the patient may need further vascular studies and should be referred to a vascular surgeon. Treatment includes pentoxifylline and, in some cases, surgery. Pseudoclaudication or neuroclaudication is a pattern of pain that is similar to that of claudication but is not caused by vascular insufficiency. Pseudoclaudication is usually caused by compression of a nerve or spinal stenosis, is worse with walking, and is relieved when the patient stops walking and sits forward or flexes and reduces the compression of the nerve.

## Systemic Diseases That Cause Pain in Extremities

*Rheumatoid arthritis* usually progresses slowly and intermittently and can be difficult to diagnose. The joints involved are symmetric and involve the metacarpal-phalangeal joints, proximal interphalangeal joints, wrists, elbows, shoulders, knees, ankles, metatarsophalangeal joints, and the cervical spine (Klippel 1997). The distribution is different in osteoarthritis. In rheumatoid arthritis the joints are stiff after prolonged immobility, for example, when the patient first wakes up in the morning. The stiffness or joint pain usually lasts longer than 1 hour. After some activity, the joints loosen up and mobility improves. Examination of the affected joints may reveal limited range of motion and swelling of the joint space. An X ray may reveal joint space narrowing or erosion of the bone. Laboratory results may include chronic anemia or elevated values for rheumatoid factor or antinuclear antibodies. If rheumatoid arthritis is suspected, the patient should be evaluated by a rheumatologist.

*Degenerative joint disease*, or osteoarthritis, is more prominent in the older population. It most commonly affects the hips, knees, cervical and lumbar spine, the distal and proximal interphalangeal joints, and the first metacarpal-phalangeal joint (Klippel 1997). The process includes degeneration of joint cartilage and bony changes at the joint. The joint pain in osteoarthritis progresses during the day and is worse at night or after extended activity. Patients usually present with slowly progressing joint pain with acute flare-ups, such as knee pain after increased activity. An X ray may show narrowing of joint spaces and osteophyte formation. Treatment is rest of the joint and acetaminophen at larger doses, such as 1,000 mg three to four times a day. Treatment also includes weight loss, physical therapy, and, in some cases, surgery, such as knee or hip replacement.

*Gout* is a disease involving overproduction or underexcretion of uric acid. The patient presents with a suddenly red-hot tender joint, most commonly the first metatarsophalangeal joint. If the patient has no previous diagnosis of gout, arthrocentesis must be done to confirm the diagnosis. Analysis of the fluid can reveal crystals. NSAIDs are used for the treatment of an acute gout attack. Other treatment options include colchicine and corticosteroids. After the acute attack subsides, some patients may receive long-term treatment. Patients with overproduction of uric acid are treated with allopurinol, and patients with underexcretion of uric acid are treated with probenecid.

The presentation of *pseudogout* is similar to that of gout, except that the knee is more commonly involved. Treatment of an acute attack of psuedogout is similar to the treatment of gout; NSAIDs such as ibuprofen or indomethacin are used, as well as the alternatives colchicine or corticosteroids.

One should be suspicious of *septic joint* in any young, sexually active patient who presents with a fever and a red, warm, tender, or edematous joint. A rheumatologist or emergency medicine physician must perform arthrocentesis in such patients as soon as feasible. The aspirated joint fluid should be sent for laboratory studies, which include white blood cell count, Gram stain culture, and crystal studies. White blood cell counts in the joint fluid may range from 10,000 to 100,000 cells/μL but are typically closer to 100,000 cells/μL in septic joints (Burton 2000). Organisms responsible include *Neisseria gonorrhoeae* or *Staphylococcus aureus* (60%), gram-negative bacilli (20%), and others (20%). If gonorrhea is suspected, throat, cervical, and urethral cultures must also be obtained, because the Gram stain plus culture. Treatment choices include ceftriaxone if gonorrhea is suspected or nafcillin plus a third-generation cephalosporin if +C is suspected not for a total of 14–28 days. NSAIDs such as ibuprofen may be used for pain control.

*Polymyalgia rheumatica* presents with pain and stiffness of the proximal joints such as the hips and shoulders (Klippel 1997). The pain and stiffness are usually worse after immobility or in the early morning. Laboratory abnormalities include an elevated erythrocyte sedimentation rate (ESR). If polymyalgia rheumatica is suspected, the patient should be referred to a rheumatologist. Treatment includes a prolonged course of prednisone.

*Polymyositis* presents as weakness that is more proximal than distal. *Dermatomyositis* is polymyositis with skin changes, such as heliotrope rash of the eyelids or Gottron's papules over the metacarpal-phalangeal joints of the hands. Laboratory abnormalities include an elevated creatine phosphokinase level. Additional tests include muscle biopsy and electromyography. If polymyositis is suspected, the patient should be evaluated by a rheumatologist. The treatment includes prednisone at high doses over a long period of time.

Patients with *fibromyalgia* present with vague complaints of weakness and of being easily fatigued, general muscle aches, and difficulty with sleep. Aches and pains are located medially and not in the joints. Other conditions must be ruled out. Although no specific tests for fibromyalgia exist, 18 symmetric points on the body are frequently tender in patients with fibromyalgia. These symmetric points of tenderness are located over muscle or tendons rather than at the joints. If fibromyalgia is suspected, the patient should be evaluated by a rheumatologist. The treatment includes tricyclic drugs (amitriptilyne or cyclobenzaprine), cognitive-behavioral therapy, and graded exercise.

Aging, decreased estrogen levels in women, decreased activity, and decreased calcium intake may lead to *osteoporosis* and increased risk for fracture, especially of the vertebrae and hips. Smoking, steroid use, and Asian ancestry are also risk factors for osteoporosis. Bone density measurements can be done to evaluate for osteopenia and risk of fracture. Preventive measures include exercise and administration of estrogen or raloxifene and calcium with vitamin D. Treatment options include alendronate, which is a bisphosphonate. Any back or hip pain in a patient with the risk factors for osteoporosis or with a diagnosis of osteoporosis should be evaluated with an X ray for possible fracture.

*Ankylosing spondylitis* most commonly presents with inflammation of the sacroiliac joints. The pain and stiffness are usually located in the sacroiliac joints, lumbar area, or buttocks. Symptoms are worse in the morning or after immobility. The symptoms may initially be limited to one side of the body but may progress to become bilateral. Laboratory abnormalities may include an elevated ESR, elevated C-reactive protein and alkaline phosphatase levels, and mild anemia. An X ray may reveal sacroiliitis or fusion of the vertebrae. Treatment begins with NSAIDs.

*Reiter's syndrome* is the triad of urethritis, conjunctivitis, and arthritis, usually presenting in that order. Reiter's syndrome is a reactive arthritis and typically follows a gastrointestinal or genitourinary infection. The arthritis typically involves lower extremity joints. The illness is self-limited, and NSAIDs may be used for the arthritis. The primary infection (often gonorrhea) must be identified and treated as soon as possible.

# References

Abeles M: Fibromyalgia syndrome, in Functional Somatic Syndromes. Edited by Manu P. New York, Cambridge University Press, 1998, pp 32–37

Burton J: Acute disorders of the joints and bursae, in Emergency Medicine: A Comprehensive Study Guide, 5th Edition. Edited by Tintinalli JE, Kelen GD, Stapczynski JS. New York, McGraw-Hill, 2000, pp 1895–1898

Dieppe PA, Lohmander LS: Pathogenesis and management of pain in osteoarthritis. Lancet 365:965–973, 2005

Elliott AM, Smith BH, Penny KI, et al: The epidemiology of chronic pain in the community. Lancet 354:1248–1252, 1999

Hellman DB: Nonarticular rheumatic disorders, in Principles of Ambulatory Medicine, 6th Edition. Edited by Barker LR, Burton JR, Zieve PD, et al. Philadelphia, PA, Lippincott Williams & Wilkins, 2003, pp 1105–1114

Klippel JH: Primer on the Rheumatic Diseases, 11th Edition. Atlanta, GA, Arthritis Foundation, 1997, pp 89–154

Linaker CH, Walker-Bone K, Palmer K, et al: Frequency and impact of regional musculoskeletal disorders. Baillieres Best Pract Res Clin Rheumatol 13:197–215, 1999

Valeriano-Marcet J, Carter JD, Vasey FB: Soft tissue disease. Rheum Dis Clin North Am 29:77–88, 2003

# PART V

# Neurological Symptoms

Section Editor:

Marc L. Gordon, M.D.

# CHAPTER 15

# The Unresponsive Psychiatric Patient

Scott Leibowitz, M.D.

Raymond E. Suarez, M.D.

## Clinical Presentation

The key to an effective evaluation of an unresponsive patient is the physician's understanding of the two elements of consciousness (arousal and awareness) and ability to pinpoint the anatomical and physiological underpinnings of the phenomenon (Samuels 1993). Arousal, the ability to be awakened, is maintained by the reticular activating system, which is located in the brainstem (Figure 15–1). A patient with a disruption in the reticular activating system, which indicates brainstem damage, appears asleep and unresponsive. Conversely, a patient who is awake and unresponsive exhibits a defect in awareness, which is an exclusively human state characterized by sensation, emotion, volition, and thought. Because awareness is a result of total cortical function, the possibility of localizing a lesion is almost naught, unless the lesion is extensive. The possibility of brainstem damage is far more concerning to the physician and is therefore a diagnosis that must be identified or excluded in a timely fashion.

In an asleep and unresponsive patient, various levels of unresponsiveness have been described. The unresponsive patient who is briefly arousable on verbal command is termed *drowsy*. *Stupor* refers to a state of unresponsiveness in which the patient cannot be aroused on verbal command but will respond to painful stimuli. *Coma* describes the condition of the patient who is asleep and unresponsive and who does not react to verbal or painful stimuli.

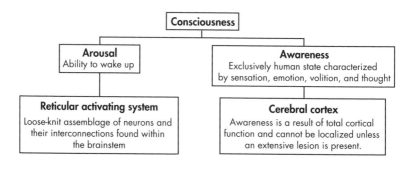

**FIGURE 15-1.**    Elements of consciousness.

## Differential Diagnosis

The differential diagnosis of an unresponsive patient is quite extensive, even among patients without psychiatric comorbidity. The medical etiologies of unresponsiveness may be classified as drug/toxin exposure, trauma, and neurological, metabolic, cardiac, and infectious causes. In the evaluation of a psychiatric patient, the physician must systematically rule out these causes of unresponsiveness, with the understanding that psychiatric causes are generally diagnoses of exclusion.

## Risk Stratification

Unresponsive patients with respiratory failure, hemodynamic compromise, focal neurological signs, severe metabolic abnormalities, head trauma, pregnancy, or evidence of infection must be immediately transferred to the nearest emergency department (see Table 5–1).

## Assessment and Management in Psychiatric Settings

The action algorithm shown in Figure 15–2 outlines a systematic method for rapid evaluation and treatment of the unresponsive psychiatric patient. The physician must first establish unresponsiveness through vocal and painful stimuli. Once unresponsiveness is determined, airway patency and breathing must be assessed, and circulation parameters such as blood pressure and pulse must be determined. For patients with cardiac arrest, the treatment team should initiate cardiopulmonary resuscitation, establish intravenous access, place an automated external defibrillator, and call 911 to have the patient transferred immediately to

**TABLE 15–1.**   Risk stratification for the differential diagnosis of an unresponsive psychiatric patient

- Myocardial infarction/hypotension
- Cardiac arrest
- Arrhythmia
- Stroke
- Herniation
- Metabolic disorder
- Hemorrhage
- Infection
- Mass lesion
- Brain abscess
- Psychiatric causes

the nearest emergency department. Low blood pressure would indicate the need for intravenous access as well as rapid transfer to a medical unit. A patient with an abnormal heart rate and normal blood pressure requires assessment with an electrocardiogram (ECG) before the decision is made to transfer the patient. Abnormal ECG findings indicate the need for a cardiac evaluation in a medical setting.

Once the initial determination is made that the unresponsive patient has stable vital signs and a patent airway with breathing, the focus of the examination shifts to assessing head trauma. The evaluation focuses on signs of head trauma such as the Battle's sign (skin discoloration along the area of the posterior auricular artery), raccoon eyes (indicating an anterior basal skull fracture), and exterior lacerations or bruises. A detailed history from witnesses or family members, if available, would also help to determine whether head trauma is a potential cause for unresponsiveness. Any patient in whom head trauma is suspected should be sent for computed tomography scan of the head to rule out subdural hematoma, epidural hematoma, subarachnoid hemorrhage, skull fractures, and/or potential brain herniations.

The hemodynamically stable, unresponsive psychiatric patient without any evidence of head trauma should then be assessed for metabolic abnormalities. Three easily reversible, yet life-threatening conditions must then be assessed and treated. A finger-stick glucose test should be performed. A finding of significant hyperglycemia indicates the possibility of diabetic ketoacidosis or nonketotic hyperosmolar coma. Immediate transfer to a facility that can provide insulin infusions and high-rate intravenous fluid infusion should be the next step. For pa-

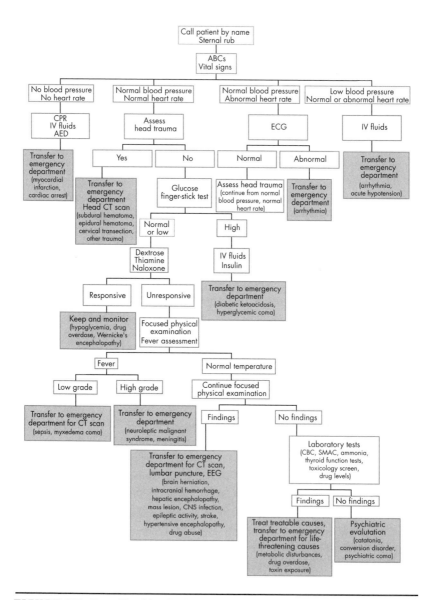

**FIGURE 15–2.** Algorithm for the assessment and treatment of an unresponsive psychiatric patient.

*Note.* ABC= airway, breathing, ciruclation; AED=automated external defibrillator; CBC=complete blood count; CNS=central nervous system; CPR=cardiopulmonary resuscitation; CT=computed tomography; ECG=electrocardiogram; EEG=electroencephalogram; IV=intravenous; SMAC=chemistry panel.

tients with a normal or low blood glucose level, the physician should proceed to administration of the "coma cocktail" (dextrose, thiamine, and naloxone), which reverses acute hypoglycemia, Wernicke's encephalopathy, and opioid overdose, respectively. It is important to note that thiamine stores may be depleted in a malnourished, alcoholic patient who receives boluses of dextrose, and the clinician must therefore administer thiamine with the dextrose (Doyon and Roberts 1994).

The systematic evaluation of an unresponsive patient should continue with the assessment of body temperature. Patients who are hypothermic or hyperthermic must be transferred to an appropriate setting where treatment modalities are possible in the event of a clinical diagnosis of sepsis, myxedema coma, neuroleptic malignant syndrome, or central nervous system infection.

A focused physical examination is the next crucial step in the algorithm. The psychiatrist must pay particular attention to findings limited to the head and neck, gastrointestinal manifestations of toxicities and liver disease, skin observations, and the sequelae of pathological neurological processes. The head and neck examination may provide many clues to life-threatening situations. A patient's breath may indicate alcohol intoxication, uremia, or liver pathology. The funduscopic examination may reveal hypertensive encephalopathy. A brief skin examination may indicate needle marks in drug users or pathognomonic rashes for specific infectious diagnoses. The neurological examination should include assessment of posture, eye abnormalities, breathing, and reflexes in order to distinguish effects of brainstem lesions from those of cortical lesions (Samuels 1993).

Normal posture, defined as a comfortable-looking body position, indicates that the brainstem is functioning well. In contrast, decerebrate posturing (extension of the lower extremities with adduction and internal rotation of the shoulders with extension of the wrists and elbows) indicates brainstem lesions, most often caused by bilateral midbrain or pontine lesions. Decorticate posturing (bilateral flexion at the elbows and wrists with shoulder adduction and extension of the lower extremities) indicates lesions above the brainstem, which require less acute treatment.

Pupil size and reactivity distinguish specific etiologies from others. Small reactive pupils may indicate thalamic lesions or metabolic disturbances. A unilateral, fixed, dilated pupil is often a sign of brain herniation from an ipsilateral cranial nerve III palsy. Reactive pinpoint pupils are often the result of a disrupted sympathetic pathway, which is seen in pontine lesions. Pinpoint pupils may also occur in opioid intoxication. While examining the pupils, the clinician may concurrently assess eye movement. Spontaneous roving eyes indicate hemispheric lesions with intact brainstem function.

Several patterns of breathing denote specific associated conditions. Hyperventilation is commonly a result of a comatose patient's efforts to correct a metabolic acidosis. Apneustic breathing (a prolonged inspiratory gasp with long pauses in between) strongly indicates brainstem damage. Ataxic breathing (mechanically ineffective, disorganized huffing and puffing) signifies that the respiratory centers in the medulla are failing. Cheyne-Stokes breathing (oscillating between hyperventilation and hypoventilation) is usually a good prognostic sign that indicates bilateral hemispheric and diencephalon insult or circulatory slowing with age.

Evaluation of spontaneous reflexes, the final component of the rapid neurological examination, also provides immediate information regarding locations of lesions in the brain (Samuels 1993). Yawning and sneezing involve neural circuitry that transcends the brainstem and thus indicate a functional brainstem. Other reflexes such as coughing, swallowing, and hiccupping may occur in the absence of brainstem lesions and are thus less prognostic.

Helpful laboratory investigations in the unresponsive patient include a complete blood count; metabolic panel; creatine phosphokinase, troponin, and ammonia levels; toxicology screening; thyroid function tests; and drug levels.

Throughout the evaluation, the psychiatric etiologies of unresponsiveness must remain in the differential diagnosis. Often, the diagnosis may "be suggested by a clinical history where the change in level of consciousness was precipitated by stress" (Baxter and White 2003, p. 318). Psychiatric etiologies of unresponsiveness are not commonly encountered among patients who fall into a coma. However, three separate diagnoses may account for unresponsiveness in patients, especially those hospitalized in a psychiatric milieu. Those three entities are catatonia, conversion disorder, and pseudocoma.

*Catatonia*, often a manifestation of schizophrenia, may also occur in a brief psychotic episode, psychotic disorder not otherwise specified, and mood disorders. Catatonia occurs in one of two forms: stuporous catatonia or excited catatonia. The most common form is stuporous, or retarded, catatonia, which is characterized by immobility, mutism, waxy flexibility (cerea flexibilitas), negativism, echopraxia or echolalia, and posturing (Moore and Jefferson 2004). Waxy flexibility refers to the tendency of a patient's limb to be moved against gravity and remain for a considerable time in the position in which it was placed despite un-

**TABLE 15-2.** Causes of catatonia

| Stuporous catatonia | Excited catatonia |
| --- | --- |
| Manic episodes of bipolar disorder | Viral encephalitis |
| Schizophrenia | Schizophrenia |
| Major depressive disorder | |
| Seizure disorder | |
| Encephalitis | |
| Focal lesions (especially of the medial or inferior aspects of the frontal lobes) | |
| Medications (antipsychotics, disulfiram, benzodiazepine withdrawal) | |
| Miscellaneous (hepatic encephalopathy, limbic encephalitis, systemic lupus erythematosus, stage III Lyme disease, subacute sclerosing panencephalitis, Wilson's disease) | |

*Source.* Adapted from Moore and Jefferson 2004.

natural and sometimes painful poses. Excited catatonia, on the other hand, is characterized by bizarre, purposeless, and frenzied hyperactivity. In severe cases, excited catatonia may merge into lethal catatonia, also known as malignant catatonia, which manifests as fever, tachycardia, hypotension, and, in some cases, death as the excitation increases (Moore and Jefferson 2004).

When catatonia is brought on by schizophrenia, there may be an alternating state between stuporous and excited catatonia. It is important to note, however, that although catatonia is a symptom of schizophrenia, as many as 20% of depressed patients have been reported to show signs of catatonia (Starkstein et al. 1996). Catatonia can also be a manifestation of other medical illnesses (Table 15–2). If medical causes of catatonia have been ruled out, psychiatric catatonia often responds to the administration of intramuscular lorazepam or electroconvusive therapy (ECT).

*Conversion disorder* is a psychiatric entity in which psychological stress translates into neurological symptoms. Involuntary psychogenic alteration of physical functioning limited to neurological symptoms is pathognomonic for this disorder, once a medical etiology has been ruled out (Table 15–3). Conversion disorder often occurs in patients with comorbid personality disorders, a substance abuse history, depression, anxiety, or a previous medical or neurological disorder. The lifetime prevalence of conversion disorder is not known with certainty but

**TABLE 15–3.**  Common conversion symptoms

| | | |
|---|---|---|
| Ageusia | Coma | Paralysis |
| Anesthesia | Convergence spasm | Parkinsonism |
| Anosmia | Deafness | Syncope |
| Aphonia | Facial weakness | Tonic-clonic pseudoseizures |
| Ataxia | Globus hystericus | Tremor |
| Blindness | Nystagmus | |

*Source.*  Adapted from Moore and Jefferson 2004.

ranges from 0.01% to 0.5% in the general population; reported estimates for the female-to-male ratio in conversion disorder range from 2:1 to as high as 10:1 (Moore and Jefferson 2004). Symptoms usually resolve spontaneously; however, a psychiatrist may use psychotherapeutic techniques that can empower the patient to overcome the symptoms.

Lastly, the psychiatrist must be able to recognize whether the patient is in a *psychogenic coma,* which is a dissociative disorder occurring as a disruption of the integrated functions of consciousness, memory, identity, or perception (Baxter and White 2003). Dissociative disorders are distinct from conversion disorders; the latter affect voluntary motor and sensory systems, and the former reflect a state of consciousness. A diagnosis of a psychogenic coma (formerly known as pseudocoma) may be suggested by a clinical history "where the change in level of consciousness was precipitated by stress and where the patient slumps to the floor without hitting his head" (Baxter and White 2003, p. 319).

Other signs manifest themselves in the patient's eyes. There may be active resistance to passive eyelid opening, and both eyelids may close quickly when the lifted upper eyelid is released. If the clinician strokes the eyelashes gently, both eyelids may flutter. Eye movements, as would be seen in the neurological examination, tend to be rapid and jerking. Bell's phenomenon, or rolled-back eyes deviated in a particular direction (usually away from the examiner), is also a manifestation of psychogenic coma.

Examination of body movements and muscle tone may also reveal signs of psychogenic coma. Patients may have active resistance when muscle tone is assessed. In bed, a patient may change his or her position or make voluntary movements. Another informal test is known as the "hand drop test." The clinician raises the patient's arm above the face (when the patient is in a supine position), and when the arm is released, it falls to the side of the patient's body in patients with psychogenic coma (Baxter and White 2003). Anxiolytic or antipsychotic medications may treat this dissociative condition and help the patient return to consciousness.

## References

Baxter CL, White WD: Psychogenic coma: case report. Int J Psychiatry Med 33:317–322, 2003

Doyon S, Roberts JR: Reappraisal of the "coma cocktail": dextrose, flumazenil, naloxone, and thiamine. Emerg Med Clin North Am 12:301–316, 1994

Moore D, Jefferson J: Handbook of Medical Psychiatry, 2nd Edition. St. Louis, Mosby, 2004

Samuels MA: The evaluation of comatose patients. Hosp Pract (Off Ed) 28:165–182, 1993

Starkstein SE, Petracca G, Teson A, et al: Catatonia in depression: prevalence, clinical correlates and validation of a scale. J Neurol Neurosurg Psychiatry 60:326–332, 1996

# CHAPTER 16

# Falls

Sung Wu Sun, M.D.

Giselle P. Wolf-Klein, M.D.

## Clinical Presentation

Falls occur frequently, particularly in elderly persons, both in community settings and in hospitals or institutional settings; and the incidence of falls among institutionalized geriatric patients is significantly higher than that among elderly people in the community (Rubenstein and Josephson 2002; Tinetti et al. 1988). However, 30%–60% of community-dwelling elderly persons have a fall each year (Campbell et al. 1989; Graafmans et al. 1996; Gross et al. 1990; Tinetti et al. 1988). A higher rate of falls has been reported in patients admitted to a psychiatry unit, compared with patients in acute care facilities (mean rate of 53.9 falls per 10,000 patient days, compared with 30.9 falls per 10,000 patient days) (Campbell 1991).

## Differential Diagnosis

### Organic Disorders

Falls are caused by a multiplicity of coexisting factors. Visual impairment, vertigo, dementia, syncope, seizure disorder, transient ischemic attacks, stroke, Parkinson's disease, or peripheral neuropathies can all contribute to falls. Cardiac factors responsible for falls include cardiac arrhythmias and acute myocardial infarction. Chronic pulmonary conditions can cause transient hypoxemia and may result in disorientation and falls. Abdominal pathology, including gastrointestinal bleeding, defecation and urination dysfunctions, and urinary incontinence, has been implicated in the pathogenesis of falls (Campbell et al. 1989; Graafmans et al. 1996; Gross et al. 1990; Rohde et al. 1990; Rubenstein and Josephson 2002; Tinetti et al. 1988). Lower extremity dysfunction caused by arthritis, musculoskeletal impairments, general weakness from acute or chronic medical illnesses including systemic and local infections, and impaired coordination may hamper the ability to fall "well" and increase the risk of injury in the fall process (Graafmans et al. 1996).

## Polypharmacy

Patients who take more than three or four medications are at increased risk of recurrent falls (deCarle and Kohn 2001). Most classes of psychotropic medications, diuretics, digoxin, and type IA antiarrhythmic agents may contribute to this risk (American Geriatrics Society 2001; Tinetti et al. 1993). Psychotropic medications that have been directly implicated in falls include antidepressants (tricyclics and selective serotonin reuptake inhibitors), antipsychotics, and benzodiazepines (long- and short-acting) (American Geriatrics Society 2001; Tinetti et al. 1994; Walker and Howland 1991). In a study by Leipzig, the odds ratio for one or more falls was 1.7 for each psychotropic drug used (American Geriatrics Society 2001). A high incidence of falls has also been reported in patients undergoing electroconvulsive therapy (Priplata et al. 2003).

## Risk Stratification

Risk factors most consistently associated with falls include older age, history of past falls, cognitive impairment, depression, impairment in activities of daily living, urinary and fecal incontinence, lower extremity weakness or other disability, impaired balance or gait, use of an ambulation assistive device, visual deficit, dizziness, higher number of medications, psychotropic medication use, arthritis, and history of stroke. An additional consideration for patients at risk for falls is the potential inability to get up from the floor without assistance, which increases the risk of developing rhabdomyolysis.

## Assessment and Management in Psychiatric Settings

### Before the Fall

Because of the high prevalence of falls and injuries in psychiatric populations, all patients should be routinely asked about their history of falls. Two questions that should be included in the assessment are 1) "Have you sustained a fall in the past year?" and 2) "Do you sometimes feel unsteady in walking?" A positive answer to either question should immediately prompt the physician to initiate a protocol to prevent falls. The patient should have a diagnostic assessment, followed by intervention to correct the primary medical problem. At all times during the process, open communication with the patient and his or her family is imperative. Lastly, the fear of falling must be acknowledged, because it results in decreased mobility and loss of independence (see Figure 16–1).

## After the Fall

When called to assess a patient who has sustained a fall, the physician should first determine whether the patient has sustained an injury. Vital signs should be measured, including pulse, blood pressure, respiratory rate, and level of consciousness. The physician should then ask the patient if he or she is in any pain and should attempt to localize the pain. It is important to remember that elderly patients may not be able to recognize, identify, and express pain in the way that younger adults do and may sometimes ambulate despite hip fractures. A thorough physical examination should be completed for any patient who has sustained a fall. Observation for abnormal positioning of the arms or legs, in particular external rotation and shortening of a leg, will help with the clinical bedside diagnosis of hip fracture. A thorough skin assessment should be done to look for ecchymoses or abrasion. Gently testing the range of motion in both arms and legs could reveal discomfort and support the suspicion of injury. Any one of these findings should lead to the immediate transfer of the patient to the nearest emergency room. In all cases, it is essential to contact the designated representative of the family in order to review the situation and discuss with them an appropriate plan of action (see Figure 16–2 for an algorithm for the assessment for treatment of a patient who has fallen).

If the patient's vital signs are unstable, the patient should remain in an unchanged position until the arrival of emergency medical service staff. If the patient does not appear to have sustained any injury, the initial treatment consists of initiating a multidisciplinary falls intervention protocol. Mechanical restraints must be reserved for extreme circumstances, because their use does not decrease the incidence of falls.

After identifying the primary reasons for the fall, clinical interventions may include adjustment of medications, provision of physical and occupational therapy, and providion of assistive devices for ambulation and safety. It is essential to reassess the patient daily for several days after

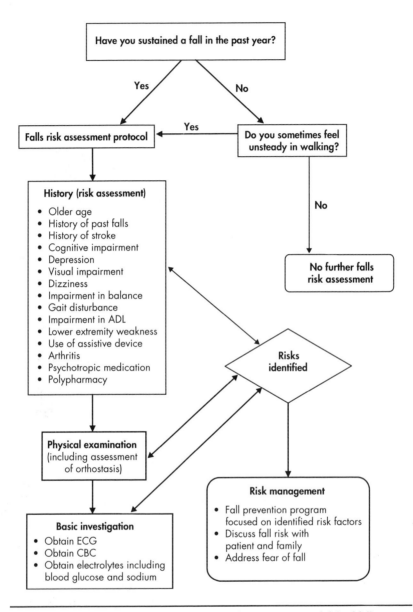

**FIGURE 16–1.**   Before the fall: algorithm for assessment of risk of falls.

*Note.*   ADL=activities of daily living; CBC=complete blood count;
ECG=electrocardiogram.

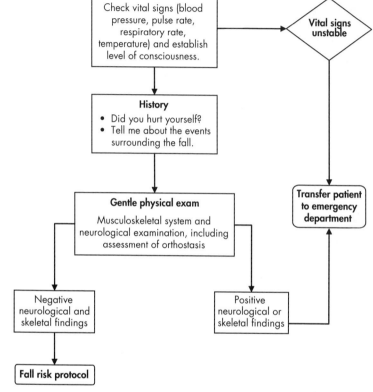

**FIGURE 16–2.** After the fall: algorithm for assessment and treatment of a patient who has fallen.

a fall to ensure that no late consequences of the fall have occurred. Ecchymoses may take as long as 48 hours to appear on the surface of the skin.

The laboratory investigations of falls include thyroid function test, urinalysis, tilt table test, 24-hour Holter monitoring, echocardiogram, and computed tomography, magnetic resonance imaging, or radiological evaluation of suspected sites. Consultations can be made according to the needs of the patient. Neurology, cardiology, ophthalmology, infectious disease, physical medicine and rehabilitation, and ear, nose, and throat services may be appropriate.

# References

American Geriatrics Society, British Geriatric Society, and American Academy of Orthopaedic Surgeons Panel on Falls Prevention: Guideline for the prevention of falls in older persons. J Am Geriatr Soc 49:664–672, 2001

Campbell AJ:Drug treatment as a cause of falls in old age: a review of offending agents. Drugs Aging 1:289–302, 1991

Campbell AJ, Borrie MJ, Spears GF: Risk factors for falls in a community-based prospective study of people 70 years and older. J Gerontol 44:M112–M117, 1989

de Carle AJ, Kohn R: Risk factors for falling in a psychogeriatric unit. Int J Geriatr Psychiatry 16:762–767, 2001

Graafmans WC, Ooms ME, Hofstee HM, et al: Falls in the elderly: a prospective study of risk factors and risk profiles. Am J Epidemiol 143:1129–1136, 1996

Gross YT, Shimamoto Y, Rose CL, et al: Why do they fall? Monitoring risk factors in nursing homes. J Gerontol Nurs 16:20–25, 1990

Priplata AA, Niemi JB, Harry JD, et al: Vibrating insoles and balance control in elderly people. Lancet 362:1123–1124, 2003

Rohde JM, Myers AH, Vlahov D: Variation in risk for falls by clinical department: implications for prevention. Infect Control Hosp Epidemiol 11:521–524, 1990

Rubenstein LZ, Josephson KR: The epidemiology of falls and syncope. Clin Geriatr Med 18:141–158, 2002

Tinetti ME, Speechley M, Ginter SF: Risk factors for falls among elderly persons living in the community. N Engl J Med 319:1701–1707, 1988

Tinetti ME, Liu WL, Claus EB: Predictors and prognosis of inability to get up after falls among elderly persons. JAMA 269:65–70, 1993

Tinetti ME, Mendes de Leon CF, Doucette JT, et al: Fear of falling and fall-related efficacy in relationship to functioning among community-living elders. J Gerontol 49:M140–M147, 1994

Walker JE, Howland J: Falls and fear of falling among elderly persons living in the community: occupation therapy interventions. Am J Occup Ther 45:119–122, 1991

# CHAPTER 17

# Head Trauma

Jerry Chang, M.D.

## Clinical Presentation

Head trauma can be classified clinically into three levels of severity on the basis of the patient's score on the Glasgow Coma Scale (GCS) after the trauma (Figure 17–1). Severe head trauma is defined as a GCS score of less than 9, moderate head trauma as a GCS score of 9–12, and mild head trauma as a GCS score of 13–15. Mild head trauma is further characterized by a loss of consciousness for no more than 30 seconds and posttraumatic amnesia that lasts no more than 24 hours.

Most cases of head trauma encountered in the psychiatric hospital or on the psychiatric ward are mild in severity and are usually precipitated by falls (see Chapter 16, "Falls").

## Differential Diagnosis

When approaching a patient with head trauma, the physician should not only address the trauma itself but also treat the cause of the trauma. A history from the patient and from witnesses of the event and a thorough physical examination will help to narrow the differential diagnosis. After evaluating and treating the patient's head trauma, the following issues should be addressed: 1) Did the patient display any seizure activity or incontinence? 2) Does the patient have any weakness or lateralizing neurological findings that may indicate a cerebrovascular event or intracranial bleeding? and 3) Did the patient recently begin taking a new medication that could cause lethargy, light-headedness, orthostatic blood pressure changes, or confusion?

Mild head trauma can cause transient headache, mild confusion, and mood changes. These symptoms can last from a few hours to a few

| Response | Score |
|---|---|
| **Eye opening** | |
| None | 1 |
| To pain | 2 |
| To verbal stimuli | 3 |
| Spontaneously | 4 |
| **Verbal response** | |
| None | 1 |
| Incomprehensible sounds | 2 |
| Inappropriate words | 3 |
| Disoriented | 4 |
| Oriented | 5 |
| **Motor response** | |
| None | 1 |
| Extension/decerebrate posturing | 2 |
| Flexion/decorticate posturing | 3 |
| Withdrawal | 4 |
| Localizes to pain | 5 |
| Obeys commands | 6 |

**FIGURE 17–1.**    Glasgow Coma Scale.

*Note.*   The sum of the points assigned in this scale is used to the assess the severity of coma and impaired consciousness (mild=13–15 points; moderate=9–12 points; severe=3–8 points). Patients with score <8 are in a coma.

weeks, but they usually cause no permanent injury. However, some patients may develop a postconcussion syndrome that may persist for months after the trauma. These patients often complain of headache, insomnia, dizziness, and impairments in memory and cognition. Some patients also report photophobia, phonophobia, increased anxiety, and mood lability. These symptoms can usually be treated conservatively, and in most cases will improve with time (Kaufman 2001; Van Dellen et al. 2003).

More worrisome in the acute setting are intracranial injuries, most notably injuries resulting in intracranial bleeding. The bleeding can cause injury to adjacent tissue and can also produce edema. If the bleeding is serious enough, it can result in increased intracranial pressure and herniation of brain tissue, potentially leading to coma and death. Epidural hematomas typically result from fractures of the temporal bone, with concomitant laceration of the middle meningeal artery. The patient commonly has a loss of consciousness, followed by a period of lucency, followed again by progressive mental status changes. Subdural hematomas occur more frequently than epidural hematomas and are caused by the tearing of the bridging veins that connect the cerebral cortex to venous sinuses. The symptoms of subdural hematomas are usually the result of injury to adjacent brain tissue or are caused by increased intracranial pressure. The patient may have headache, vomiting, changes in mental status, and papilledema.

## Risk Stratification

The use of computed tomography (CT) scans of the head to screen for intracranial injury in patients with head trauma is becoming the standard of care in hospitals that have CT equipment. However, concern has been raised about use of unnecessary CT scans in patients with mild head trauma, because such use increases medical costs.

Age has been considered a risk factor for intracranial bleeding in many studies. As people age, the brain atrophies, which increases the risk of subdural hematoma. Most studies have recommended obtaining a CT scan for all patients ages 60 years and older who have head trauma (Haydel et al. 2000; Mack et al. 2003; Stiell et al. 2001). Patients with a GCS score less than 15 within 2 hours of the trauma are at increased risk for positive CT scan findings (Holmes et al. 1997; Stiell et al. 2001). A review of the literature identified coagulopathy, including the use of warfarin, a history of chronic liver failure, and renal dialysis, as a risk factor for chronic subdural hematoma (Chen and Levy 2000). Patients with alcohol or drug intoxication have been found to be at increased risk for intracranial bleeding after head trauma (Falimirski et al. 2003; Haydel et al. 2000).

The significance of a loss of consciousness or the presence of amnesia for the time surrounding the traumatic event is debated in the literature. Earlier studies found that patients who sustained a loss of consciousness or had amnesia were at increased risk for intracranial injury, and the researchers encouraged physicians to obtain a CT scan for all patients with these characteristics (Moran et al. 1994; Stein and Ross 1992). However, more recent reports suggested that loss of consciousness or amnesia without signs of skull fracture or symptoms of headache, somnolence, mental status changes, nausea/emesis, seizure, perseveration, neurological deficit, blurred/double vision, vertigo, or hemotympanum is not an indication for a CT scan of the head, because the management of these patients would not be affected by CT findings (Miller et al. 1996; Falimirski et al. 2003).

To help standardize the management of head trauma, Stiell et al. (2001) identified suspected skull fracture, signs of a basal skull fracture, vomiting more than twice, failure to reach a GCS score of 15 within 2 hours, and age greater than 65 years as risk factors that increase the likelihood of positive CT scan findings. A second set of criteria indicated the following factors as predictors of positive CT scan findings after head injury: age 60 years and older, drug or alcohol intoxication, headache, vomiting, deficits in short-term memory, physical evidence of trauma above the clavicles, and seizure (Haydel et al. 2000). In both of these studies, all patients with positive CT scan findings had at least one of the identified risk factors (Haydel et al. 2000; Stiell et al. 2001).

Although debate continues about which patients with mild head trauma should have a CT scan of the head, increased vigilance may be indicated in psychiatric patients. Many patients, because of their illness, may already have questionable changes in mental status or lower GCS scores, which make accurate assessment difficult. Rarely, a subdural hematoma can mimic or worsen psychiatric symptoms and therefore may be missed in this population or misdiagnosed as an exacerbation of the preexisting psychiatric illness. Subdural hematomas have been known to mimic dementia, mood symptoms, and even psychosis (Black 1984, 1985; Ishikawa et al. 2002; Marik et al. 2002).

## Assessment and Management in Psychiatric Settings

When called to evaluate a patient with head trauma, the physician must decide whether the patient can be managed safely on the unit or whether a more complete evaluation, including a CT scan of the head to rule out an intracranial injury, is needed. Patients older than age 60 years who sustain a head trauma should always be sent for a CT scan to rule out occult bleeding, even if they are asymptomatic. Patients with chronic liver failure or renal failure treated with dialysis have impaired coagulation and may be at risk for intracranial bleeding. Many medications also predispose patients to intracranial bleeding, including platelet inhibitors and warfarin (Chen and Levy 2000).

The physician should determine if the fall was witnessed, and, if so, should ask the witnesses how the patient fell and why. Witnesses should be asked about any seizure activity or weakness, which may indicate a cerebrovascular event and requires further treatment, and asked whether the patient lost consciousness. Patients with a loss of consciousness after head trauma have a higher likelihood of intracranial bleeding and should be sent for a CT scan (Moran et al. 1994; Stein and Ross 1992).

Patients with amnesia for the time surrounding the trauma are also at higher risk for intracranial bleeding and should also be sent for a CT scan (Stein and Ross 1992). The physician should determine if there is any change in the patient's mental status and should calculate the patient's GCS score. A patient with any change in mental status or a GCS score less than 15 should be sent for further evaluation with a CT scan to rule out intracranial injury (Holmes et al. 1997; Stiell et al. 2001). For some psychiatric patients, it may be difficult to determine if there has been a change in mental status, or it may even be difficult to calculate a GCS score. Patients with dementia or disorganized thoughts and speech may be especially difficult to evaluate accurately. The physician should err on the side of caution and should ask the patient if he or she has any symptoms that may indicate increased intracranial pressure or brain injury, such as nausea and vomiting, severe headache, vertigo, somnolence, and blurred or double vision. Any of these symptoms may be an indication of intracranial injury, and a CT of the head is warranted in patients with these symptoms (Falimirski et al. 2003).

A thorough physical examination, including a full neurological assessment, is also necessary. The physician should look for focal or lateralizing neurological deficits that would require further evaluation and should look for any signs of trauma above the clavicles or for signs of a skull fracture such as retromastoid ecchymoses (Battle's sign), periorbital ecchymoses (raccoon eyes), cerebrospinal fluid (CSF) rhinorrhea, CSF otorrhea, or hemotympanum. Any of these signs indicate an increased risk of intracranial injury and the need for an evaluation in the emergency department and a CT scan of the head (Falimirski et al. 2003; Haydel et al. 2000; Stiell et al. 2001) (see Figure 17–2).

If, after a careful history and physical examination, no further evaluation or CT scan of the head is required, the physician may consider asking the nursing staff to evaluate the patient with a neurological examination every 2–4 hours for the next few days. Acute subdural hematomas may present up to 72 hours after head trauma with signs and symptoms of increased intracranial pressure, changes in mental status, or exacerbations of psychiatric illness. The physician should be sensitive to any changes in the mental status of a patient with recent head trauma, even if the patient's initial CT scan had negative findings. A repeat scan may be indicated.

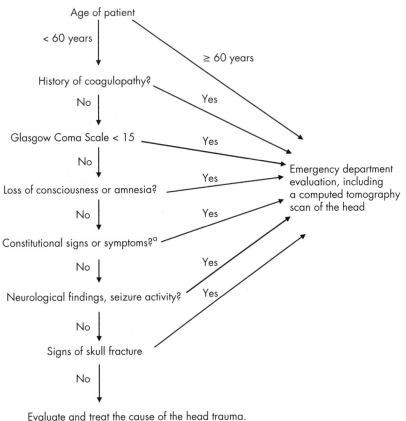

**FIGURE 17–2.**    Algorithm for assessment and treatment of a patient with head trauma.

[a]Headache, somnolence, mental status changes, nausea/emesis, blurred or double vision, vertigo.

# References

Black DW: Mental changes resulting from subdural hematoma. Br J Psychiatry 145:200–203, 1984

Black DW: Subdural hematoma. a retrospective study of the "great neurologic imitator." Postgrad Med 78:107–111, 1985

Chen JC, Levy ML: Causes, epidemiology, and risk factors of chonic subdural hematoma. Neurosurg Clin N Am 11:399–406, 2000

Falimirski ME, Gonzalez R, Rodriguez A, et al: The need for head computed tomography in patients sustaining loss of consciousness after mild head injury. J Trauma 55:1–6, 2003

Haydel MJ, Preston CA, Mills TJ, et al: Indications for computed tomography in patients with minor injury. N Engl J Med 343:100–105, 2000

Holmes JF, Baier ME, Derlet RW: Failure of the Miller criteria to predict significant injury in patients with a Glasgow Coma Scale score of 14 after minor head trauma. Acad Emerg Med 4:788–792, 1997

Ishikawa E, Yanaka K, Sugimoto K, et al: Reversible dementia in patients with chronic subdural hematomas. J Neurosurg 96:680–683, 2002

Kaufman DM: Clinical Neurology for Psychiatrists, 5th Edition. Philadelphia, PA, WB Saunders, 2001

Mack LR, Chan SB, Silva JC, et al: The use of head computed tomography in elderly patients sustaining minor head trauma. J Emerg Med 24:157–162, 2003

Marik PE, Varon J, Trask T: Management of head trauma. Chest 122:699–711, 2002

Miller EC, Derlet RW, Kinser D: Minor head trauma: is computed tomography always necessary? Ann Emerg Med 27:290–294, 1996

Moran SG, McCarthy MC, Uddin DE, et al: Predictors of positive CT scans in the trauma patient with minor head injury. Am Surg 60:533–535, 1994

Stein SC, Ross SE: Mild head injury: a plea for routine early CT scanning. J Trauma 3:11–13, 1992

Stiell IG, Wells GA, Vandemheen K, et al: The Canadian CT Head Rule for patients with minor head injury. Lancet 357:1391–1396, 2001

Van Dellen JR, Becker DP, Bradley WG, et al: Trauma of the nervous system, in Neurology in Clinical Practice. Edited by Bradley WG, Daroff RB, Fenichel GM, et al. Newton, MA, Butterworth-Heinemann, 2003, pp 861–892

# Headache

Sassan Naderi, M.D.

Marc L. Gordon, M.D.

## Clinical Presentation

New or unusually severe headaches are cause for concern. Likewise, the quality of the headache (throbbing, stabbing, pressure-like, or steady) is important in the diagnosis of its etiology. The area of greatest pain intensity often gives clues to the etiology of the headache. Unilateral temple pain may be a clue that the patient has temporal arteritis. Likewise, pituitary apoplexy often presents with intense pain between the eyes. Pain in the occiput and nuchal rigidity may be indicators of meningitis or subarachnoid hemorrhage. A headache that reaches maximal intensity within minutes is a danger sign and warrants aggressive investigation to rule out intracranial hemorrhage. Likewise, headaches that awaken the patient from sleep or have a nocturnal pattern should raise suspicion of increased intracranial pressure. Pain duration also provides diagnostic clues. The patient should be asked how often headaches occur and asked about the duration of the longest headache-free period in the last 6 months. Any activities that may have triggered or worsened the headache should be noted, as well as associated activities and recent trauma. Patients with space-occupying lesions or increased intracranial pressure may have increased pain with Valsalva's maneuver or change in cranial position.

Associated symptoms that may indicate that the patient has a dangerous secondary headache include changes in the patient's baseline mental status, nuchal rigidity, changes in vision, fever, or focal neurological deficits. Likewise, family history may help delineate the etiology of the patient's headache, particularly for cerebral aneurysms and arteriovenous malformations (AVMs).

## Differential Diagnosis

The physician must distinguish serious and life-threatening presentations from those that are less serious. Often, dangerous headaches are secondary to another process, of which the headache is only a symptom. Primary headaches, although sometimes debilitating, do not cause significant mortality or permanent morbidity. It is exceedingly important to distinguish between primary and secondary headaches (Table 18–1). The distinction is best accomplished with a thorough history and physical examination that are supported by ancillary testing.

**TABLE 18–1.**    Differential diagnosis of secondary and primary headaches

**Secondary headaches**
Mass lesions
   Brain tumors
   Brain abscess
Intracranial hemorrhage
Subdural hematoma
   Epidural hematoma
   Subarachnoid hemorrhage
   Parenchymal cerebral hemorrhage
   Postconcussive headaches
Increased intracranial pressure
   Pseudotumor cerebri
Decreased intracranial pressure
   Post-lumbar puncture headache
Inflammatory/vasculitic headaches
   Temporal arteritis
Infectious causes
   Meningitis
   Sinusitis

**Primary headaches**
Migraine headache
   Migraine without aura
   Migraine with aura
   Basilar artery migraine
   Ophthalmoplegic migraine
Cluster headache
Tension-type headache

---

**TABLE 18-2.** Symptoms that aid in risk stratification of headache

**Alarming attributes of a headache**
Abrupt onset
High level of severity
Progressive course
Nocturnal worsening
Awakening from sleep because of pain
Increased pain with Valsalva's maneuver
Recent head trauma

**Alarming associated symptoms**
Change in baseline mental status
Nuchal rigidity
Change in vision
Fever
Focal neurological deficits

---

## Risk Stratification

In evaluating the patient's headache, the physician must first determine if the headache is primary, and probably benign, or secondary, and possibly dangerous (Table 18–2).

## Assessment and Management in Psychiatric Settings

The physical examination should include assessment of vital signs, a detailed neurological examination, and examination of the eyes, as well as examination of the head, face, and neck. The clinician should be looking for alarming signs that indicate that the patient may be experiencing a serious and dangerous secondary headache (Table 18–3).

Documentation of elevated temperature is critical. Fever suggests the possibility of meningitis, encephalitis, or brain abscess, as well as intracranial hemorrhage or an etiology involving the hypothalamus. Likewise, acute sinusitis or temporal arteritis may present with a headache and fever. Diastolic blood pressure >110 mm Hg increases the likelihood that hypertension is the etiology of the headache. Elevated blood pressure becomes a hypertensive emergency if it is accompanied by focal neurological deficits or a change in mental status (Fisher and Williams 2005). Likewise, hypertension may be the result of any process

**TABLE 18–3.** Signs that aid in risk stratification of headache

Change in gait
Change in mental status
Dysconjugate gaze
Fever
Focal neurological deficits
Inability to touch finger to nose
Nuchal rigidity (Kernig's sign, Brudzinski's sign)
Papilledema
Significant hypertension (especially with bradycardia)
Stigmata of recent head trauma (Battle's sign, raccoon eyes)
Tender, indurated, pulseless temporal artery
Unequal pupils
Visual field abnormalities

causing increased intracranial pressure, especially if hypertension is accompanied by bradycardia. Any focal neurological deficits may be indicative of structural intracranial pathology. Abnormal gait, inability to touch finger to nose, or difficulty with tandem gait may be clues to a posterior fossa mass. On funduscopic examination, spontaneous venous pulsations in the upright patient indicate normal intracranial pressure. Papilledema indicates increased intracranial pressure. Flame hemorrhages, hard exudates, and arteriovenous nicking are seen in patients with malignant hypertension. Subhyaloid or preretinal hemorrhages may be suggestive of subarachnoid hemorrhage. Other alarming signs include unequal pupils, visual field abnormalities, and dysconjugate gaze.

Palpation of the head may show areas of tenderness that may indicate trauma or muscle spasm. Tenderness, induration, and loss of pulsatility of the temporal arteries may indicate temporal arteritis. Tenderness to percussion over the sinuses may indicate sinusitis, and tenderness of the teeth may indicate a dental infection or abscess. The temporomandibular joints must be examined as a possible source of headache. Stiffness of the neck may be a manifestation of meningeal irritation. A positive Kernig's sign and/or Brudzinski's sign may be elicited in patients with meningitis or subarachnoid hemorrhage. The test for Kernig's sign is performed by having the patient lie supine while the examiner flexes the thigh at a right angle to the trunk. The test is positive if complete extension of the leg at the knee joint elicits pain. Brudzinski's

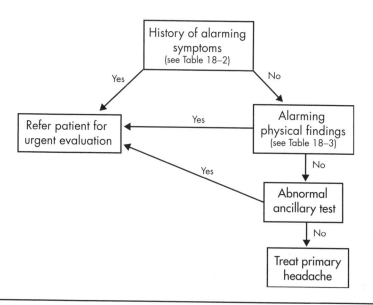

**FIGURE 18–1.**    Algorithm for assessment and treatment of a patient with headaches.

sign consists of involuntary flexion of the patient's hips and knees when the neck is passively flexed.

New-onset headache in patients age 50 years or older should be further evaluated with laboratory analysis of erythrocyte sedimentation rate (ESR). Suspicion of temporal arteritis should be increased if the patient's ESR is elevated. Computed tomography (CT) is a sensitive test for finding intracranial hemorrhages. If there is a high level of clinical suspicion of subarachnoid hemorrhage, a lumbar puncture to check for xanthochromia is indicated if the CT scan is negative. CT or magnetic resonance imaging (MRI) is the diagnostic study of choice if intracranial mass or AVM is suspected. CT may also show an aneurysm if it is greater than 0.5–1.0 cm in size, but magnetic resonance angiography (MRA) or angiography would better define an aneurysm. Lumbar puncture is also indicated if there is suspicion of meningitis (see Figure 18–1).

## Secondary Headaches

### Hypertensive Headache

Hypertensive headaches are throbbing occipital headaches that do not generally occur until the diastolic pressure exceeds 110 mm Hg. Hypertension is an overdiagnosed cause of headaches, but if the headache is due to hypertension, control of the blood pressure with appropriate antihypertensive agents will alleviate the pain.

## Mass Lesion

**Brain tumor.**   The index of suspicion for brain tumors is raised if there is pain on awakening, if the pain is worse with Valsalva's maneuver, or if there is a new or unfamiliar headache associated with nausea and vomiting. The initial examination may be without focal findings. Follow-up must be arranged, and the diagnosis can be made by using a CT scan with contrast or an MRI scan.

**Brain abscess.**   Brain abscess is similar to other space-occupying lesions, except that the patient usually also has a fever and, in some cases, may have a history of sinusitis. Diagnosis is made with a CT or MRI scan.

## Intracranial Hemorrhage

Patients with intracranial bleeding (subdural, epidural, or subarachnoid) often present with headache. Diagnosis can be made with a CT scan. A high level of suspicion of intracranial hemorrhage is appropriate in elderly patients who have experienced even a minor trauma. Postconcussive headaches may follow trauma within hours to days (see Chapter 17, "Head Trauma").

## Increased Intracranial Pressure

Pseudotumor cerebri (idiopathic intracranial hypertension) typically occurs in young obese females with irregular menstruation. Usual complaints are of visual problems with severe headache. The physical examination shows papilledema, and the CT scan reveals slit-like ventricles. Treatments may include acetazolamide for reduction of cerebrospinal fluid (CSF) production, ventriculoperitoneal shunt, optic nerve sheath fenestration, or serial lumbar punctures and administration of steroids.

## Decreased Intracranial Pressure

Headache caused by decreased intracranial pressure may occur after lumbar puncture. The size of the needle used in lumbar puncture, the amount of fluid withdrawn, and the number of punctures are causative factors in this bicranial, pulsatile, frontal headache, which is exacerbated when the patient is in the upright position. Prophylactic treatments include rest, analgesics, avoidance of lifting, and adequate hydration. In cases of intractable pain, a blood patch may be placed at the site of the lumbar puncture. Likewise, high-dose caffeine has shown some efficacy in treating these headaches.

## Inflammatory/Vasculitic Headaches

Temporal arteritis is a disease in which branches of the external carotid artery, most often the temporal artery, become infiltrated with lymphocytes, plasma cells, and multinucleated giant cells. It is a disease of people age 50 years and older, and women are four times more likely to be affected than men (Silberstein et al. 2001). Temporal arteritis is often associated with polymyalgia rheumatica. The headache may be unilateral or bilateral, with a piercing or burning quality. Frequent jabs, often excruciating, are experienced at night. The inflamed artery is tender and pulseless and can sometimes be rolled between the fingers and the skull. Patients with temporal arteritis have an elevated ESR. Biopsy of the involved artery will yield a definitive diagnosis. Treatment should not be withheld while awaiting diagnosis, because blindness is the most common sequela and can develop rapidly secondary to ischemic pathological papillitis. Treatment includes long-term use of corticosteroids.

## Infectious Causes of Headache

**Meningitis.**   Headache caused by meningitis usually involves the entire head and is associated with fever. As mentioned earlier, Kernig's sign and/or Brudzinski's sign may be present. Diagnosis is made with a lumbar puncture and examination of the CSF for white blood cells and measurement of glucose and protein levels with concomitant cultures. Antibiotics are used for treatment of bacterial meningitis; viral meningitis is treated symptomatically.

**Sinusitis.**   Sinusitis is an acute infection of the nasal, paranasal, or mastoid sinuses and may be associated with severe headaches. The pain is either stabbing or aching. Often the pain is made worse when the patient bends over or coughs and is lessened when the patient is supine. In a physical examination, the patient may report tenderness with palpation of the affected sinus. Sinusitis is treated with antibiotics and decongestives.

## Toxic Headaches

A wide variety of chemical substances have been reported to induce headaches, especially in patients with underlying primary headache disorders. Substances that have been implicated include monosodium glutamate, aspartame, alcohol, carbon monoxide, nitrites, and many medications. For example, headaches have been reported in patients taking histamine type 2 blockers, nonsteroidal anti-inflammatory drugs (NSAIDs), oral nitrates, antibiotics, dipyridamole, and psychotropic medications such as selective serotonin reuptake inhibitors. Because headache is such a common complaint, it is listed as a potential adverse effect in the package insert for numerous medications, although causality is not necessarily established. It is important for the clinician to evaluate patients for other causes of headache, rather than simply attribute the headache to medication.

## Primary Headaches

### Migraine Headache

Migraine headaches are characterized by recurrent attacks of headaches that are usually unilateral but that vary in intensity, frequency, and duration. They may be associated with anorexia, photophobia, phonophobia, nausea, and vomiting. Migraines are often familial. They may be precipitated by ingestion of chocolate, nuts, cheese, alcohol, or monosodium glutamate, as well as by exposure to perfumes and by fatigue, stress, oversleeping, and use of vasodilators. Women are more likely to be afflicted than men, and there may be an association with the woman's menstrual cycle. Migraines may start in childhood, but more often they begin in puberty. More than 80% of patients with migraine headaches had their first attack before age 30 years. Migraine without aura accounts for more than 80% of all migraine headaches. In contrast to migraine with aura (formerly known as classic migraine), migraine without aura has no sharply defined neurological symptoms. Vague prodromes such as irritability may precede the headache by hours or days. Migraine with aura occurs in about 15% of patients with migraine and is characterized by a sharply defined, reversible neurological deficit that precedes or accompanies the migraine (Cologno et al. 2002). The aura of a migraine may consist of focal neurological symptoms such as visual scintillations (bright zigzag lines) or scotomas, numbness, weakness, or aphasia. The International Headache Society has used specific diagnostic criteria to define migraine with aura, which include a) one or more fully reversible aura symptoms indicating brain dysfunction, b) at least one aura symptom developing gradually over more than 4 minutes or two or more symptoms occuring in succession, c) no single aura symptom lasting more than 1 hour, and d) headache following aura in less than 1 hour and possibly beginning before or occuring simultaneously with aura. The diagnosis of migraine with aura is made in patients with at least two attacks having at least three of the four features listed and no other explanation for the symptoms (Silberstein et al. 2001).

Mild to moderate migraine headache attacks may be treated acutely with acetaminophen or NSAIDs. For patients with more debilitating pain, selective serotonin receptor agonists (triptans) have been shown to be efficacious and are the drugs of choice. Ergotamine preparations and dihydroergotamine may also be used. Vasoconstrictive medications, such as triptans and ergotamine preparations, are contraindicated in patients with hemiplegic or basilar migraine, because of concerns that these medications could predispose the patient to stroke (Silberstein et al. 2001). Similarly, use of triptans may be contraindicated in patients with Prinzmetal's angina or ischemic heart disease. Use of triptans is generally contraindicated in patients who are taking monoamine oxidase inhibitors. Other medications that maybe used for debilitating headaches include barbiturates and opiates. Care should be taken in dispensing these medications, because of their addictive and abuse potential.

Preventive treatment is indicated for patients with debilitating headaches that do not respond to abortive therapy, patients who cannot tolerate treatment regimens, and patients with a high frequency of headaches. Prevention may consist of pharmacological or nonpharmacological interventions. Nonpharmacological prevention of migraines involves avoiding identifiable triggers such as chocolate and alcohol. Pharmacological prevention of migraines should be discussed with a neurology consultant.

### Cluster Headache

Cluster headache occurs primarily in men and has onset between age 20 and 30 years. It consists of unilateral intense ocular or retro-orbital pain lasting less than 2 hours but occurring several times a day for periods of weeks to months. There may be facial flushing, forehead sweating, lacrimation, rhinorrhea, or conjunctival injection on the side of the pain. The headache may follow the ingestion of alcohol or the use of histamine-containing compounds.

Acute abortive treatment of cluster headache may include inhalation of 100% oxygen, sumatriptan injection, use of ergotamines, and instillation of 4% lidocaine solution into the ipsilateral nostril. Medications that may be used as preventive measures include lithium carbonate, prednisone, verapamil, and the antiepileptic medication divalproex sodium.

*Tension-Type Headache*

Tension-type headache is often bilateral and is characterized by constant, nonthrobbing, viselike pain. There may be focal areas of pain in the bioccipital regions, the bitemporal regions, and the vertex of the head alone or in combination. Tension-type headaches are classified as episodic and chronic. In a physical examination, the patient may have scalp tenderness as well as localized nodules that can be detected by manual palpation in the pericranial or cervical muscles. In general, patients with tension-type headaches have muscle tenderness. Treatment consists of mild analgesics such as acetaminophen and NSAIDs. Relaxation techniques and biofeedback are also helpful. If the headache becomes chronic in nature, tricyclics such as nortriptyline may be helpful.

# References

Cologno D, Torelli P, Manzani GC: Transient visual disturbances during migraine without aura attacks. Headache 42:930–933, 2002

Fisher N, Williams G: Hypertensive vascular disease, in Harrison's Principles of Internal Medicine, 16th Edition. Edited by Kasper DL, Braunwald E, Fauci AS, , et al. New York, McGraw-Hill, 2005, pp 1463–1480

Silberstein SD, Saper J, Freitag F: Migraine: diagnosis and treatment, in Wolff's Headache and Other Head Pain, 7th Edition. Edited by Silberstein SD, Lipton RB, Dalessio D. New York, Oxford University Press, 2001, pp 121–137

# CHAPTER 19

# Syncope

Michael E. Bernstein, M.D.

Kumar Alagappan, M.D.

## Clinical Presentation

Syncope is a sudden, transient loss of consciousness associated with the inability to maintain postural tone. The loss of consciousness generally lasts 15–20 seconds, and cognitive function returns as cerebral perfusion increases. Approximately 12%–48% of the population experience syncope at some time in their lives (De Lorenzo 2002). Elderly persons are particularly susceptible because of the physiological changes of aging (Forman and Lipsitz 1997). Syncope most commonly is a manifestation of a benign self-limiting process that can be accurately discerned from a comprehensive history and physical examination. However, because it can also be the first presentation of many life-threatening conditions, a comprehensive diagnostic evaluation is indicated in selected cases. The evaluation of a patient with syncope is the same as that for a patient with *presyncope,* which is defined as the prodromal symptoms of fainting (dizziness, nausea, vomiting, etc.) without a loss of consciousness (Krahn et al. 2001).

## Differential Diagnosis

There is an extensive differential diagnosis for the patient presenting with syncope. Causes can be broadly divided into the following categories: reflex-mediated, neurogenic, cardiac, other organic causes, pharmacological, and psychogenic (Table 19–1).

**TABLE 19—1.**   Differential diagnosis of syncope

| Reflex-mediated causes | Cardiac causes |
|---|---|
| Vasovagal | Structural cardiopulmonary disease |
| Situational |    Valve stenosis/incompetence |
|   Micturition |    Cardiomyopathies |
|   Defecation |    Congenital heart disease |
|   Posttussive |    Atrial myxoma |
|   Deglutition |    Pericardial disease |
|   Neuralgia |    Cardiac tamponade |
| Carotid sinus hypersensitivity |    Pulmonary hypertension |
| Orthostatic hypotension |    Aortic dissection |
| **Psychogenic causes** |    Pulmonary embolism |
| Stress |    Vertebrobasilar insufficiency |
| Hyperventilation | Myocardial ischemia/infarction |
| Anxiety disorder | Dysrhythmias |
| Panic disorder |   Bradydysrhythmias |
| Conversion disorder |    Sick sinus syndrome |
| Major depression |    Second- and third-degree heart block |
| **Neurogenic causes** |    Prolonged Q–T syndrome |
| Transient ischemic attacks |    Pacemaker/defibrillator malfunction |
| Cerebrovascular accident |   Tachydysrhythmias |
| Subclavian steal |    Ventricular tachycardia |
| Peripheral neuropathy |    Ventricular fibrillation |
| Migraine |    Torsades de pointes |
| Seizure |    Supraventricular tachycardia |
| **Other organic causes** |    Wolff-Parkinson-White syndrome |
| Pregnancy | **Medications/drugs[a]** |
| Narcolepsy | |
| Hypoxia | |
| Hypoglycemia | |
| Unknown | |

[a]The most commonly implicated medications include antihypertensives, β-blockers, calcium channel blockers, cardiac glycosides, diuretics, nitrites, antidysrhythmics, antipsychotics, antidepressants, sedative-hypnotics, phenothiazines, antiparkinsonian drugs, alcohol, and cocaine.
*Source.*   Adapted from Blok 2000.

## Organic Disorders

### Reflex-Mediated Syncope

Reflex-mediated syncope is also referred to as neurocardiogenic syncope because it represents the failure of the circulatory system to produce

---

**TABLE 19–2.**    Factors resulting in neurocardiogenic dysfunction

---

Cardiovascular deconditioning

Comorbid conditions

Decreased endocrine response after volume depletion

Decreased baroreceptor sensitivity

Decreased basilar levels of renin and aldosterone

Decreased cardiac output in response to hypotension, exercise, and postural changes

Less sensitive thirst mechanisms

Polypharmacy

---

or maintain adequate tone in certain situations (Kenny 2002). A disruption in the *neurogenic feedback loop* (for pathophysiology, see below) is responsible for the syncopal event. This process is the most common cause of syncope in the general population (Sarasin et al. 2002). Postural changes, dehydration, physiological changes, and emotional stress are often implicated. Reflex-mediated syncope rarely occurs without warning signs or symptoms, and this diagnosis should not be made if prodromal symptoms (dizziness, nausea, diaphoresis) are not present. *Vasovagal* syncope is the most common type of reflex-mediated syncope; its prevalence is inversely related to age, which is believed to be the result of a decrease in vagal tone with age (Weimer and Williams 2003). Situational syncopal episodes (syncope related to micturition or deglutition, posttussive syncope), on the other hand, are more common in elderly people. Elderly people are particularly susceptible to neurocardiogenic dysfunction secondary to the factors listed in Table 19–2 (Consensus Committee of the American Autonomic Society 1996).

Orthostatic hypotension is defined as a fall in systolic blood pressure of at least 20 mm Hg or a fall in diastolic blood pressure of at least 10 mm Hg within 3 minutes of standing up from a supine position (Olshansky 2003). Orthostatic hypotension is caused most commonly by volume depletion and/or medications that blunt the physiological response of the heart to postural changes. Other predisposing factors not necessarily related to age are pregnancy, physical exhaustion, and prolonged recumbency.

### Neurogenic Syncope

Cerebrovascular disorders are rarely the primary cause of syncope. Instead, when strokes and transient ischemic attacks occur, there generally are focal neurological defects that do not resolve in a brief period of time, as occurs in the true syncopal episode (Olshansky 2003). Seizures, on the other hand, can present in a similar manner as syncope, especially if the seizure is atypical or is not witnessed. In addition, compromised cerebral blood flow from any cause may result in tonic-clonic movements (Linzer et al. 1997). However, true syncope and a change in consciousness from neurological pathology can be differentiated through electroencephalogram (EEG) monitoring or by the observation of a postictal state, which precludes a quick, complete recovery. A final diagnostic puzzle can occur with brainstem ischemia from decreased blood flow to the reticular activating system. This pathological state leads to sudden brief episodes known as "drop attacks." However, these attacks are typically associated with other neurological signs and symptoms such diplopia, vertigo, and nausea (Blok 2000).

## Cardiac Syncope

Cardiac syncope accounts for about 18% of all cases of syncope; the causes can be divided into arrhythmias and structural cardiopulmonary lesions (Turnbull and Bono 2002). Arrhythmias account for the majority of cardiac-related syncope and often present with sudden syncope or palpitations without the typical prodrome seen in the reflex-mediated syncopal events. The paroxysmal nature of arrhythmias makes it extremely difficult to diagnose this condition in the emergency department. In fact, the electrocardiogram (ECG) has a diagnostic yield of less than 5% in these cases (Cherin et al. 1997). Therefore, further outpatient testing is generally indicated in cases in which there is any suspicion of cardiac syncope. Aortic stenosis is the most common structural cardiac abnormality that causes syncope, but any structural abnormality in which there is obstruction to blood flow can result in a syncopal episode.

## Other Organic Causes

In syncope studies that included patients with seizures, metabolic abnormalities were identified in less than 3% of cases (Roden 2004). In addition, hypoglycemic patients and hypoxic patients with syncope will not return to baseline without dextrose and oxygen administration, respectively. An "unknown" cause, which is diagnosed after a comprehensive evaluation does not reveal a source, accounts for about 39% of cases and is associated with a 1-year mortality rate of approximately 6% (Roden 2004).

## Drug Effects, Toxicities, and Withdrawal

Medications have the potential to induce syncope through their specific pharmacological properties. For instance, antihypertensives can blunt the sympathetic reflex (increased heart rate) to postural changes, diuretics can deplete intrathoracic volume, and antiarrhythmics can be proarrhythmic. In addition, many medications can either cause or predispose patients to arrhythmias that may cause presyncope, syncope, or sudden death (Ellison et al. 1990). One large study, in an elderly population, identified nontricyclic antidepressants, neuroleptic drugs, and antiparkinsonian drugs as particularly dangerous in this population (Grubb et al. 1994). Specifically, fluoxetine, promethazine, haloperidol, and L-dopa were associated with an excess risk of syncope. Fluoxetine therapy is generally regarded as benign but has been associated with bradycardia and consequent faintness, presyncope, and syncope. The mechanism is believed to be a direct central nervous system effect in which increased serotonin influences medullary cardiovascular regulation (Hewetson et al. 1986). The effect is highly variable, and fluoxetine has been used as an effective therapy for some patients with orthostatic hypotension that is refractory to other forms of therapy (Kouakam et al. 2002). Finally, sick sinus syndrome has been found to be aggravated by carbamazepine (Hewetson et al. 1986).

## Psychiatric Disorders

Psychiatric disorders account for approximately 2% of all syncopal episodes; the typical psychiatric patient with syncope is 20–40 years old and has frequent fainting episodes (Turnbull and Bono 2002). These patients have multiple associated symptoms, including nausea, lightheadedness, numbness, and intense fear or dread. Psychiatric disorders may represent a susceptibility to syncope, and psychiatric disorders should be considered in assessing patients with syncope without other diagnoses. The psychiatric conditions most commonly implicated are major depression, anxiety disorders, and panic disorder (American College of Emergency Physicians 2001). The symptoms can be reproduced with hyperventilation maneuvers and positive tilt table testing without a concurrent change in vital signs.

## Risk Stratification

The goal of the evaluation after a syncopal episode is to determine if the patient is at increased risk of sudden death. Recent studies have recog-

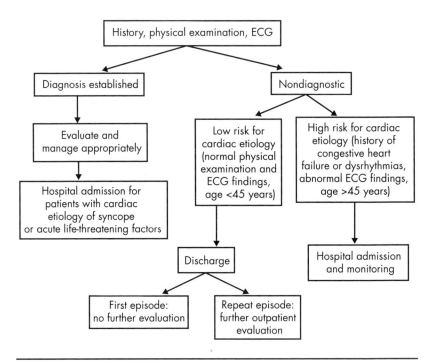

**FIGURE 19–1.**    Algorithm for assessment and treatment of patient with syncope.
*Note.*   ECG=electrocardiogram.

nized four significant predictors of sudden cardiac death or significant dysrhythmia within 1 year of a syncopal episode: abnormal ECG findings (all except nonspecific ST-T changes), age >45 years, history of ventricular dysrhythmia, and history of congestive heart failure (Calkins and Zipes 2001). An increasing number of risk factors for a given patient exponentially increases the risk of dysrhythmias. Hospitalization is required for patients with any of the following characteristics: abnormal ECG findings, chest pain, history of arrhythmia, age >70 years, and any acute neurological abnormalities (see Figure 19–1).

## Assessment and Management in Psychiatric Settings

A thorough history and physical examination (and an ECG) focused on symptoms, chronology, and current clinical status provide the basis for a diagnosis in 45%–85% of patients with syncope (De Lorenzo 2002).

**TABLE 19-3.** Essential components of history and physical examination in a patient with syncope

Events leading up to the syncopal episode
Antecedent illness and past medical history
Patient position and setting in which the syncopal event took place
Prodromal symptoms
Duration of unconscious period
Time until patient was fully awake
Vital signs

The essential components of a history and physical examination for patients with syncope are shown in Table 19–3.

Dyspnea immediately before a syncopal episode may be a manifestation of a pulmonary embolism. A sudden event without warning should raise suspicion of an arrhythmia, and a sudden event associated with exertion should raise suspicion of a structural cardiopulmonary lesion. Angina or sudden intense chest pain may suggest an acute myocardial infarction, cardiac tamponade, aortic stenosis, or aortic dissection. Focal neurological abnormalities may suggest a neurological process. Loss of bowel or bladder function may suggest a seizure. The worst headache of a patient's life should raise suspicion of subarachnoid hemorrhage. Abdominal or back pain should raise suspicion of an abdominal aortic aneurysm or a ruptured ectopic pregnancy. Diaphoresis, pallor, and light-headedness immediately preceding the syncopal event may suggest neurocardiogenic or vasovagal syncope. A syncopal event precipitated by a change in position (supine to upright) may suggest orthostatic hypotension.

The laboratory investigations most useful after syncope are pulse oximetry, ECG, tests for levels of all electrolytes (including magnesium and calcium), 24-hour ECG monitoring to assess the presence of arrhythmias or conduction abnormalities, echocardiography to determine the presence of outflow tract obstruction, and a tilt table test. Patients ages 65 years and older and those with any risk factors for coronary artery disease, a history of cardiovascular disease, hypoxia, or neurological deficits must be transferred immediately to the nearest emergency department. In the absence of neurological findings, routine computed tomography scanning, EEG, and lumbar puncture are very rarely useful.

# References

American College of Emergency Physicians: Clinical policy: critical issues in the evaluation and management of patients presenting with syncope. Ann Emerg Med 37:771–776, 2001

Blok BK: Syncope, in Emergency Medicine: A Comprehensive Study Guide, 5th Edition. Edited by Tintinalli JE, Kelen GD, Stapczynski JS. New York, McGraw-Hill, 2000, pp 352–356

Calkins H, Zipes DP: Hypotension and syncope, in Heart Disease: A Textbook of Cardiovascular Medicine, 6th Edition. Edited by Braunwald E, Zipes DP, Libby P. Philadelphia, PA, WB Saunders, 2001, pp 932–940

Cherin P, Colvez A, Deville de Periere G, et al: Risk of syncope in the elderly and consumption of drugs: a case-control study. J Clin Epidemiol 50:313–320, 1997

Consensus Committee of the American Autonomic Society and the American Academy of Neurology: Consensus statement on the definition of orthostatic hypotension, pure autonomic failure, and multiple system atrophy. Neurology 46:1470, 1996

De Lorenzo RA: Syncope, in Rosen's Emergency Medicine: Concepts and Clinical Practice, 5th Edition. Edited by Marx JA, Hockberger R, Walls R, et al. St. Louis, MO, Mosby, 2002, pp 174–178

Ellison JM, Milofsky JE, Ely E: Fluoxetine-induced bradycardia and syncope in two patients. J Clin Psychiatry 51:385–386, 1990

Forman DE, Lipsitz LA: Syncope in the elderly. Cardiol Clin 15:295–311, 1997

Grubb BP, Samoil D, Kosinski D, et al: Fluoxetine hydrochloride for the treatment of severe refractory orthostatic hypotension. Am J Med 97:366–368, 1994

Hewetson KA, Pitch AE, Watson RD: Sick sinus syndrome aggravated by carbamazepine therapy for epilepsy. Postgrad Med J 62:497–498, 1986

Kenny RA: Neurally mediated syncope. Clin Geriatr Med 18:191–210, vi, 2002

Kouakam C, Lacroix D, Klug D, et al: Prevalence and prognostic significance of psychiatric disorders in patients evaluated for recurrent unexplained syncope. Am J Cardiol 89:530–535, 2002

Krahn AD, Klein GJ, Yee R, et al: Predictive value of presyncope in patients monitored for assessment of syncope. Am Heart J 141:817–821, 2001

Linzer M, Yang EH, Estes NA 3rd, et al: Diagnosing syncope: part 1. value of history, physical examination, and electrocardiography. Clinical Efficacy Assessment Project of the American College of Physicians. Ann Intern Med 126:989–996, 1997

Olshansky B: Evaluation of the patient with syncope [UpToDate Patient Information Web site]. 2003. Available at: http://patients.uptodate.com. Accessed January 15, 2003.

Roden DM: Drug-induced prolongation of the QT interval. N Engl J Med 350:1013–1022, 2004

Sarasin FP, Louis-Simonet M, Carballo D, et al: Prevalence of orthostatic hypotension among patients presenting with syncope in the ED. Am J Emerg Med 20:497–501, 2002

Turnbull CL, Bono MJ: Evaluating syncope in the acute setting. Emerg Med 34:14–20, 2002

Weimer LH, Williams O: Syncope and orthostatic intolerance. Med Clin North Am 87:835–865, 2003

# CHAPTER 20

# Seizures

Alexandra E. McBride, M.D.

## Clinical Presentation

A seizure can be defined as a paroxysmal episode of abnormal neuronal activity. A diagnosis of epilepsy indicates recurrent paroxysmal episodes of brain dysfunction manifested by stereotyped alterations in behavior (Engel and Pedley 1998). Seizures are mainly differentiated as either partial or generalized, and these categories indicate the electrographic correlation with seizure onset.

Partial seizures arise from a focal area of the brain, and the continuation or spread from that region determines the characteristics of the seizure. Preserved consciousness distinguishes simple partial seizures from complex partial seizures, in which there is loss of or alteration in consciousness. In a complex partial seizure, the patient may continue some normal behavior yet have impaired response to and memory of ongoing events. A partial seizure may continue and spread throughout the brain, becoming a secondarily generalized tonic-clonic seizure. Once generalization occurs, this seizure may appear similar to a primary generalized tonic-clonic seizure. Careful questioning by the clinician for any motor, sensory, or behavioral symptoms immediately before the generalized tonic-clonic activity can help to distinguish between these two seizure types.

Primary generalized seizures have a nonfocal onset. They may be brief and nonconvulsive or longer in duration and convulsive (see Table 20–1). *Status epilepticus* is defined as continuous seizure activity or recurrent seizures with incomplete interictal recovery lasting 30 minutes or longer (Leppik 2001).

**TABLE 20–1.**    Overview of seizure characteristics

| Seizure type | Duration | Loss or alteration in consciousness | Postictal confusion |
|---|---|---|---|
| Generalized seizures | | | |
| Generalized tonic-clonic | 1–2 minutes | Yes | Yes |
| Absence | <10 seconds | Yes | No |
| Myoclonic | 1 second | No | No |
| Tonic | 10–30 seconds | Yes | No |
| Partial seizures | | | |
| Simple partial | 5–10 seconds | No | No |
| Complex partial | 1–2 minutes | Yes | Yes |
| Secondary generalized tonic-clonic | 1–2 minutes | Yes | Yes |

*Source.*   Modified from Commission on Classification and Terminology of the International League Against Epilepsy 1981; Leppik 2001, p. 13.

## Differential Diagnosis

Paroxysmal alterations in cognitive, motor, or sensory functions may mimic a seizure yet have various nonepileptic etiologies. These events are termed nonepileptic seizures, and they may be physiological or psychological in nature. A comprehensive history of the circumstances surrounding the event must be obtained. The clinician should inquire about prodromal symptoms, clinical features during and after the event, use of medications or drugs of abuse, comorbid illnesses, provoking factors, and history of similar or other paroxysmal events.

### Organic Disorders

Seizure-like phenomena include syncope, cardiac dysfunction, effects of drug use, and metabolic disturbance (Day et al. 1982).

   One of the most common of these phenomena is syncope, which causes sudden transient loss of consciousness and postural tone. Accompanying myoclonic jerks or tonic contraction of the extremities during syncope may be interpreted by witnesses as evidence of a convulsive seizure; however, a full tonic-clonic seizure is less common in syncope. Other features that distinguish seizures include lack of postictal confusion, urinary incontinence (which is rare in syncope), and lack of neurological sequelae after the event (Kaufmann 1997).

Although seizures are sudden in onset, cerebrovascular events such as ischemic stroke and transient ischemic attacks (TIAs) are similarly paroxysmal in nature. The potentially repetitive nature of TIAs and their effect of compromising regional cerebral blood supply and thereby causing motor or sensory deficits, aphasia, or cognitive dysfunction may mimic epileptic events. Loss of consciousness, vertigo, ataxia, and visual disturbance may occur both in vertebrobasilar insufficiency or TIAs and in seizures (Feldmann and Wilterdink 1991). TIAs may last up to 24 hours, but 50% resolve within 30 minutes (Scheinberg 1991). Todd's paralysis can cause transient postictal deficits such as weakness or atonic seizures (Luciano 2002). Unilateral or bilateral tonic or clonic movements, tremor, and decerebrate posturing have been described in brainstem lesions and stroke (Saposnik and Caplan 2001).

Transient global amnesia is a sudden temporary loss of both anterograde and retrograde memory without other neurological signs or symptoms that lasts less than 24 hours. Although the etiology is unclear, proposed mechanisms include cerebrovascular perfusion changes, migraine, and epilepsy (Lewis 1998).

Because of their involuntary nature, recurrence, and paroxysmal features, a number of movement disorders may be mistaken for seizures. These paroxysmal movement disorders may have dystonic, dyskinetic, or choreoathetotic features. Some are kinesigenic, or movement induced, and others are not related to movement (Bhatia 1999). The abnormal movement may affect one extremity or be bilateral with preserved consciousness, which may be interpreted as evidence of a simple partial seizure (Goodenough et al. 1978). Other various abnormal movements such as myoclonus, tics, spasm, and tremor may also mimic seizures, but identification of the associated symptoms and a detailed history can confirm the diagnosis of a movement disorder.

Other than sleep disturbance, sleep disorders may include behavioral phenomena that appear similar to seizures. In narcolepsy, cataplexic attacks or sudden drop attacks, sleep paralysis, and hypnagogic hallucinations may appear as a loss or alteration of consciousness and may be interpreted as evidence of generalized or complex partial seizures (see Table 20–2).

Patients with classic migraine experience an aura followed by headache. The aura has variable presentations, such as visual disturbance, olfactory hallucination, or sensory changes, and may appear to be a simple partial seizure. However, the longer duration of migraine aura (min-

**TABLE 20–2.**    Differential diagnosis of seizures

Cerebrovascular disease
Endocrine dysfunction
Ingestion of toxin
Metabolic disturbance
Migraine
Movement disorder
Psychiatric disorder
Sleep disorder
Syncope
Transient global amnesia

utes rather than seconds, as in an epileptic aura) helps to distinguish migraine aura from a seizure. Basilar artery or posterior circulation migraine may have an aura that includes confusion, ataxia, or vertigo. In addition, headaches may occur before, during, or after a seizure. Electroencephalogram (EEG) abnormalities can be seen during a migraine, and these nonspecific EEG changes distinguish migraine and its accompanying aura from a seizure (Bazil 1994).

Ingestion of potentially toxic substances may cause delirium, psychosis, and confusional states that mimic complex partial seizures. Alcohol ingestion may cause behavioral changes and impaired responsiveness. Alcoholic blackouts appear as an episode of amnesia with preserved consciousness. Drugs of abuse such as lysergic acid diethylamide (LSD), phencyclidine hydrochloride, cocaine, amphetamines, methylenedioxymethamphetamine (Ecstasy), and mescaline, among others, may alter consciousness; however, the longer duration of drug effects helps to distinguish these effects from a seizure. Poisoning with strychnine causes generalized motor activity with rigidity, extension of the extremities, or fasciculations, and these effects may appear as tonic, clonic, or tonic-clonic seizures, but an intact sensorium is a distinguishing feature. Camphor poisoning initially may cause variable symptoms, such as vertigo, change in vision, abdominal pain, and later confusion, that mimic partial seizures; true tonic-clonic seizures may occur in later stages of poisoning (Luciano 2002).

Metabolic and endocrine disorders can cause sudden changes in sensation or behavior, stupor or confusion, and abnormal movements, and these symptoms may be mistaken for seizures. Common metabolic disturbances that may have the appearance of seizures include hypo- or

---

**TABLE 20-3.**   Differential diagnosis of psychiatric disorders with nonepileptic psychogenic episodes

Anxiety disorder
Conversion disorder
Dissociative disorder
Intermittent explosive disorder
Panic disorder
Posttraumatic stress disorder
Psychosis
Somatoform disorder

---

hyperglycemia, hypocalcemia, and hyponatremia. Thyroid dysfunction can cause cognitive changes and movement disorders that mimic seizures and can also cause actual seizures (Kothbauer-Margreiter et al. 1996). Pheochromocytoma and carcinoid syndrome may have autonomic symptoms, such as palpitations, sweating, flushing, epigastric sensation, and anxiety, and these symptoms can be interpreted as simple partial seizures (So and Andermann 1998). Acute intermittent porphyria causes sudden autonomic symptoms and may also lead to focal or generalized seizures (Glaser and Pincus 1987).

## Psychiatric Disorders

Some psychiatric disorders may have paroxysmal features that can be difficult to distinguish from seizures. In addition, nonepileptic events that are psychogenic—often called pseudoseizures—may resemble various seizure types yet have no clinical or electrical features consistent with epileptic events. Table 20–3 lists some psychiatric disorders that may have symptoms similar to seizures.

Anxiety disorders such as panic disorder and posttraumatic stress disorder have prominent autonomic features such as tachycardia, sweating, and hyperventilation that can also be seen in simple partial seizures. Other symptoms, such as confusion, derealization, numbness, blindness, vertigo, visual changes, and occurrence out of sleep, suggest a seizure (Stonnington 1994). However, environmental triggers or phobic stimuli and a longer duration of up to 20 minutes, rather than the few minutes characterized by typical ictal events, help to distinguish anxiety disorder features from epileptic seizures (Luciano 2002).

Intermittent explosive disorder, also known as episodic dyscontrol, manifests as directed or undirected aggressive behavior that may be unprovoked or out of proportion to a provoking stimulus (American Psychiatric Association 2000). The duration can be minutes to hours, and patients may be remorseful after the event. The features of directed aggression, duration, distractibility from the abnormal behavior, and lack of stereotypy of these events differentiate episodic dyscontrol syndrome from epileptic seizures (Luciano 2002).

Dissociative episodes may be mistaken for seizures. In dissociative fugue, which may last hours to months, patients become confused about their personal identity and travel away from their home (American Psychiatric Association 2000). However, patients with dissociative fugue have no change in consciousness, as in a complex partial seizure, and the duration of the dissociative state is much longer than that of a typical seizure. Patients with dissociative identity disorder have independent personalities, some of whom may have fugues that are mistaken for complex partial seizures. Dissociative amnesia is characterized by selective memory loss. Overall, the features that distinguish dissociative disorders from seizures include prolonged duration, lack of altered consciousness, absence of automatisms, abrupt resolution of amnesia, disruption of personal identity without altered sensorium, and resolution of symptoms with suggestion or an amobarbital (Amytal) interview (Stonnington 1994).

Psychotic disorders with symptoms of hallucinations include schizophrenia and psychotic depression. Hallucinations may also be associated with seizures. Ictal hallucinations may occur during a simple partial seizure; they are brief, commonly auditory or visual, and perceived by the patient to be unreal (Gloor et al. 1982). Postictal psychosis may include hallucinations. Postictal psychosis usually occurs 24–48 hours after a cluster of seizures and may also feature paranoid delusions (Szabo et al. 1996).

Pseudoseizures (nonepileptic events of psychogenic origin) may be seen in conversion disorder or factitious disorders. Pseudoseizures have a variety of clinical manifestations and can mimic simple partial, complex partial, and generalized tonic-clonic seizures. Some common clinical features may distinguish these events from epileptic seizures; however, further diagnostic testing is needed for a definitive diagnosis and appropriate treatment. Distinguishing features of pseudoseizures include lack of stereotypy, fluctuating or irregular movements, pelvic thrusting, opisthotonos, facial grimacing, and unresponsiveness for more than 5 minutes with motor arrest (Alper 1994). In addition, urinary incontinence and injury have been seen in up to 20% of patients with nonepileptic events. A history of physical or sexual abuse, substance abuse, or other psychiatric illness is more likely in patients with nonepileptic events (Morrell 1993).

## Drug Effects

In some circumstances, psychotropic medication is associated with seizures in patients with and without epilepsy. In addition, significant potential drug interactions must be considered when antiepileptic medications and psychotropic medications are combined. Further, some cognitive and psychiatric side effects may be seen with antiepileptic medication.

Various theories have been proposed to explain the occurrence of seizures with use of antipsychotic medications, including a proconvulsant effect related to dopamine and histamine receptor blocking activity (Torta and Monaco 2002). Seizures are associated with both the new atypical and the older antipsychotic medications (Koch-Stoecker 2002). Of the antipsychotics, clozapine has been associated with the highest incidence of seizures (3.5%). This effect is dose dependent; a 4.4% incidence of seizures has been associated with higher doses (600–900 mg/day), and a 1.0% incidence with doses <300 mg/day. Of the atypical antipsychotic medications, risperidone was associated with the lowest incidence of seizures (0.3%) in premarketing trials. Olanzapine and quetiapine were associated with equivalent risks of 0.9% for incidence of seizures. A study of seizure incidence associated with phenothiazine use found that 1.2% of the patients had seizures and that greater risk was associated with higher doses. Haloperidol is associated with a lower risk of seizures, compared with phenothiazines. Rapid titration and higher doses increase the probability of seizures associated with antipsychotic medications.

The overall incidence of seizures associated with therapeutic doses of antidepressants ranges from 0.1% to 4% (Harden 2002). In general, selective serotonin reuptake inhibitors (SSRIs) present the lowest risk of seizures, followed by monoamine oxidase inhibitors, and then tricyclic antidepressants (TCAs). Of the SSRIs, fluoxetine may have a higher seizure frequency at 0.2%, compared with paroxetine at 0.1% (Gupta et al. 2002). Clomipramine is associated with a higher risk of seizures, and its use should be avoided in patients with epilepsy. In a comparison of patients receiving imipramine and amitriptyline, the incidence of seizures was 0.1%–0.6% and 0.1%, respectively (Rosenstein 1993). The risk of seizures with buproprion is dose related. At doses of less than 450 mg/day, the risk is 0.35%–0.86%, similar to that with other antidepressant medications, but the risk increases with higher doses (Van Wyck 1983). Similar to antipsychotic medications, antidepressants at higher doses and those given with rapid titration are associated with a higher risk of seizures (Harden 2002). One must be aware, however, that the risk of seizure in the overall community population is 0.8%.

Some antiepileptic medications may affect the metabolism and consequently the drug levels and efficacy of psychotropic medications. Antiepileptic medications that induce cytochrome P450 enzyme activity may increase the metabolism of risperidone and antidepressants such as the TCAs and paroxetine (Spina and Perucca 2002). Carbamazepine may decrease the levels of psychotropic medications, including haloperidol, olanzapine, risperidone, and TCAs. Phenytoin may decrease the levels of clozapine and TCAs. Valproic acid, a cytochrome P450 enzyme inhibitor, may increase the levels of some neuroleptics. Lithium levels may be increased by carbamazepine and phenytoin (Gupta et al. 2002).

## Risk Stratification

Urgent assessment and return to consciousness is necessary for any patient with a seizure. Most partial seizures with secondary generalization and generalized tonic-clonic seizures last between 1 and 2 minutes and not more than 5 minutes (Lowenstein 1999). Afterward, the patient typically has a postictal state lasting for a few minutes. Status epilepticus is defined as continuous seizure activity or recurrent seizures with incomplete recovery of consciousness for 20–30 minutes. This duration has been estimated as the time in which neuronal injury begins to occur. In practice, continuous seizures or recurrent seizures within a 5-minute period should be treated emergently, because their prolonged duration indicates the potential for status epilepticus. Status epilepticus differs from recurrent seizures that take place over a number of hours, during which the patient fully regains consciousness between the events (Lowenstein and Alldredge 1998). In a patient with long-standing epilepsy, a breakthrough seizure is evaluated in relation to the patient's history of epilepsy, use of antiepileptic medications, and provoking factors. Consultation with the patient's neurologist is needed to address these issues. In a patient without a history of epilepsy or prior similar events, emergent medical attention is indicated.

Common accidents related to seizures include head trauma, burns, and falls. Head injury is the most common type of seizure-related accident (Spitz 1998). In addition to assessment of the patient for resolution of a seizure and return to consciousness, examination for injury that may have occurred during the seizure is indicated, and evaluation in an emergency department may be required to complete this examination.

## Assessment and Management in Psychiatric Settings

The approach to the patient with a paroxysmal event begins with a detailed history of the episode and the surrounding circumstances. Seizures with identifiable provoking factors, such as hypoglycemia, imply a direct remediable cause. Recurrent unprovoked events warrant further evaluation to prevent future events. In addition to the patient's experience, accounts from any witnesses to the event will significantly assist in determining if the event appears most consistent with a seizure and, if so, what type of seizure. A rapid review of the patient's medical record will help clarify prior history of seizure disorder, seizure types, diagnostic evaluations, and treatments. Other illnesses should be reviewed for any relationship with the patient's seizures. For example, 3%–10% of patients who experience a stroke also develop epilepsy (Bladin et al. 2000). Medication use, as well as use of over-the-counter medications and drugs of abuse, should be determined. A thorough physical examination should be done and should include assessment to identify any injury sustained from the seizure, evaluation for general medical abnormalities that may indicate a nonepileptic etiology for the event, and a detailed neurological examination (see Table 20–4).

Laboratory evaluations assist in determining the cause of a seizure or paroxysmal event and in determining future treatment. Common blood tests include complete blood count, electrolyte panel, and liver function tests. If epilepsy is diagnosed, these studies provide a baseline prior to initiation of treatment with antiepileptic medications. Lumbar puncture is not routinely performed, but it is indicated if a central nervous system infection or head trauma with possible subarachnoid hemorrhage is suspected.

An EEG is useful in determining if a paroxysmal event was a seizure and in classifying the type of seizure and epilepsy syndrome. As patients return to a normal neurological baseline after a seizure, the EEG findings may similarly be normal between events. A review of EEG findings in patients with definite epilepsy found that 56% had an initial abnormal EEG finding, and subsequent EEGs increased this proportion to 82%, leaving only a minority of epilepsy patients with normal EEG findings (Daly 1997). The gold standard for diagnosing seizures is con-

**TABLE 20–4.**　Approach to the management of a patient with paroxysmal events

**Circumstances of the event**

History of the event

Relevant past medical history of prior events and comorbid illnesses

Current medication use/substance abuse

**Physical examination**

Vital signs during and after the event

Assessment for injury

**Neurological examination**

Evaluation of return to consciousness

Assessment for focal neurological deficits

**Diagnostic testing**

Finger-stick glucose test during the event (if possible) or immediately after

Routine laboratory tests (complete blood count, measurement of serum electrolytes, magnesium, calcium)

Measurement of antiepileptic medication levels, if indicated

Toxicology screen, if indicated

Neuroimaging (computed tomography, magnetic resonance imaging, electroencephalogram)

**Neurology consultation**

For determination of management in a patient with established epilepsy

For detailed examination, analysis of diagnostic testing, and determination of further management

**Transfer to emergency department**

Transfer a patient with recurrent seizures or suspected status epilepticus.

Transfer a patient with injury incurred during the event.

Consider transfer for a patient with new-onset seizure.

tinuous video-EEG monitoring. It can be performed in a hospital or ambulatory setting. For example, nonepileptic psychogenic events would fail to demonstrate an electrographic seizure pattern, and review of the video recording would demonstrate clinical manifestations that are atypical for epileptic seizures. Some patients with a diagnosis of nonepileptic events by video-EEG recording have interictal EEG abnormalities that are most likely related to comorbidities such as stroke (McBride et al. 2002). A computed tomography or magnetic resonance imaging scan of the brain should be performed on all patients with new-onset

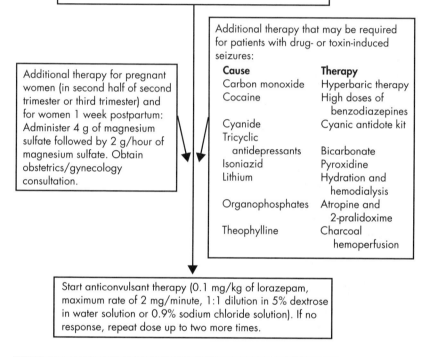

- Assess and control airway. Obtain vital signs and pulse oximetry measurements. Administer oxygen by means of nonrebreather mask calibrated to deliver 100% oxygen.
- Perform finger-stick glucose test, and obtain blood sample for analysis of serum electrolytes, calcium, magnesium, and drug levels.
- Administer thiamine (100 mg), then glucose (50 mL of a 50% dextrose solution).

Additional therapy for pregnant women (in second half of second trimester or third trimester) and for women 1 week postpartum: Administer 4 g of magnesium sulfate followed by 2 g/hour of magnesium sulfate. Obtain obstetrics/gynecology consultation.

Additional therapy that may be required for patients with drug- or toxin-induced seizures:

| Cause | Therapy |
|---|---|
| Carbon monoxide | Hyperbaric therapy |
| Cocaine | High doses of benzodiazepines |
| Cyanide | Cyanic antidote kit |
| Tricyclic antidepressants | Bicarbonate |
| Isoniazid | Pyroxidine |
| Lithium | Hydration and hemodialysis |
| Organophosphates | Atropine and 2-pralidoxime |
| Theophylline | Charcoal hemoperfusion |

Start anticonvulsant therapy (0.1 mg/kg of lorazepam, maximum rate of 2 mg/minute, 1:1 dilution in 5% dextrose in water solution or 0.9% sodium chloride solution). If no response, repeat dose up to two more times.

**FIGURE 20−1.** Algorithm for initial treatment of a patient with a seizure.

seizures, adults with febrile seizures, patients with seizures followed by neurological deficits, patients with seizures after head trauma, and in the immunocompromised and anticoagulated hosts who present with seizures. If the clinical and diagnostic assessment leads to a determination of recurrent epileptic seizures or a single seizure with diagnostic indicators of risk for seizure recurrence, then treatment with antiepileptic medications is indicated.

After obtaining vital signs and checking for airway patency, intravenous access with normal saline shold be established and a finger-stick glucose test must be performed. Thiamine 100 mg and hypertonic glucose solution should be immediately administered if glucose level is less than 80 mg/dL. The specific therapeutic interventions required for pregnant women and patients with drug- or toxin-induced seizures are presented in Figure 20–1. Anticonvulsant therapy is initiated with intravenous lorazepam at a maximum rate of 2 mg/minute.

# References

Alper K: Nonepileptic seizures. Neurol Clin 12:153–173, 1994

American Psychiatric Association: Diagnostic and Statistical Manual of Mental Disorders, 4th Edition, Text Revision. Washington DC, American Psychiatric Association, 2000

Bazil CW: Migraine and epilepsy. Neurol Clin 12:115–127, 1994

Bhatia KP: The paroxysmal dyskinesias. J Neurol 246:149–155, 1999

Bladin CF, Alexandrov AV, Bellavance A, et al: Seizures after stroke, a prospective multicenter study. Arch Neurol 57:1617–1622, 2000

Commission on Classification and Terminology of the International League Against Epilepsy: Proposal for revised clinical and electroencephalographic classification of epileptic seizures. Epilepsia 22:489–501, 1981

Daly DD: Epilepsy and syncope, in Current Practice of Clinical Electroencephalography, 2nd Edition. Edited by Daly DD, Pedley TA. Philadelphia, PA, Lippincott-Raven, 1997, pp 269–334

Day SC, Cook EF, Funkenstein H, et al: Evaluation and outcome of emergency room patients with transient loss of consciousness. Am J Med 73:15–23, 1982

Engel J, Pedley TA: Introduction: what is epilepsy? in Epilepsy: A Comprehensive Textbook, Vol 1. Edited by Engel J, Pedley TA. Philadelphia, PA, Lippincott-Raven, 1998, pp 1–13

Feldmann E, Wilterdink JL: The symptoms of transient cerebral attacks. Semin Neurol 11:135–145, 1991

Glaser GH, Pincus JH: Neurologic complications of internal disease, in Clinical Neurology, Vol 4. Edited by Baker AB, Baker LH. Philadelphia, PA, Harper & Row, 1987, pp 1–57

Gloor P, Olivier A, Quesney LF, et al: The role of the limbic system in experiential phenomena of temporal lobe epilepsy. Ann Neurol 12:129–144, 1982

Goodenough DJ, Fariello RG, Annis BL, et al: Familial and acquired paroxysmal dyskinesias. Arch Neurol 35:827–831, 1978

Gupta AK, Ettinger AB, Weisbrot DM: Psychiatric comorbidity in epilepsy, in Managing Epilepsy and Co-Existing Disorders. Edited by Ettinger AB, Devinsky O. Boston, MA, Butterworth-Heinemann, 2002, pp 343–387

Harden CL: The co-morbidity of depression and epilepsy: epidemiology, etiology, and treatment. Neurology 59 (suppl 4):S48–S55, 2002

Kaufmann H: Syncope, a neurologist's viewpoint. Cardiol Clin 15:177–194, 1997

Koch-Stoecker S: Antipsychotic drugs and epilepsy: indications and treatment guidelines. Epilepsia 43 (suppl 2):19–24, 2002

Kothbauer-Margreiter I, Sturzenegger M, Komor J, et al: Encephalopathy associated with Hashimoto thyroiditis: diagnosis and treatment. J Neurol 243:585–593, 1996

Leppik IE: Contemporary Diagnosis and Management of the Patient With Epilepsy, 5th Edition. Newton, PA, Handbooks in Health Care, 2001

Lewis SL: Aetiology of transient global amnesia. Lancet 352:397–399, 1998

Lowenstein DH: Status epilepticus: an overview of the clinical problem. Epilepsia 40 (suppl 1): S3–S8, 1999

Lowenstein DH, Alldredge BK: Status epilepticus. N Engl J Med 338:970–976, 1998

Luciano DJ: Nonepileptic paroxysmal disorders, in Managing Epilepsy and Co-Existing Disorders. Edited by Ettinger AB, Devinsky O. Boston, MA, Butterworth-Heinemann, 2002, pp 3–35

McBride AE, Shih TT, Hirsch LJ: Video-EEG monitoring in the elderly: a review of 94 patients. Epilepsia 43:165–169, 2002

Morrell MJ: Differential diagnosis of seizures. Neurol Clin 11:737–754, 1993

Rosenstein DL, Nelson CC, Jacobs SC: Seizure associated with antidepressants: a review. J Clin Psychiatry 54:8, 1993

Saposnik G, Caplan LR: Convulsive-like movements in brainstem stroke. Arch Neurol 58:654–657, 2001

Scheinberg P: Transient ischemic attacks: an update. J Neurol Sci 101:133–140, 1991

So NK, Andermann F: Differential diagnosis, in Epilepsy: A Comprehensive Textbook, Vol 1. Edited by Engel J, Pedley TA. Philadelphia, PA, Lippincott-Raven, 1998, pp 791–797

Spina E, Perucca E: Clinical significance of pharmacokinetic interactions between antiepileptic and psychotropic drugs. Epilepsia 43 (suppl 2):37–44, 2002

Spitz MD: Injuries and death as a consequence of seizures in people with epilepsy. Epilepsia 39:904–907, 1998

Stonnington CM: Psychiatric imitators of epilepsy, in Imitators of Epilepsy. Edited by Fisher RS. New York, Demos, 1994, pp 255–281

Szabo CA, Lancman M, Tagno S: Postictal psychosis: a review. Neuropsychiatry Neuropsychol Behav Neurol 9:258–264, 1996

Torta R, Monaco F: Atypical antipsychotics and serotoninergic antidepressants in patients with epilepsy: pharmacodynamic considerations. Epilepsia 43 (suppl 2):8–13, 2002

Van Wyck F, Manberg PJ, Miller LL, et al: Overview of clinically significant adverse reactions to bupropion. J Clin Psychiatry 44:191–196, 1983

# CHAPTER 21

# Extrapyramidal Syndromes Related to Neuroleptics

Brian Koo, M.D.

Mark F. Gordon, M.D.

Marc L. Gordon, M.D.

Extrapyramidal syndromes (EPS) are a group of movement disorders that result from dysfunction of the basal ganglia or closely related structures. Primary EPS are disorders that result from direct dysfunction of the involved structures. Secondary EPS are disorders related to the effect of drugs, infections, inflammation, vascular insults, or metabolic abnormalities. The syndromes most often seen in conjunction with administration of neuroleptics are parkinsonism, acute dystonia, tardive dyskinesia, acute akathisia, postural tremor, and neuroleptic malignant syndrome (NMS).

## Neuroleptic-Induced Parkinsonism

### Clinical Presentation

Parkinsonism is characterized by muscular rigidity, bradykinesia/hypokinesia, rest tremor, and postural instability. Parkinsonism is caused by decreased dopaminergic activity in the basal ganglia. It is most commonly seen in idiopathic Parkinson's disease, in which a degeneration of the nigrostriatal neurons produces a decrease in dopamine production. Any agent with dopamine receptor–blocking or dopamine-depleting properties can induce parkinsonism. Medications are the most commonly implicated parkinsonism-inducing agents, and neuroleptics, especially the typical antipsychotics, are the most frequent cause of drug-induced parkinsonism.

About 15% of patients who chronically take neuroleptic medication develop parkinsonism (Janno et al. 2004). The syndrome typically emerges 1–10 weeks after the initiation of neuroleptic therapy. Women are about twice as likely to develop the syndrome, compared with men. Higher neuroleptic doses and longer periods of neuroleptic usage increase the risk of neuroleptic-induced parkinsonism.

Patients age 40 years and older are more likely than younger patients to develop neuroleptic-induced parkinsonism, possibly suggesting that this disorder is an expression of preclinical Parkinson's disease. According to this theory, the dopamine receptor–blocking effects of neuroleptic medication may exacerbate a preexisting depletion of dopamine stores (latent Parkinson's disease). The mechanism underlying the development of neuroleptic-induced parkinsonism appears to be the blockade of postsynaptic dopamine $D_2$ receptors in the basal ganglia. The likelihood that a particular neuroleptic will induce parkinsonism is related to the agent's affinity for blocking $D_2$ receptors. High-potency neuroleptics likely to cause neuroleptic-induced parkinsonism include haloperidol and fluphenazine. Neuroleptics less likely to cause this disorder include low-potency antipsychotics, such as chlorpromazine and thioridazine, and the atypical antipsychotics, such as clozapine and quetiapine.

Selective serotonin reuptake inhibitors (SSRIs) have also been implicated in the development of secondary parkinsonism. It is postulated that this effect may be due to increased activity of serotonergic neurons in the raphe nucleus, which project to and inhibit striatal dopaminergic neurons.

The clinical syndrome of parkinsonism resulting from neuroleptic use is virtually indistinguishable from idiopathic Parkinson's disease. Symptoms include drooling, hypophonic dysarthria, rigidity (i.e., cogwheeling), akinesia or bradykinesia, tremor, stooped posture, shuffling gait, and imbalance. Tremor is often less prominent in neuroleptic-induced parkinsonism than in Parkinson's disease. The pill-rolling tremor characteristic of Parkinson's disease is rarely seen in neuroleptic-induced parkinsonism. The tremor of neuroleptic-induced parkinsonism is often coarse and similar to essential tremor.

## Differential Diagnosis

When considering the diagnosis of neuroleptic-induced parkinsonism, the clinician must rule out depression; idiopathic Parkinson's disease; other forms of secondary parkinsonism, such as those resulting from a basal ganglia stroke, neoplasm, or infection; the effects of medications such as centrally acting calcium channel blockers, metoclopramide, and reserpine; and the effects of toxins such as manganese and carbon monoxide.

## Assessment and Management in Psychiatric Settings

Withdrawal of the offending drug, if possible, is the treatment of choice. Neuroleptic withdrawal, however, may worsen the underlying condition (such as psychosis in schizophrenia) for which the drug is being prescribed. Mild neuroleptic-induced parkinsonism in patients with good control of psychotic symptoms while taking a stable does of a neuroleptic may require only observation and no intervention. For more significant cases of neuroleptic-induced parkinsonism, the clinician may lower or discontinue the offending agent, add an antiparkinsonian medication (such as an anticholinergic drug or amantadine), or substitute an atypical neuroleptic for the offending agent. In the majority of cases of neuroleptic-induced parkinsonism, the symptoms of parkinsonism cease within weeks of discontinuation of the causative agent, but in rare cases, symptoms may persist for more than a year, and some patients may require treatment with anticholinergics or amantadine. Patients should continue taking these medicines for a few months and then should be reassessed to determine the utility of continued treatment.

# Neuroleptic-Induced Acute Dystonia

## Clinical Presentation

Dystonia refers to a group of movement disorders with repetitive twisting movements or abnormal postures. Dystonia often involves large muscle groups such as those of the neck, trunk, and proximal limbs. Smaller muscle groups may be involved as well, including the muscles that control eye movements, swallowing, facial expression, and fine motor coordination. Dystonic movements may be sustained or intermittent. Furthermore, they may be jerky, rhythmic, or tremulous. Emotional stress and purposeful action often activate or worsen dystonic movements. Neuroleptics are the most frequent cause of drug-induced dystonia.

The reported incidence of neuroleptic-induced acute dystonia ranges from 2.3% to 64%, with the lower limit being a more realistic figure (Tarsy 1983). The dystonic reaction is acute, occurring shortly after the introduction or dose elevation of a neuroleptic medication. Fifty percent of cases occur within 24 hours and 90% within 5 days of the medication introduction or dose change (Ayd 1961). Neuroleptic-induced acute dystonia is 15 times more likely in patients younger than age 35 years than in their older counterparts and twice as likely in men younger than age 50 years than in women in that age group. In patients age 50 years and older, the incidence is similar for men and women (Perry and Lund 1988). There is some suggestion that neuroleptic-induced acute dystonia occurs at a higher rate in patients with mania, compared with patients with schizophrenia (Nasrallah et al. 1988). Other risk factors include alcohol and cocaine usage.

Medication-induced acute dystonic reactions can occasionally be dose related, but the majority of these reactions are idiosyncratic. Neuroleptic-induced acute dystonia appears to result from an alteration of dopaminergic-cholinergic balance in the basal ganglia. High-potency $D_2$ receptor blockers, such as haloperidol, are more likely than low-potency ones to trigger acute dystonic reactions. This preferential block of the $D_2$ receptor leads to an excess of striatal cholinergic output. Agents that balance dopamine blockade with muscarinic $M_1$ receptor blockade are less likely to produce dystonic reactions. Paradoxically, dystonic reactions may be caused by an increase of nigrostriatal dopaminergic activity that occurs as a compensatory response to dopamine receptor blockade.

Although high-potency antipsychotics most often trigger neuroleptic-induced acute dystonia, this reaction has been described with virtually every neuroleptic. Antiemetics and certain antidepressants (such as SSRIs) may also cause acute dystonia.

The clinical features depend on the muscle groups involved, the most common being the cranial, axial, and nuchal muscle groups. *Oculogyric crisis* is characterized by an involuntary tonic deviation of the eyes. The eyes are most often conjugately deviated upward and less often laterally or obliquely. The crisis is accompanied by fear, restlessness, or compulsive thoughts. *Buccolingual crisis* is characterized by twisting movements of the tongue, forced jaw opening or closing, or facial grimacing. This crisis often results in dysarthria and dysphagia. *Torticollis* involves spasm of the neck muscles that causes deviation of the neck laterally (*lateral torticollis*), anteriorly (*anterocollis*), or posteriorly (*retrocollis*). *Opisthotonic crisis* is characterized by spasm of the paravertebral muscles that causes back hyperextension. *Tortipelvic crisis* involves spasm in the muscles of the abdominal wall, pelvis, and hip that causes truncal torsion and inability to stand.

## Differential Diagnosis

Local infection of the oropharyngeal or peritonsillar region may result in trismus, mimicking an acute dystonic reaction. Conditions that cause ophthalmoplegia, such as stroke, need to be differentiated from oculogyric crisis. Some infections and effects of toxins can mimic neuroleptic-induced acute dystonia. Such toxins include tetanus, rabies, lysergic acid, strychnine, and the venom of the black widow spider (Kipps et al. 2005). Disorders of metabolism, such as hypocalcemia and hypomagnesemia, can cause diffuse muscle cramping and spasm. In addition, because acute dystonia may be seen in NMS, the latter disorder should be considered in the differential diagnosis.

## Assessment and Management in Psychiatric Settings

Acute treatment of neuroleptic-induced dystonia involves stabilization and monitoring of vital signs. Rarely, airway protection is required. The natural history of neuroleptic-induced acute dystonia without discontinuation of the offending neuroleptic is characterized by a self-limiting course over a 1-week period. However, because the reaction is almost always distressing and uncomfortable for the patient, drug therapy should be initiated promptly. Anticholinergic medications, such as diphenhydramine or benztropine, are the medications of choice. The preferred route is intravenous administration, which allows the medication to take effect in less than 5 minutes. The intramuscular route may be used if intravenous administration is not possible. Therapy given intramuscularly takes up to 10 times longer to have an effect than similar medicines given intravenously. Oral anticholinergics should not be given in the acute setting because of the delayed onset of action and the danger of aspiration. Benzodiazepines are also effective in the treatment of neuroleptic-induced acute dystonia.

With severe or frequent recurrence of dystonia, discontinuation of the neuroleptic and institution of another psychotropic agent may be needed. Patients younger than age 35 years, the group with the highest risk for development of neuroleptic-induced acute dystonia, benefit from prophylaxis with oral benztropine or diphenhydramine when they begin taking a high-potency neuroleptic. The duration of the prophylactic treatment is about 1 week.

# Neuroleptic-Induced Acute Akathisia

## Clinical Presentation

Akathisia is a movement disorder characterized by a subjective feeling of inner restlessness and various motor manifestations associated with this feeling. Akathisia may cause dysphoria or agitation. Motor manifestations range from mild finger or toe tapping to pacing or even running. It is considered a separate entity in the classification of movement disorders. One of the most common movement disorders caused by neuroleptics, akathisia occurs in 20%–75% of patients taking neuroleptic medication (Chung 1996). Like neuroleptic-induced acute dystonia, acute akathisia occurs in hours to days of neuroleptic initiation. High-potency neuroleptics are most often associated with the induction of acute akathisia. Other medications that can cause acute akathisia include antiemetics and antidepressants, especially the SSRIs.

The risk of developing akathisia is higher with the use of high-potency drugs, high doses of neuroleptics, rapid dose escalation, and the presence of other extrapyramidal side effects. The pathogenesis of akathisia is poorly understood. Its common association with neuroleptic medication suggests a dopamine receptor–blocking mechanism in the mesocortex. There appears to be overactivity in both the noradrenergic and serotonergic systems. Neuroleptics with potent serotonin (5-HT) receptor antagonism are less likely to cause akathisia. Furthermore, some $5\text{-HT}_2$ antagonists, such as cyproheptadine, and β-blockers, such as propranolol, help treat neuroleptic-induced acute akathisia.

Akathisia has subjective and objective clinical components. The patient experiences an overwhelming restlessness and inability to remain still. This sensation results in the objective motor manifestations of the syndrome. The sitting patient may constantly shift positions, cross and uncross the legs, or perform rocking motions. The standing patient may pace frantically about or repetitively shift from one foot to the other. In its milder form, akathisia may cause the patient to appear anxious, leading to an erroneous diagnosis of generalized anxiety. Severe akathisia is associated with severe dysphoria, anxiety, and irritability and rarely may lead to akathisia-induced violence and suicide.

Akathisia may be classified as acute, tardive, chronic, or withdrawal akathisia or pseudoakathisia. Acute akathisia has an onset within hours or days of initiating a neuroleptic. Tardive akathisia has a delayed onset of approximately 3 months. In chronic akathisia, symptoms usually persist for at least 3 months irrespective of the type of onset. Withdrawal akathisia begins within 6 weeks of medication discontinuation or dose decrement. In pseudoakathisia, objective movements resembling akathisia are present in the absence of subjective awareness or distress.

## Differential Diagnosis

Acute akathisia should be differentiated from restless leg syndrome and catatonic agitation, both of which occur in the absence of medication administration. Restless leg syndrome shares both the subjective and objective qualities of akathisia but has a distinct day-night variation in the intensity of the symptoms, with worsening in the evening and nighttime. The agitation of catatonia often includes purposeless movement and is unrelated to external stimuli.

## Assessment and Management in Psychiatric Settings

Anticholinergics are most effective when neuroleptic-induced acute akathisia is accompanied by parkinsonism. β-Blockers may be more effective. Propranolol is the drug of choice, at a starting dose of 10 mg three times a day. It may be increased to a total of 120 mg/day. The onset of action is rapid and often occurs in 4–40 hours. Benzodiazepines may be used on a short-term basis. Benzodiazepine effects include sedation and hypotension.

To treat acute akathisia, the dosage of the neuroleptic should be lowered before adding another medication. If symptoms persist, the neuroleptic may be discontinued and replaced with a lower-potency neuroleptic, unless the replacement is contraindicated.

# Neuroleptic-Induced Tardive Dyskinesia

## Clinical Presentation

Tardive dyskinesia is a movement disorder that manifests 6 months or more after treatment with a neuroleptic medication. The movements are involuntary and often involve the tongue, lips, face, trunk, and limbs. The movements are often stereotyped (patterned and repetitive) and sometimes resemble choreoathetosis.

Of patients treated with a neuroleptic for more than 1 year, 10%–20% develop tardive dyskinesia. In a large prospective study, Kane et al.

(1985) showed that the incidence of tardive dyskinesia was cumulative over several years. In the 850 subjects treated with neuroleptic medication in that study, the incidence of tardive dyskinesia was 5% at 1 year, 10% at 2 years, 15% at 3 years, 19% at 4 years, and 23% at 5 years.

Older age is a risk factor for the development of tardive dyskinesia. Patients older than age 50 years have significantly increased risk, and elderly patients are more likely to develop severe and persistent forms of tardive dyskinesia. Women may be more susceptible to tardive dyskinesia, compared with men (Yassa and Jeste 1992). Schizophrenic patients with predominantly negative symptoms may have increased risk of developing tardive dyskinesia.

Dopamine hypersensitivity is the most widely accepted explanation of tardive dyskinesia. This hypothesis proposes that in response to chronic dopamine receptor blockade induced by neuroleptics, the nigrostriatal dopamine system develops greater sensitivity to dopamine, which leads to production of dyskinesias. This theory may explain why a greater number of drug-free periods or *drug holidays* is a risk factor for tardive dyskinesia. Alternatively, tardive dyskinesia may arise from overactivity of the adrenergic system, which produces large amounts of neurotoxic free radicals, resulting in peroxidation of lipid membranes. The basal ganglia, which have high levels of oxidative metabolism, are exposed to greater concentrations of these free radicals and are preferentially damaged.

Chronic treatment with dopamine antagonists often causes tardive dyskinesia. The atypical antipsychotics are associated with less risk of tardive dyskinesia than the typical antipsychotics. Tardive dyskinesia has also have been reported in patients treated with metoclopramide, antihistamines, fluoxetine, and tricyclic antidepressants (Kane et al. 1985).

Tardive dyskinesia occurs late in the setting of antipsychotic usage. The abnormal movements resemble choreoathetosis. However, unlike true chorea, the movements are stereotypic and repetitive. The most common movements are perioral, including tongue twisting or protrusion, jaw lateral and thrusting movements, facial grimacing, and lip puckering. Hand clenching and finger movements are also common. If the trunk or limbs are affected, the movements include pelvic thrusting or limb chorea. Often the movements are not distressing to the patient, especially if limited to the perioral region. The dyskinesias may be suppressed by voluntary movements of the affected areas but are worsened by movements of other body parts.

## Differential Diagnosis

Consideration should be given to other movement disorders induced by neuroleptics, especially dystonia and akathisia. The stereotyped dyskinesias (as in classic tardive dyskinesia), dystonia, and akathisia at times coexist in a patient and may represent a spectrum of delayed neuroleptic-induced abnormal movements. Edentulous dyskinesia may mimic the classic orobuccolingual dyskinesias of tardive dyskinesia. Other diagnoses to consider include Huntington's disease, Wilson's disease, Sydenham's chorea, hyperthyroidism, hypoparathyroidism, Tourette's disorder, and spasmodic torticollis.

## Assessment and Management in Psychiatric Settings

Once tardive dyskinesia has been detected, the neuroleptic dose should be lowered. If lowering the dosage is ineffective, the neuroleptic may need to be discontinued. Possible worsening of the dyskinesias on reduction or cessation of the neuroleptic is called withdrawal dyskinesias. Benzodiazepines or baclofen may be tried to lessen tardive dyskinesia. To avoid withdrawal dyskinesias in severe tardive dyskinesia, reserpine may be given while the offending medication is discontinued. The antioxidant properties of vitamin E may be helpful in the treatment and prevention of tardive dyskinesia.

# Neuroleptic-Induced Tremor

Tremor is a rhythmic oscillating movement. It is a common adverse effect of many medications, including psychotropics. Tricyclic antidepressants and SSRIs can enhance physiological tremor. Lithium induces an 8–12 Hz fine postural and action tremor affecting the hands. With prolonged lithium usage or toxicity, damage to the cerebellum may occur, exacerbating the tremor. Valproic acid can induce or worsen a postural and action tremor.

Neuroleptic agents are associated with a parkinsonian-type tremor. The tremor may exist in isolation or may be accompanied by other features of parkinsonism, such as rigidity and bradykinesia.

Treatment of neuroleptic-induced tremor consists of using the lowest dose of neuroleptic that is effective in treating the psychiatric illness. Patients can take the medication at bedtime to minimize daytime tremor. Patients should eliminate caffeine intake, because it can increase the tremors. If needed, low-dose β-adrenergic antagonists may be used.

## Neuroleptic Malignant Syndrome

### Clinical Presentation

NMS is the most feared complication of neuroleptic therapy. It has a highly unpredictable course and may occur at any time during treatment. Motor and behavioral symptoms include muscular rigidity, akinesia, agitation, and obtundation. Autonomic symptoms are also prominent and include hyperpyrexia (up to 107°F), sweating, tachycardia, and hypertension. Immediate treatment is imperative because NMS can result in death.

The reported incidence of NMS ranges from 0.5% to 3% among patients chronically taking antipsychotics (Bottoni 2002). NMS is an idiosyncratic reaction and is not directly related to the dose or duration of neuroleptic treatment. NMS is thought to result from an overwhelming dopamine receptor blockade or from depletion of dopamine. It can be considered a state of acute dopamine deficiency. In the corpus striatum of the basal ganglia, decreased activity in the dopaminergic system results in muscle rigidity that then produces a large amount of heat energy and ultimately hyperpyrexia. Fever may also occur from the effects of dopamine receptor blockade on the thermoregulatory centers in the preoptic region of the anterior hypothalamus. Delirium is exacerbated by dopamine receptor blockade in the mesocortical and nigrostriatal systems. Dysautonomia results from decreased dopaminergic activity in the sympathetic nervous system of the spinal cord.

NMS can occur at any time during the use of a dopaminergic agent, but it most often occurs with initiation or dosage increase of the neuroleptic drug. NMS has also been triggered by abrupt cessation of dopaminergic therapy in patients with Parkinson's disease. NMS can occur with any neuroleptic agent, but it is most commonly associated with butyrophenones, phenothiazines, and thioxanthenes. It has been reported to occur during treatment with clozapine, olanzapine, and risperidone. Initiation of neuroleptic therapy at a high dose, rapid titration of the neuroleptic, use of long-acting depot preparations, and concomitant use of lithium increase the risk of developing NMS.

Possible risk factors include preexisting organic brain disease, dehydration, heat exposure, hyponatremia, and exhaustion. Young men seem to be at highest risk for developing NMS. There is a bimodal distribution of NMS, with the vast majority of cases occurring in patients ages 20–40 years and a second peak occurring in patients ages 70 years and older. The vast majority of the younger cohort includes schizophrenic patients being treated for psychosis. The older population includes patients receiving neuroleptics for behavioral reasons and Parkinson's disease patients abruptly withdrawing from levodopa.

Before 1984 the mortality rate in patients with NMS was nearly 40%. In more recent years the mortality rate has decreased to 11.6%, largely because of early detection of NMS (Bottoni 2002).

The classic features of NMS include muscular rigidity, hyperthermia (>100.4°F), autonomic instability, and altered sensorium. The muscular rigidity is often associated with rhabdomyolysis. The core temperature in patients with NMS generally ranges from 101.3°F to 107.6°F, but rarely it can be normal. Autonomic instability is characterized by diaphoresis, tachycardia, tachypnea, labile blood pressure, diaphoresis, cardiac dysrhythmias, and incontinence. The level of consciousness often waxes and wanes. The altered mental status may include confusion, agitation, delirium, stupor, and coma. The creatine kinase level is usually significantly increased and reflects myonecrosis. Myoglobin in the urine and rising creatinine levels suggest renal insufficiency. Leukocytosis and elevated serum transaminase levels may occur. Electrolyte abnormalities and metabolic acidosis are common.

The clinical course of NMS usually begins with rigidity and autonomic changes, followed by fever within several hours of onset. Symptoms of NMS usually evolve over 24–72 hours. If left untreated, symptoms persist for up to 2 weeks. Early detection is imperative.

Complications of NMS include myocardial infarction, rhabdomyolysis, renal failure, aspiration pneumonia, respiratory failure, pulmonary embolism, coagulopathy, and sepsis. Death early in the course of NMS often results from respiratory failure or cardiac disease, whereas death late in the course often results from renal failure.

## Differential Diagnosis

Because the symptoms of NMS are rather nonspecific, NMS is not easily diagnosed. In any patient with altered mental status and fever, both systemic and central nervous system infections (meningoencephalitis) should be ruled out. Cerebrospinal fluid analysis in NMS reveals no abnormality. The serotonin syndrome shares several clinical manifestations with NMS and may be caused by similar medications, namely tricyclic antidepressants and monoamine oxidase inhibitors. Like NMS, serotonin syndrome is characterized by agitation, fever, and autonomic symptoms, including tachycardia and diaphoresis. Unlike NMS, serotonin syndrome often occurs within hours of medication administration. Serotonin syndrome is characterized by anxiety and agitation and very rarely by stupor or coma. Rhabdomyolysis and rigidity are rarely seen in serotonin syndrome. Common muscular abnormalities seen in serotonin syndrome include myoclonus and tremor. Fever is often less pronounced in serotonin syndrome than in NMS.

Malignant hyperthermia shares several features with NMS, including fever, muscular rigidity, rhabdomyolysis, and altered sensorium. It may be distinguished from NMS by its abrupt onset and by its association with inhaled anesthetics or succinylcholine, not neuroleptics.

Distinguishing lethal catatonia syndrome from NMS may be particularly challenging. Lethal catatonia syndrome and NMS occur in similar patient populations. Severe cases of lethal catatonia syndrome may proceed to stuporous exhaustion, autonomic instability, rigidity, and fever. The prodrome of lethal catatonia syndrome distinguishes it from NMS. Lethal catatonia syndrome begins with psychotic excitement, including labile mood, anorexia, insomnia, bizarre repetitive mannerisms, and disorganized thought processes.

Drug withdrawal syndromes, such as from alcohol (acute delirium tremens) and benzodiazepines, may cause fever, altered consciousness, and autonomic instability and may be confused with NMS. Although rigidity may occur in drug withdrawal syndromes, severe parkinsonism is unlikely. An accurate history should clarify this diagnosis. Heatstroke with fever and altered consciousness is usually obvious from the clinical setting. Neuroleptic drugs, however, by altering sweating, may contribute to the risk of heatstroke. Thyroid storm and anticholinergic toxicity should also be considered.

## Assessment and Management in Psychiatric Settings

The diagnosis of NMS should be followed immediately by discontinuation of the neuroleptic agent. Supportive medical care includes hydration and reduction of fever. Patients require close monitoring of vital signs, neurological status, electrolytes, and fluid balance. Hemodialysis may be needed for patients in acute renal failure. If NMS has resulted from an abrupt withdrawal of a dopamine agonist, the agent(s) should be promptly reinstituted. Dantrolene (1.0–3.0 mg/kg iv every 6 hours) can be used to treat muscle rigidity; the medication acts directly on the sarcoplasmic reticulum. Dantrolene also lessens fever, presumably by affecting the component of fever related to peripheral heat production. Bromocriptine mesylate (2.5–10 mg iv every 8 hours) reduces parkinsonism and may shorten the duration of NMS. Bromocriptine can be administered alone or in combination with dantrolene. Other agents used less commonly include amantadine, levodopa, and diphenhydramine. Electroconvulsive therapy may be effective in some cases but should not be used as a primary therapy for NMS.

## References

Ayd F: A survey of drug-induced extrapyramidal reactions. JAMA 175:1054–1060, 1961

Bottoni TN: Neuroleptic malignang syndrome: a brief review. Hosp Physician 3:58–63, 2002

Chung WS, Chiu HP: Drug-induced akathesia revisited. Br J Clin Pract 50:270–278, 1996

Janno S, Holi M, Tuisku K, et al: Prevalence of neuroleptic-induced movement disorders in chronic schizophrenia inpatients. Am J Psychiatry 161:160–163, 2004

Kane JM, Woerner M, Lieberman J: Tardive dyskinesia: prevalence, incidence, and risk factors. Psychopharmacology Suppl 2:72–78, 1985

Kipps CM, Fung VS, Grattan-Smith P, et al: Movement disorder emergencies. Mov Disord 20:323–334, 2005

Nasrallah HA, Churchill CM, Hamdan-Allan GA: Higher frequency of neuroleptic-induced dystonia in mania than in schizophrenia. Am J Psychiatry 145:1455–1456, 1988

Perry P, Lund BC: Early-onset extrapyramidal side effects. Clinical Psychopharmacology Seminar. October 1999.

Tarsy D: Neuroleptic-induced extrapyramidal reactions: classification, description, and diagnosis. Clin Neuropharmacol 6 (suppl 1):S9–S26, 1983

Yassa R, Jeste DV: Gender differences in tardive dyskinesia: a critical review of the literature. Schizophr Bull 18:701–715, 1992

# PART VI

# Gastrointestinal Abnormalities

Section Editor:

Nakechand Pooran, M.D.

# CHAPTER 22

# Dysphagia

Nakechand Pooran, M.D.

S. Devi Rampertab, M.D.

## Clinical Presentation

Dysphagia is the term used to describe the sensation of food being hindered in its passage from the mouth to the stomach. Dysphagia can be broadly divided into oropharyngeal dysphagia and esophageal dysphagia. The first is caused by disorders that affect the neuromuscular mechanics of the pharynx and upper esophageal sphincter, and the latter results from an array of disorders affecting the esophageal body.

*Oropharyngeal dysphagia* is the result of a wide variety of conditions. Neuromuscular causes include cerebrovascular accident, Parkinson's disease, multiple sclerosis, brainstem tumors, amyotrophic lateral sclerosis, and peripheral neuropathies. It has been shown that 50% of residents in long-term care facilities have dysphagia (Lin et al. 2002). Other causes of oropharyngeal dysphagia include mechanical etiologies such as Zenker's diverticulum, cervical osteophyte, thyromegaly, and retropharyngeal abscess, as well as skeletal muscle etiologies such as muscular dystrophies and myasthenia gravis. With oropharyngeal dysphagia, the food bolus cannot be pushed from the hypopharyngeal area through the upper esophageal sphincter into the esophageal body. Clinically, the patient complains of the inability to initiate a swallow and localizes symptoms to the region of the cervical esophagus. A liquid bolus may enter the trachea or the nose, and in severe cases, saliva cannot be swallowed, resulting in drooling. Dysphagia within 1 second of swallowing is highly suggestive of oropharyngeal dysphagia (Bruckstein 1989).

*Esophageal dysphagia* can be subdivided into two basic categories: mechanical obstruction and motility disorders. Mechanical obstruction may be a consequence of a benign stricture (usually secondary to chronic gastroesophageal reflux), esophageal webs and rings (Schatzki's ring), esophageal neoplasm, and vascular anomalies such as an aberrant subclavian artery or an enlarged aorta (Bruckstein 1989). Motility disorders include achalasia, spastic motility disorders, scleroderma, and Chagas' disease. Three questions become crucial in identifying the likely cause of esophageal dysphagia: 1) What type of food causes the symptoms (solid or both liquid and solid)? 2) Is the dysphagia intermittent or progressive? and 3) Does the patient have heartburn?

Patients who report dysphagia with both solids and liquids most likely have an esophageal motility disorder. Intermittent episodes of dysphagia associated with chest pain and sensitivity to hot or cold liquids are characteristic of diffuse esophageal spasm. On the other hand, *achalasia* presents as progressive dysphagia with regurgitation of bland material and weight loss. Likewise, *scleroderma* is a progressive dysphagia; however, its associated symptoms include chronic heartburn and Raynaud's phenomenon. *Mechanical obstruction* is suspected in patients who report dysphagia only with solids. Episodic and nonprogressive dysphagia without weight loss is a key feature of an *esophageal web* or *ring*. Progressive dysphagia in the setting of weight loss raises concern for *carcinoma*, whereas progressive dysphagia associated with heartburn is more likely to be the result of a *peptic stricture*.

*Functional dysphagia* is characterized by difficulty swallowing solids or liquids without evidence of anatomical abnormalities. It is interesting to note that patients with functional dysphagia have high rates of psychiatric comorbidity, particularly anxiety disorders, depressive disorders, somatization disorder, and phobias. Functional dysphagia must be distinguished from *globus*, which describes a feeling of having a lump or tightness in the throat. Globus is seen most commonly in middle-aged women, especially as a transient response to emotional stress. It is unrelated to swallowing and is present between meals.

*Xerostomia*, particularly in the setting of anticholinergic drug use, can also result in dysphagia because of loss of moistening and lubrication.

*Drug-induced dysphagia* is common among psychiatric patients, and there have been multiple reports of sudden death in patients taking phenothiazines and tranquilizers (Farber 1957; Fioritti et al. 1997; Hollister 1957; Hollister and Kosek 1965; Kahrilas and Pandolfino 2002). Risperidone has been reported to induce dysphagia by causing a dystonic reaction with uvular swelling (Stewart 2003) and disruption of the oral and pharyngeal phases of swallowing (Yates 2000). In both cases, the dysphagia was reversed with the cessation of risperidone. Clozapine commonly induces hypersalivation (Davydov and Botts 2000). The cause of this hypersalivation is unknown, although a number of mechanisms are proposed. Patients with excessive salivation may have difficulty with swallowing, especially at night.

## Differential Diagnosis

A classification of dysphagia in psychiatric populations was proposed by Bazemore et al. (1991) and was later validated by Fioritti et al. (1997). *Bradykinetic dysphagia* is associated with a delay in the initiation of the swallow reflex. There is also a delay in the oral phase of swallowing. This type of dysphagia is associated with the use of neuroleptic agents and is similar in pathophysiology to the dysphagia of Parkinson's disease. This type of dysphagia has been associated with the most morbidity and mortality. *Dyskinetic dysphagia* is associated with long-term use of psychotropic agents. Dysphagia occurs secondary to involuntary movements of tongue and oral muscles. *Fast eating dysphagia* is the most common form of dysphagia in the psychiatric population. Patients with this form of dysphagia have normal oral motor activity but take large bites and consume food rapidly. Because of psychosis or mental retardation, they are restless and have poor attention to eating. *Medical dysphagia* is due to a specific medical condition. *Paralytic dysphagia* is the result of a neurological process, such as a cerebrovascular accident, that results in asymmetry or weakness of the tongue, palate, or pharynx.

## Risk Stratification

Acute food impaction is a true medical emergency. Although the majority of food bolus impactions pass spontaneously, 10%–20% require non-operative intervention, and 1% or fewer require surgery (Richter 2002). Patients who present with food bolus impaction commonly have underlying esophageal pathology and a history of dysphagia. They report acute onset of drooling, vomiting, and inability to tolerate their secretions. Patient localization of the level of impaction is unreliable. The physical examination should focus on evaluating for evidence of stridor (indicating airway obstruction) and perforation (evinced by swelling, erythema, crepitus in the cervical or mediastinal regions, tachycardia, or fever). Patients who are in severe distress or unable to swallow oral secretions require immediate transfer to a medical unit.

For patients with complaints of dysphagia who are at risk for aspiration, the order should be given that the patient should receive nothing by mouth, and the patient should be evaluated in a speech and swallow consultation to determine the feasibility of oral feedings.

Patients with chronic gastroesophageal reflux may develop Barrett's esophagus (Kahrilas and Pandolfino 2002) and are at risk of esophageal adenocarcinoma. Dysphagia and a long-standing history of heartburn should be evaluated with upper gastrointestinal endoscopy. In addition, patients presenting with a history of weight loss associated with progressive dysphagia should also be evaluated for potential malignancy.

## Assessment and Management in Psychiatric Settings

A careful history, the first step in the clinical evaluation of swallowing disorders, may determine the cause of dysphagia in more than 80% of patients (Castell and Donner 1987). The history can help distinguish between oropharyngeal and esophageal causes of dysphagia and can also determine whether the cause is a mechanical (structural) disorder or a motor disorder.

The physical examination is not as useful, except to determine neuromuscular dysfunction in patients with oropharyngeal dysphagia. A complete neurological examination is essential. Body weight and general appearance may suggest disease duration and severity. An examination of the head and neck to look for signs of lymphadenopathy or thyroid or oropharyngeal masses may also be useful.

If the history and physical examination suggest that oropharyngeal dysphagia is the cause of the patient's discomfort, the first step is to assess whether the patient is at high risk for choking and aspiration. If so, the patient must be put on a non-oral diet immediately and transferred to a medical unit. A speech and swallow evaluation should be obtained for all patients in whom oropharyngeal dysphagia is suspected. If, however, the etiology is felt to be esophageal in origin, a gastroenterology consultation should be requested. A gastroenterology evaluation is emergent for patients who complain that food has not gone down after eating (food impaction).

If oropharyngeal dysphagia is suspected, a multidisciplinary approach, including input from speech and swallow, radiology, otolaryngology, neurology, and gastroenterology consultations, is beneficial. The best initial test for suspected oropharyngeal dysphagia is the videofluoroscopic or cineradiographic study of swallowing, often referred to as the "modified barium study" (Bazemore 1991). A series of swallows of varying volumes and consistencies are imaged in the lateral position. This study is highly sensitive for the detection of oropharyngeal dysfunction as well as risk for aspiration and can aid in determining the management of patients with this disorder. If a structural lesion is detected, the otolaryngologist performs a nasoendoscopy using a small videoendoscope. If a motor abnormality is found through the modified barium swallow, and there is evidence of aspiration, a nonoral means of feeding, such as use of a percutaneous endoscopic gastrostomy tube, is recommended. On the other hand, if there is evidence of abnormal upper esophageal sphincter function, patients may benefit from esophageal dilation or myotomy. If neuromuscular dysfunction is identified, swallowing therapy with diet modification and adjustment of swallowing posture and swallowing technique may improve the patient's symptoms.

The initial management of suspected esophageal dysphagia may include either a standard barium swallow or upper gastrointestinal endoscopy. Upper gastrointestinal endoscopy is almost always necessary in the evaluation of esophageal dysphagia, because it allows both for diagnosis and possible therapy with potential for endoscopic dilation. A barium swallow, however, may be more sensitive than endoscopy in detecting subtle narrowing of the esophagus from extrinsic compression, peptic strictures, or esophageal rings. It can also be useful in characterizing esophageal motility disorders such as achalasia. If a structural lesion is found, endoscopy with dilation may be required. If a patient with esophageal dysphagia has a nondiagnostic barium study or upper gastrointestinal endoscopy, the patient can be assessed with esophageal manometry, which can be used to detect motility abnormalities in most subjects (Lind 2003).

The management of functional dysphagia is not well delineated. Reassurance is a key component, particularly with emphasis on the nonprogressive and benign nature of this condition. A trial of anti-reflux therapy can be attempted (Lind 2003).

Several measures can be taken to help reduce the potential for complications in the management of dysphagia. Crushing pills and ensuring that a soft or pureed diet is followed in patients with dysphagia may help to prevent complications of acute esophageal impaction. Moreover, if a patient is suspected of having oropharyngeal dysphagia, a strict nothing-by-mouth status is essential in preventing aspiration pneumonia. Alternative non-oral methods of feeding should be considered, and the patient may require an endoscopic percutaneous gastrostomy.

# References

Bazemore PH, Tonkonogy J, Ananth R: Dysphagia in psychiatric patients: clinical and videofluoroscopic study. Dysphagia 6:2–5, 1991

Bruckstein AH: Dysphagia. Am Fam Physician 39:147–156, 1989

Castell DO, Donner MW: Evaluation of dysphagia: a careful history is crucial. Dysphagia 2:65–71, 1987

Davydov L, Botts SR: Clozapine-induced hypersalivation. Ann Pharmacother 34:662–665, 2000

Farber IJ: Drug fatalities. Am J Psychiatry 114:371–372, 1957

Fioritti A, Giaccotto L, Melega V: Choking incidents among psychiatric patients: retrospective analysis of thirty-one cases from the west Bologna psychiatric wards. Can J Psychiatry 42:515–530, 1997

Hollister LE: Unexpected asphyxial death and tranquilizing drugs. Am J Psychiatry 114:366–367, 1957

Hollister LE, Kosek JC: Sudden death during treatment with phenothiazine derivatives. JAMA 192:1035–1038, 1965

Kahrilas PJ, Pandolfino JE: Gastroesophageal reflux disease and its complications, including Barrett's metaplasia, in Sleisenger and Fordtran's Gastrointestinal and Liver Disease, 7th Edition, Vol 1. Edited by Feldman M, Friedman LS, Sleisenger MH. Philadelphia, PA, WB Saunders, 2002, pp 561–598

Lin LC, Wu SC, Chen HS, et al: Prevalence of impaired swallowing in institutionalized older people in Taiwan. J Am Geriatr Soc 50:1118–1123, 2002

Lind CD: Dysphagia: evaluation and treatment. Gastroenterol Clin North Am 32:553–575, 2003

Richter JR: Dysphagia, odynophagia, heartburn and other esophageal symptoms, in Sleisenger and Fordtran's Gastrointestinal and Liver Disease, 7th Edition, Vol 1. Edited by Feldman M, Friedman LS, Sleisenger MH. Philadelphia, PA, WB Saunders 2002, pp 93–101

Stewart JT: Dysphagia associated with risperidone therapy. Dysphagia 18:274–275, 2003

Yates WR: Gastrointestinal disorders, in Kaplan and Sadock's Comprehensive Textbook of Psychiatry, 7th Edition, Vol 2. Edited by Sadock BJ, Sadock VA. Philadelphia, PA, Lippincott Williams & Wilkins, 2000, pp 1175–1786

# CHAPTER 23

# Heartburn

Nakechand Pooran, M.D.

S. Devi Rampertab, M.D.

## Clinical Presentation

Heartburn, the classic symptom of gastroesophageal reflux disease (GERD), is described as a retrosternal burning sensation that typically starts inferiorly in the epigastrium and travels upward to the neck. Patients may also describe the feeling as indigestion, acid regurgitation, sour stomach, or a hot feeling in the chest or may describe pain that is relieved with antacids.

## Differential Diagnosis

Heartburn is the result of the presence of acid in the esophagus. Therefore, GERD is the most common diagnosis. The symptoms of GERD are quite characteristic; therefore, the diagnosis is usually made with much certainty. In the psychiatric population, functional heartburn may be more prevalent than erosive esophageal disease. Erosive esophageal disease typically responds to acid suppression medication, but functional heartburn does not. Other conditions that can produce heartburn and mimic GERD are infectious esophagitis, pill-induced esophagitis, peptic ulcer disease, biliary colic, coronary artery disease, and esophageal motor disorders.

*Infectious esophagitis* is most commonly secondary to infection with *Candida albicans,* cytomegalovirus, or herpes simplex. Patients with infectious esophagitis may have a history of prior esophageal infection or clinical evidence of immunosuppression. Candidal esophagitis can also occur in diabetic patients, alcoholic patients, and patients who are taking inhaled corticosteroids (Baehr and McDonald 1994; Rome II International Working Team 2000).

*Pill-induced esophagitis* is the result of irritation of the mucosa by certain medications, leading to mucosal injury (Kikendall 1999). Antibiotics (especially doxycycline), bisphosphonates, and potassium chloride are commonly implicated. Other medications such as iron sulfate, nonsteroidal anti-inflammatory agents (NSAIDs), and antiretrovirals have also been associated with pill-induced esophagitis. Laker and Cookson (1997) reported on a series of four patients who developed reflux esophagitis after they began taking clozapine. The mechanism is unknown, although changes in gastric motility and anticholinergic effects are implicated.

It can be difficult to differentiate reflux disease from *peptic ulcer disease*. The patient with peptic ulcer disease may provide a history of peptic ulcers or use of ulcerogenic medications such as NSAIDs or may report symptoms confined to the epigastric region. It is not critical to differentiate peptic ulcer disease from reflux disease, because the treatment of the two disorders is similar.

*Biliary colic* can rarely produce symptoms of heartburn. Like peptic ulcer disease, the discomfort of biliary colic is localized to the epigastrium or right upper quadrant. The patient may also complain of nausea and/or vomiting. Symptoms usually have their onset after a meal, especially a meal with a high fat content.

## Risk Stratification

Heartburn can rarely be an atypical presentation for acute coronary syndrome (Goyal 1996; Nebel et al. 1976). Patients with this presentation do not have a history of heartburn, or their current symptoms are different from their usual reflux symptoms. In addition, symptoms associated with acute coronary syndrome, such as dyspnea, diaphoresis, or lightheadedness, may be present. This presentation is most likely to occur in elderly patients, as well as in female and diabetic patients. These patients should have a cardiac evaluation before having a gastrointestinal evaluation.

Heartburn can also be the first symptom in a patient with esophageal cancer. This presentation is most likely to occur in elderly patients with new-onset heartburn. These patients are more likely to have dysphagia and weight loss, and their symptoms do not respond to empirical treatment with acid suppression. Patients whose symptoms warrant rapid endoscopic evaluation are those with a history of dysphagia, weight loss, anemia or gastrointestinal bleeding, and long-standing heartburn (>10 years) (DeVault and Castell 1999).

## Assessment and Management in Psychiatric Settings

The aim of treatment for heartburn is to reduce the exposure of the esophagus to gastric acid. This reduction is accomplished by combining lifestyle modifications and acid suppression therapy (Castell 1999; DeVault and Castell 1999). Lifestyle modifications include elevation of the head of the bed. Having the patient lie on extra pillows does not help. In addition, smaller and more frequent meals and not lying down within 3 hours of eating may help prevent heartburn. Avoidance of certain foods, such as chocolate, coffee, caffeinated beverages, fatty foods, and citrus products, may reduce heartburn (Castell 1999). These foods decrease the resting lower esophageal sphincter pressure, thereby increasing reflux episodes.

Acid suppression is accomplished by using medications that block gastric acid production. The first available medications were histamine receptor type 2 ($H_2$) antagonists (DeVault and Castell 1994). Histamine is a major stimulus for acid production. These medications block the histamine receptors on the acid-producing cells (parietal cells) in the stomach. Cimetidine should be used cautiously in patients with psychiatric disorders, because it can cause delirium in addition to increasing the blood levels of tricyclics, carbamazepine, valproic acid, and selective serotonin reuptake inhibitors (SSRIs). Patients develop tachyphylaxis to $H_2$ antagonists after prolonged usage (Jones et al. 1988). The $H_2$ antagonists have been supplanted by the proton pump inhibitors (PPIs) as the drug of choice for acid suppression. PPIs inhibit the $H^+/K^+$ ATPase pumps on parietal cells (Lind 1997). These pumps are involved in the final step of acid production. Omeprazole, used in treatment of reflux, has been reported to lower serum levels of clozapine (Frick et al. 2003). This reduction is due to induction of the cytochrome P450 isoenzymes by omeprazole. In addition to antisecretory medication, some clinicians would add a prokinetic agent such as metoclopramide to facilitate gastric emptying, with the hope of decreasing gastric content reflux into the esophagus (see Figure 23–1).

Most patients are treated empirically. Patients whose symptoms are well controlled with medications do not require any further investigations. Patients whose symptoms are not controlled with empirical acid suppression therapy are initially evaluated with upper endoscopy and ambulatory pH monitoring. Upper endoscopy evaluates for the pres-

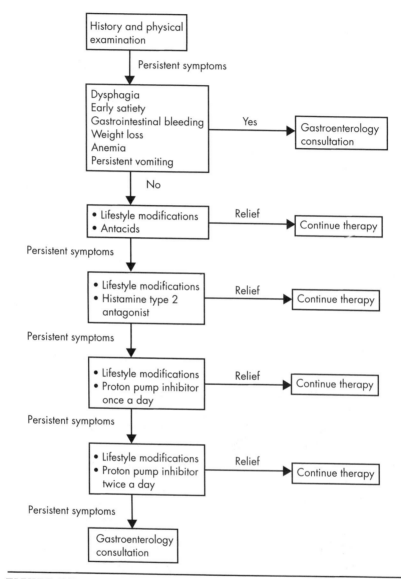

**FIGURE 23–1.**    Algorithm for the assessment and treatment of a patient with heartburn.

ence, extent, and severity of mucosal inflammation. Etiologies of heartburn are investigated by upper endoscopy, and possible complications of reflux such as scarring, stricture, and Barrett's esophagus are assessed. Twenty-four-hour ambulatory pH monitoring is the most definitive test to determine whether a patient has abnormal reflux. If patients are intolerant of endoscopy and pH monitoring, a barium esophagram can be substituted to ascertain some information.

Psychiatric patients have a high prevalence of heartburn. Avidan et al. (2001) found that patients with psychiatric disorders were 2.7 times more likely to have heartburn than patients who were not psychiatrically ill. The higher prevalence has been attributed to a few mechanisms. Psychiatric disease may directly affect the enteric nervous system and, as a consequence, alter esophageal motility. This alteration may result in prolonged esophageal acid exposure. Psychotropic medications with anticholinergic effects such as tricylic antidepressants and neuroleptics may precipitate heartburn by changing esophageal motor function (Mohammed et al. 2005). These medications also delay acid clearance from the esophagus by decreasing salivary secretion of bicarbonate. Lastly, patients with psychiatric disorders have a high rate of consumption of alcohol and tobacco (Andersen and Jensen 1991; Kahrilas and Gupta 1990). Both of these substances can decrease the resting pressure of the lower esophageal sphincter and, therefore, increase the likelihood of having reflux disease.

## References

Andersen LI, Jensen G: Risk factors for benign oesophageal disease in a random population sample. J Intern Ed 230:5–10, 1991

Avidan B, Sonnenberg A, Giblovich H, et al: Reflux symptoms are associated with psychiatric disease. Aliment Pharmacol Ther 15:1907–1912, 2001

Baehr PH, McDonald GB: Esophageal infections: risk factors, presentation, diagnosis, and treatment. Gastroenterology 106:509–532, 1994

Castell DO: A practical approach to heartburn. Hosp Pract 34:89–94,97–98, 1999

DeVault KR, Castell DO: Current diagnosis and treatment of gastroesophageal reflux disease. Mayo Clin Proc 69:867–876, 1994

DeVault KR, Castell DO: Updated guidelines for the diagnosis and treatment of gastroesophageal reflux disease. Am J Gastroenterol 94:1434–1442, 1999

Frick A, Kopitz J, Bergemann N: Omeprazole reduces clozapine plasma concentrations: a case report. Pharmacopsychiatry 36:121–123, 2003

Goyal RK: Changing focus on unexplained esophageal chest pain. Ann Intern Med 124:1008–1011, 1996

Jones DB, Howden CW, Burget DW, et al: Alteration of H2 receptor sensitivity in duodenal ulcer patients after maintenance treatment with an H2 receptor antagonist. Gut 29:890–893, 1988

Kahrilas PJ, Gupta RR: Mechanisms of acid reflux associated with cigarette smoking. Gut 31:4–10, 1990

Kikendall JW: Pill esophagitis. J Clin Gastroenterol 28:298–305, 1999

Laker MK, Cookson JC: Reflux oesophagitis and clozapine. Int Clin Psychopharmacol 12:37–39, 1997

Lind T, Havelund T, Carlsson R, et al: Heartburn without oesophagitis: efficacy of omeprazole therapy and features determining theraputic response. Scand J Gastroenterol 32:974–979, 1997

Mohammed I, Nightingale P, Trudgill NJ: Risk factors for gastro-oesphageal reflux disease symptoms: a community study. Aliment Pharmacol Ther 21:821–827, 2005

Nebel OT, Fornes MF, Castell DO: Symptomatic gastroesophageal reflux: incidence and precipitating factors. Am J Dig Dis 21:953–956, 1976

Rome II International Working Team: Functional heartburn, in Rome II: The Functional Gastrointestinal Disorders, 2nd Edition. Edited by Drossman DA, Corazziari E, Talley NJ, et al. McLean, VA, Degnon Associates, 2000, pp 275–278

# CHAPTER 24

# Nausea and Vomiting

## Prasun Jalal, M.D.

## Clinical Presentation

Vomiting must be differentiated from *regurgitation,* which is passive retrograde flow of gastric contents into the mouth without any associated muscle contraction (Hasler 2001). *Rumination* is the repeated regurgitation of gastric contents, which are often rechewed and reswallowed with some volitional control. Although originally described among mentally retarded children and persons with psychiatric illness, rumination can occur in adults and in persons without psychiatric illness. *Dyspepsia* is a chronic or recurrent upper abdominal discomfort or pain that sometimes may be associated with postprandial fullness, bloating, and early satiety. *Indigestion* is a nonspecific term that includes a variety of upper abdominal complaints, such as nausea, vomiting, heartburn, regurgitation, and dyspepsia.

## Differential Diagnosis

### Disorders of Gut and Peritoneum

*Obstruction of hollow viscera* produces vomiting as the main symptom. Gastric outlet obstruction is usually caused by ulcer disease, but it can be associated with bezoars or malignancy and is often intermittent. Small bowel obstruction is usually acute and is associated with abdominal pain. Small bowel and large bowel obstructions result from adhesions, tumors, volvulus, intussusception, or inflammatory disease such as Crohn's disease. Peptic ulcer disease, cholecystitis, pancreatitis, biliary colic, and appendicitis can also cause nausea and vomiting. *Enteric infections* with viruses and bacteria such as *Staphylococcus aureus* and *Bacillus cereus* may present with vomiting as the predominant symptom. *Impaired motor function* of the gastrointestinal tract from gastroparesis, intestinal pseudo-obstruction, and mesenteric ischemia may present with unexplained nausea and vomiting.

## Extra-Abdominal Disorders

*Cardiac diseases* such as congestive heart failure may lead to nausea and vomiting, and nausea and vomiting may be the presenting symptoms of acute myocardial infarction. Many *diseases of central nervous system* present with nausea and vomiting. Increased intracranial pressure caused by tumor, infarction, hemorrhage, abscess, meningitis, and obstruction of cerebrospinal fluid outflow may lead to vomiting with or without concomitant nausea.

*Labyrinthine disorders* present with nausea and vomiting, often accompanied by vertigo. Motion sickness, labyrinthitis, tumors, and Meniere's disease can also present with vomiting.

*Cyclic vomiting syndrome* is a rare disorder that causes episodes of intractable nausea and vomiting, usually in children and predominantly in females (Pfau et al. 1996). It is often associated with migraine headaches, motion sickness, and atopy.

*Endocrine and metabolic causes* of nausea and vomiting include uremia, hepatic failure, hypoxia, sepsis, prolonged starvation, ketoacidosis, Addison's disease, hypo- and hyperthyroidism, hypercalcemia, and acute intermittent porphyria. Pregnancy is the most common endocrinological cause of nausea and vomiting; these symptoms are present in approximately 70% of pregnant women during the first trimester.

## Drugs and Toxins

Drugs are common causes of vomiting, and symptoms are likely to present early in the course of the use of the drug. Drugs that produce vomiting include dopaminergic agonists, nicotine, digoxin, and opiates. Other medications, such as nonsteroidal anti-inflammatory drugs and antibiotics such as erythromycin, can cause nausea. Other drugs that cause nausea and vomiting include antihypertensives, diuretics, antiarrhythmics, oral hypoglycemics, oral contraceptives, gastrointestinal medications such as sulfasalazine, and cancer chemotherapy agents. Anticipatory nausea has been described during chemotherapy.

## Psychiatric Disorders

A variety of psychiatric disorders, including anorexia nervosa, bulimia, depression, and anxiety disorders, may be associated with nausea and vomiting. Psychogenic vomiting occurs most commonly in young women with emotional problems who often have a history of psychiatric illness or social difficulties. Emotional responses to unpleasant thoughts, tastes, or smells may induce vomiting, suggesting a role of the cerebral cortex in these effects.

# Risk Stratification

In the clinical approach, the following questions can be addressed to outline the etiology and determine the management priority.

## Is the Onset Acute?

Acute nausea and vomiting are usually associated with gastrointestinal infections, ingestion of toxins (such as food poisoning), and use of medications, or, more significantly, with mechanical obstruction, perforation, inflammation, and ischemia. It is important to identify these more significant problems, for which the patient would require immediate hospital admission and, in some cases, surgery. In contrast, chronic nausea and vomiting would indicate a medication-related side effect, metabolic disorders, pregnancy, motility problems, or a gradually progressive partial obstruction of the gastrointestinal tract.

## What Are the Characteristics of Vomiting Episodes?

Vomiting soon after eating is usually psychogenic in etiology; delayed vomiting ($\geq 1$ hour after eating) is usually related to mechanical obstruction or a motility disorder. Vomiting in the morning before food is taken occurs in patients with elevated intracranial pressure or metabolic disorders and in pregnant women. Relief of pain after vomiting is seen in peptic ulcer disease and small bowel obstruction but not in pancreatitis or cholecystitis. Projectile vomiting (vomiting unaccompanied by nausea or retching) is suggestive of but not specific for elevated intracranial pressure. The presence of old food suggests gastric outlet obstruction, gastroparesis, or small bowel obstruction. The presence of bile excludes gastric outlet obstruction. Feculent material in vomitus indicates distal intestinal or colonic obstruction. Vomiting of undigested food is suggestive of esophageal disorder such as achalasia, esophageal stricture, or Zenker's diverticulum. Blood in vomitus should raise suspicion of an ulcer or malignancy. Hematemesis with repeated vomiting or retching suggests Mallory-Weiss syndrome, which results from a tear of the gastroesophageal junction.

## Are There Any Associated Symptoms?

The presence of fever suggests inflammation. Significant weight loss should raise concern about malignancy. Vertigo or tinnitus indicates labyrinthine disease. A presentation with headache, neck stiffness, or focal neurological deficits suggests a central cause of vomiting. Associated abdominal pain is common in inflammation or obstruction. Early satiety and postprandial fullness with abdominal discomfort are consistent with gastroparesis. In pregnant women, the duration of amenorrhea helps to differentiate between hyperemesis, which generally occurs early in pregnancy, and acute fatty liver of pregnancy, which occurs in the last trimester.

## Is the Nausea Related to the Introduction of a Psychtropic Drug?

Nausea and vomiting are uncommon with standard tricyclic antidepressant drugs, in view of the drugs' anticholinergic effects. With newer antidepressants such as selective serotonin reuptake inhibitors (SSRIs), monoamine oxidase inhibitors, and other drugs such as venlafaxine and nefazodone, nausea and vomiting are the most frequently reported adverse effects and appear to be dose dependent. In a study comparing newer antidepressants, fluoxetine and sertraline were associated with relatively lower rates of nausea and vomiting (26% and 35%, respectively) and venlafaxine was associated with the highest rate (72%) in 1,000 patient-months of treatment (Mackay et al. 1999). Nausea may be minimized by beginning with a lower dosage of the drug and gradually titrating to achieve the desired therapeutic effect.

All antipsychotics are potential antiemetics. Traditional antipsychotics are dopamine $D_2$ receptor antagonists and are associated with significant adverse events, including extrapyramidal syndromes (parkinsonian features, acute dystonic reaction, akathisia, and tardive dyskinesia) and hyperprolactinemic effects (galactorrhea and sexual dysfunction). The second-generation antipsychotics, such as clozapine, risperidone, quetiapine, and olanzapine, are serotonin-dopamine antagonists with greater activity at serotonin 5-HT$_{2A}$ receptors and greater specificity for the mesolimbic than for the striatal dopamine system and thus have fewer extrapyramidal side effects. Olanzapine has been reported to be an effective antiemetic in the treatment of nausea and vomiting that is refractory to other medications, including phenothiazines, metoclopramide, butyrophenones, corticosteroids, and 5-HT$_3$ antagonists, in patients with advanced malignancy (Srivastava et al. 2003) and has been associated with significantly fewer adverse events than clozapine (Tollefson et al. 2001).

## Assessment and Management in Psychiatric Settings

In the presence of nausea and vomiting, the clinician performing the abdominal examination should look for distention, specific areas of tenderness, involuntary guarding, and palpable masses and should determine the character of bowel sounds by auscultation. The general examination may reveal evidence of anemia, jaundice, mucosal pigmentation, lymphadenopathy, and hernia. The patient's fingernails should be inspected to detect evidence of self-induced vomiting. The loss of dental enamel may indicate bulimia. Neurological examination may show cranial nerve deficits, including papilledema, visual field loss, nystagmus, or focal motor abnormalities. The cardiovascular system may show evidence of congestive heart failure. An electrocardiogram must be rapidly obtained for patients with risk factors for coronary artery disease.

Apart from providing information to identify the etiology, the history and physical examination are also important for assessment of the consequences of vomiting. Light-headedness, orthostatic hypotension, tachycardia, and reduced skin turgor point toward significant fluid loss.

Initial laboratory tests include a complete blood count to test for anemia and leukocytosis and a chemistry profile to check for electrolyte imbalance, metabolic alkalosis, azotemia, and liver function abnormalities. In women of childbearing age, a pregnancy test should be obtained. An abdominal radiograph may be indicated. Serum drug levels should be measured if drug toxicity is suspected (see Figure 24–1).

The aim of therapy is to correct the consequences of vomiting, such as fluid, electrolyte, or nutritional deficiencies; identify and treat the underlying disease; and provide empirical treatment if a primary cause cannot be promptly eliminated (Quigley et al. 2001). If the patient can tolerate oral intake, a low-fat, low-residue, and preferably liquid diet in small frequent meals is recommended to minimize the delay in gastric emptying. Carbonated beverages should be eliminated to reduce gastric distention. Hydration is essential, and patients with moderate to severe

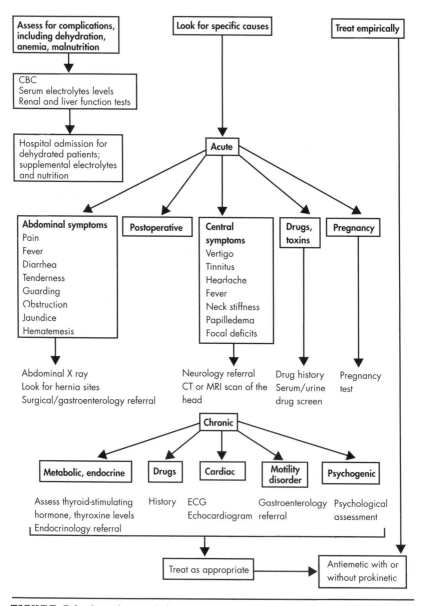

**FIGURE 24–1.**    Approach for management of nausea and vomiting.

*Note.*    CBC=complete blood count; CT=computed tomography;
ECG=electrocardiogram; MRI=magnetic resonance imaging.

dehydration and protracted vomiting should be hospitalized. Intravenous fluid replacement is usually done with a normal saline solution infusion and potassium supplementation.

The two classes of pharmacological agents used in treatment are *antiemetics* and *prokinetics*. *Antiemetics* act on the central nervous system to suppress nausea and vomiting. Antihistaminics, such as meclizine and diphenhydramine, and anticholinergics, such as scopolamine, are used for the treatment of motion sickness and inner ear disorders acting through the labyrinth-activated pathways (Hasler 2001). Phenothiazines and butyrophenones act through a central antidopaminergic mechanism in the area postrema and are used to treat nausea and vomiting induced by drugs and toxic and metabolic etiologies, including postoperative and postchemotherapy nausea and vomiting. Prochlorperazine, promethazine, and droperidol are widely used antiemetic drugs from these two groups. Serotonin 5-HT$_3$ antagonists, such as ondansetron and granisetron, are particularly useful in treatment of postchemotherapy nausea and vomiting and other causes of refractory emesis. *Prokinetics* are used in motility disorders, including gastroparesis and functional dyspepsia. Cholinergic agonists acting on muscarinic M$_2$ receptors are modestly effective and associated with significant side effects. Cisapride, a 5-HT$_4$ agonist, is a very effective promotility agent; however, concern has been raised regarding its rare proarrhythmic effect, and it should never be used in conjunction with psychotropic drugs that prolong the Q–Tc interval (Hill et al. 1998). Metoclopramide, a combined 5-HT$_4$ agonist and D$_2$ antagonist, acts predominantly on peripheral receptors in the gastrointestinal tract, but its use is limited in view of central adverse effects in 10%–20% of treated patients (Tonini et al. 2004).

Additional tests should be performed as indicated by the consulting gastroenterologist and may include endoscopic and radiological studies to evaluate the gastrointestinal tract. Ultrasound or an abdominal computed tomography (CT) scan with oral and intravenous contrast can be used to diagnose intra-abdominal inflammatory and neoplastic processes. If the search for anatomical abnormalities has negative findings, gastrointestinal motility testing, such as gastric emptying studies and electrogastrography, may detect a functional gastrointestinal disorder. Imaging of the head with CT or magnetic resonance imaging is used to identify a central cause of vomiting.

# References

Hasler WL: Nausea, vomiting, and indigestion, in Harrison's Principles of Internal Medicine, 15th Edition, Vol 1. Edited by Braunwald E, Fauci AS, Kasper DL, et al. New York, McGraw-Hill, 2001, pp 236–238

Hill SL, Evangelista JK, Pizzi AM, et al: Proarrhythmia associated with cisapride in children. Pediatrics 101:1053–1056, 1998

Mackay FR, Dunn NR, Martin RM, et al: Newer antidepressants: a comparison of tolerability in general practice. Br J Gen Pract 49:892–896, 1999

Pfau BT, Li BU, Murray RD, et al: Differentiating cyclic from chronic vomiting patterns in children: quantitative criteria and diagnostic implication. Pediatrics 97:364–368, 1996

Quigley EM, Hasler WL, Parkman HP: AGA technical review on nausea and vomiting. Gastroenterology 120:263–286, 2001

Srivastava M, Brito-Dellan N, Davis MP, et al: Olanzapine as an entiemetic in refractory nausea and vomiting in advanced cancer. J Pain Symptom Manage 25:578–582, 2003

Tollefson GD, Birkett MA, Kiesler GM, et al: Double-blind comparison of olanzapine versus clozapine in schizophrenic patients clinically eligible for treatment with clozapine. Biol Psychiatry 49:52–63, 2001

Tonini M, Cipollina C, Poluzzi E, et al: Review article: clinical implications of enteric and central D2 receptor blockade by antidopaminergic gastrointestinal prokinetics. Aliment Pharmacol Ther 19:379–390, 2004

# CHAPTER 25

# Diarrhea

Robert J. Brunner, M.D.

## Clinical Presentation

Most patients consider the consistency of the stool (i.e., increased fluidity) to be the essential characteristic of diarrhea. Because stool consistency is very difficult to measure objectively, stool frequency and stool weight have been used as surrogate markers to define diarrhea. Three or more bowel movements per day are considered to be abnormal, and the upper limit of stool weight is agreed to be 200 g/day in Western countries (Schiller and Sellin 2002). Nevertheless, diarrhea should not be defined solely on the basis of fecal weight. Patients with a high-fiber diet may have increased fecal weight without any complaints of abnormal bowel habitus. Conversely, other patients have normal stool weights but complain of diarrhea because their stools are loose or watery. Chronic diarrhea is generally defined as increased frequency of defecation (three or more times per day or at least 200 g/day of stool) lasting more than 14 days (Fine and Schiller 1999).

## Differential Diagnosis

Most cases of diarrhea have an organic cause that can be classified by several schemes, including by time course (acute or chronic), by volume (large or small), by epidemiology, and by stool characteristics (watery, fatty, or inflammatory).

Acute diarrhea (<2 weeks), which often has an infectious cause, is usually self-limited or easily treated. Although there are rare infectious agents that can cause prolonged diarrhea in the immunocompetent host (such as *Giardia lamblia* and *Yersinia*), chronic diarrhea usually has a noninfectious etiology. Most cases of acute diarrhea are a result of viral pathogens. The most common viruses implicated are adenovirus, rotavirus, and Norwalk virus. Common bacterial infections include various strains of *Escherichia coli, Campylobacter, Salmonella,* and *Shigella.* One clinical approach in narrowing the differential diagnosis is to relate the diarrhea to its setting. In a recent traveler, one should consider acute bacterial or protozoal infections, such as amebiasis or giardiasis. Epidemics are for the most part viral, although a small percentage are the result of ingestion of a preformed bacterial food toxin.

If the source of the diarrhea is proximal to the left colon but leaves the rectosigmoid reservoir intact, bowel movements are few but have a large volume (Schiller and Sellin 2002). Frequent, small painful stools point to a distal source of pathology, whereas painless, large-volume stools suggest a right colon or small bowel source. Many processes, such as *Clostridium difficile* infection, can involve both the small and the large bowel or both the left and right colon. Diarrhea that is accompanied by clinical signs or symptoms of dehydration often involves the small bowel.

Determining if the diarrhea is produced by osmotic or secretory mechanisms helps to determine the cause; the small number of osmotic causes can be distinguished from the much larger number of secretory causes (Powell 2003). This assessment is based on calculation of the stool electrolyte composition. In secretory diarrhea, sodium, potassium, and the accompanying anions account entirely for the stool osmolality, whereas in osmotic diarrhea, unabsorbable solutes within the lumen of the gut account for much of the osmotic activity of the bowel. Examples of unabsorbed solutes include laxatives, sorbitol, and magnesium salts.

In hospitalized patients, the clinician must strongly consider drug side effect as a possible cause. Almost *any drug* can induce diarrhea, regardless of whether the agent was recently introduced (Chassany et al. 2000). New drugs may also interact with previously well-tolerated drugs to produce clinically significant diarrhea. Liquid preparations containing sorbitol may cause osmotic diarrhea. *C. difficile* colitis must be considered in patients who have taken even a single dose of antibiotics within the previous 6 weeks (Bartlett 2002). In HIV/AIDS patients, diarrhea may result from opportunistic infections such as *Cryptosporidium* or cytomegalovirus, as well as from the side effects of the antiretroviral drug regimen. Lastly, in the diabetic population, the clinician might consider the diagnosis of change in intestinal motility, which may be related to the patient's glycemic drug regimen or to diseases associated with diabetes, such as celiac disease, pancreatic exocrine insufficiency, or small bowel bacterial overgrowth.

In cases of chronic diarrhea, the differential diagnosis can be enormous. One way to help limit this wide range is to characterize the stools as fatty, watery, or inflammatory on the basis of a simple stool test (e.g., Sudan stain for fat, test for presence of fecal leukocytes). Each of these stool characteristics is associated with a particular spectrum of diseases (see Table 25–1).

**TABLE 25–1.** Likely causes of diarrhea, by patients' epidemiological characteristics

**Travelers**
Bacterial infection (mostly acute)
Protozoal infections (e.g., amebiasis, giardiasis)
Tropical sprue

**Patients affected by epidemics/outbreaks**
Bacterial infection
Viral infection (e.g., rotavirus)
Protozoal infections (e.g., cryptosporidiosis)
Epidemic idiopathic secretory diarrhea (Brainerd diarrhea)

**Diabetic patients**
Altered motility (increased or decreased)
Drugs (especially acarbose, metformin)
Associated diseases
  Celiac disease
  Pancreatic exocrine insufficiency
  Small bowel bacterial overgrowth

**AIDS patients**
Opportunistic infections (e.g., cryptosporidiosis, cytomegalovirus, herpes, *Mycobacterium avium* complex)
Drug side effect
Lymphoma

**Institutionalized and hospitalized patients**
Drug side effects
*Clostridium difficile* toxin-mediated colitis
Tube feeding
Ischemia
Fecal impaction with overflow diarrhea

*Source.* Modified from Thielman and Guerrant 2004.

Psychiatric disorders resulting in diarrhea are rare. For the most part, besides reviewing the patient's drug regimen, which may include cholinergic or anticholinergic agents, the clinician should consider the possibility of surreptitious use of laxatives or other agents such as thyroid-stimulating medication. There has also been an association between irritable bowel syndrome (IBS) and several psychiatric disorders, including depression and anxiety disorders (Schiller and Sellin 2002). The diagnosis of IBS should be considered for a patient with chronic diarrhea only after all organic causes have been ruled out.

## Risk Stratification

A careful medical history should be the first step in evaluating a patient with diarrhea and in determining risk stratification. Patients often have a good idea of stool frequency but are less aware of stool weight. Patients with diarrhea who also have dry mouth, increased thirst, decreased urine output, or weakness are dehydrated because of the increased level of stool output. Dehydration is a marker for increased severity of diarrhea.

Stool characteristics, such as the presence of blood, mucus, oil, or food droplets, are a very important part of the initial history. The presence of blood suggests the possibility of malignancy or inflammatory bowel disease, although blood is often a result of acute infectious diarrhea with mucosal ulcerations. The presence of oil or food particles suggests malabsorption, maldigestion, or increased intestinal transport. Urgency and incontinence suggest a problem with rectal compliance or with the muscles regulating defection. Nocturnal diarrhea is strongly suggestive of an organic cause rather than a functional problem such as IBS (Schiller and Sellin 2002). Coexisting symptoms, such as flatulence, pain, bloating, and fever, should be noted.

Iatrogenic causes of diarrhea are very common, and the history can often elicit clues. Drugs, previous surgery, and radiation therapy are common causes and should be noted in the history. Use of over-the-counter agents should also be documented. A dietary history is also very important and may reveal the ingestion of poorly absorbable carbohydrates such as fructose, sorbitol, or mannitol. These substances are found in a variety of fruit juices and sodas, as well as in "sugar-free" candies.

A common cause of diarrhea in psychiatric patients who are taking anticholinergic medication is "overflow" diarrhea from fecal impaction. Patients who are not ambulatory are at particularly high risk of fecal impaction and overflow diarrhea. Patients who are ambulatory should be encouraged to walk as often as possible, and constipation should be treated early.

The history is essential in differentiating patients with IBS from those with other functional or organic conditions that cause diarrhea. Factors that suggest IBS are a long history that may extend back to adolescence, passage of mucus, or exacerbation of symptoms by stress. Factors that argue against a diagnosis of IBS include a recent onset of symptoms, diarrhea that awakens the patient from sleep, weight loss, the presence of blood in the stool, and stool weights greater than 400–500 g/day (Schiller and Sellin 2002).

Physical findings are useful in determining the severity of the diarrhea rather than its cause. Intravascular volume status should be assessed by measurement of vital signs, including orthostatic blood pressure measurements. A careful examination of the abdomen, including auscultation for the presence and quality of bowel signs and checking for abdominal distention and tenderness or rebound, should be performed. A rectal examination must be done, and the presence of mucus and stool consistency should be noted. A stool guaiac smear test should also be performed. Sphincter tone should be assessed.

Rarely, the physical examination may provide direct evidence of the cause of the diarrhea. The characteristic skin changes of dermatitis herpetiformis may be seen in patients with gluten intolerance. Flushing may indicate the rare finding of carcinoid (Schiller and Sellin 2002). In a patient with tremor, hyperthyroidism may be considered. New-onset arthritis may be seen in inflammatory bowel disease as well as in Whipple's disease and severe enteric infections. Lymphadenopathy suggests HIV or lymphoma (see Figure 25–1).

## Assessment and Management in Psychiatric Settings

Most cases of acute diarrhea are caused by infectious diseases that have a self-limited course of a few days to a few weeks, and these patients do not require any intervention unless there are signs or symptoms of dehydration or systemic involvement. If these signs or symptoms are present, a more detailed evaluation must be performed. If the patient appears extremely ill or appears to be having toxic reaction, he or she should be immediately transferred to an emergency department for evaluation and therapy.

For the nontoxic patient with acute diarrhea, the initial assessment is followed by therapy to accomplish fluid and electrolyte repletion. Oral rehydration solutions may be used in patients who are not vomiting.

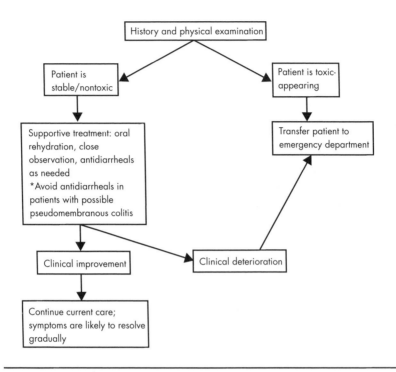

**FIGURE 25–1.**    Algorithm for assessment and treatment for a patient with diarrhea.

Fluid intake should be adjusted to maintain a normal resting heart rate as well as to ensure that the patient produces at least 750 mL/day of urine. In the patient who is vomiting, intravenous fluid is required. In a patient with normal renal function, a saline-based fluid, combined with dextrose if the patient does not have diabetes, may be used if intravenous therapy is available.

Because infection is a frequent cause of acute diarrhea, physicians often consider treating the patient empirically with antibiotics. Such therapy should be reserved for very ill patients and is best administered on a medical unit. Nonspecific antidiarrheal agents such as loperamide and codeine can reduce symptoms and may benefit patients with acute diarrhea. Antimotility agents should not be prescribed in patients with infectious diarrhea, including *C. difficile* colitis, because of the risk of toxic megacolon and bowel perforation. Patients with bloody diarrhea should be transferred to the nearest emergency department.

# References

Bartlett G: Antibiotic-associated diarrhea. N Engl J Med 346: 334–339, 2002

Chassany O, Michaux A, Bergmann JF: Drug-induced diarrhea. Drug Saf 22:53–72, 2000

Fine KD, Schiller LR: AGA technical review on the evaluation and management of chronic diarrhea. Gastroenterology 116:1464–1486, 1999

Powell DW: Approach to the patient with diarrhea, in Textbook of Gastroenterology, 5th Edition. Edited by Yamada T. Philadelphia, PA, Lippincott, 2003, pp 732–738

Schiller L R, Sellin JH: Diarrhea, in Sleisenger and Fordtran's Gastrointestinal and Liver Disease, 7th Edition, Vol 1. Edited by Feldman M, Friedman LS, Sleisenger MH. Philadelphia, PA, WB Saunders, 2002, pp 131–151

Thielman NM, Guerrant RL: Acute infectious diarrhea. N Engl J Med 350:38–47, 2004

# CHAPTER 26

# Constipation

## Kostas Sideridis, D.O.

## Clinical Presentation

Constipation means many things to patients, including hard stool, infrequent passage of stool, straining, or incomplete evacuation. A careful history is needed to clearly define what patients mean when they complain of constipation. An international working group defined constipation according to the Rome II criteria to includes the presence of two or more of the following five symptoms for 12 weeks within the last year: straining during 25% of bowel movements, lumpy and hard stools during 25% of bowel movements, incomplete evacuation during 25% of bowel movements, sensation of anorectal blockage during 25% of bowel movements, and manual maneuvers performed to facilitate passage of stool during 25% of bowel movements (Thompson and Longstreth 2000).

## Differential Diagnosis

The differential diagnosis for constipation is vast. One way to remember the causes is by classifying them into three broad categories: normal-transit constipation, slow-transit constipation, and disorders of defecation and anorectal evacuation. These categories may overlap, and the cause of constipation may be multifactorial. Normal-transit constipation or functional constipation is the most common, occurring about 60% of the time (Pare et al. 2001). Patients who complain of this disorder have normal transit time and stool frequency but consider themselves to have constipation. These patients have low-fiber diets and poor oral intake of fluids, especially water (Pare et al. 2001). The symptoms commonly respond to an increase in dietary fiber and osmotic laxatives. If no improvement occurs with this treatment, another cause, such as a disorder of defecation or slow-transit constipation, is sought.

Disorders of defecation and anorectal evacuation, the second most common type of causes of constipation, commonly occur in female patients secondary to trauma caused by childbearing, previous pelvic surgeries, and weakness of pelvic musculature. Anatomical abnormalities such as rectocele, anal fissures, rectal abscesses, thrombosed hemorrhoids, rectal or vaginal prolapse, and solitary rectal ulcers may be present. Patients with rectocele tend to complain of a lump in the rectum and an inability to complete evacuation. Anismus, caused by pelvic floor dysfunction with abnormal perineal descent, also causes constipation. Patients with anorectal disorders are commonly found to have eating disorders and/or a history of physical and sexual abuse (Camilleri et al. 1994). Evacuation disorders occur after passage of hard stool with resultant anal fissures or thrombosed hemorrhoids. Secondary to the pain, patients avoid defecation, which makes the constipation much worse. Neuromuscular diseases implicated in causing constipation include spinal cord lesions, multiple sclerosis, Parkinson's disease, and cerebrovascular disease. Immobility and medications such as dopamine agonists and muscle relaxants are used in the treatment of these neurological disorders and may further worsen constipation. Hirschsprung's disease, caused by a loss of ganglion cells in the distal bowel, results in atonic bowel and subsequent constipation. Patients with this disorder usually present with childhood constipation. Metabolic disorders, such as uremia, hypokalemia, hypercalcemia, porphyria, diabetes mellitus, hypothyroidism, and hyperparathyroidism, can slow the bowel transit.

Medications, including those commonly used for hospitalized psychiatric patients, are a common cause of slow-transit constipation. Clozapine and olanzapine are notorious for their anticholinergic properties, which worsen constipation (Chengappa et al. 2000). Clozapine-induced constipation has even resulted in death (Levin et al. 2002). Pain medications such as opioids and nonsteroidal anti-inflammatory medications commonly cause constipation. Other causes of constipation include phenothiazines, tricyclic antidepressants, anticonvulsants, serotonin receptor antagonists, and antiparkinsonian medications (Garvey et al. 1990). Most anticholinergic medications, including antihistamines and antispasmodics, have also been implicated. Calcium channel blockers, especially verapamil, frequently cause constipation. Nutritional supplements such as iron and calcium, aluminum, most antacids, and the resin binder cholestyramine commonly cause constipation.

Personality clearly affects stool size and consistency (Camilleri et al. 1994). Persons who are energetic and possess an outgoing personality have larger stool weights and less constipation than withdrawn, depressed patients (Lembo and Camilleri 2003). Patients with severe delayed colonic transit tend to be older women with depressed mood and poor anger control (Camilleri et al. 1994). In a study by Eammanuel et al. (2001), women with constipation scored higher on measures of somatization and anxiety, compared with healthy control subjects. These psychological scores correlated inversely with the rectal blood flow to the distal gut. Constipation may be the sole presenting symptom of depression in primary care and a prominent feature of schizophrenia and bipolar disorder. Patients with eating disorders commonly have pelvic floor dysfunction and slow transit time. Suspicion for anorexia nervosa should be high when a young, underweight woman presents with constipation. These patients may be found to be abusing laxatives as part of their psychiatric disorder and as a treatment for their constipation.

## Risk Stratification

Acute onset of constipation is worrisome because it may indicate bowel pathology, such acute bowel obstruction. The cause of the obstruction may be a malignancy of the colon or adjacent organs with metastasis. Rarely, a volvulus may be present. In elderly debilitated patients, acute onset of constipation may be a sign of colonic pseudo-obstruction (Ogilvie's syndrome) (Camilleri et al. 1994). An immediate abdominal X ray will help in distinguishing acute colonic obstruction. If acute obstruction is present, immediate transfer to an emergency department and surgical consultation are necessary. Patients age 40 years and older with weight loss, gross or occult blood in the stool, loss of appetite, change in stool caliber and pattern, or new-onset constipation should have a colonoscopic evaluation as soon as possible to rule out a colorectal malignancy.

## Assessment and Management in Psychiatric Settings

The patient with constipation should be assessed with a thorough history and complete physical examination (see Figure 26–1). The duration (acute vs. chronic), severity, onset, frequency, and consistency (hard, formed, soft) of bowel movements; the stool size (small, pellet-like, long column); and the degree of straining should be established. The patient's family history of colorectal carcinoma and the patient's dietary history of fiber and water intake should be determined. The number of meals per day, time when the meals are consumed, and the amount of water drunk each day should be noted. A record of daily physical activity is also important. The history provides the most useful information about the etiology of constipation. It is important to rule out a systemic process or a neurological disorder. A complete medication history, including use of over-the-counter medications and dietary or herbal supplements, must be obtained. Patients may also complain of other gastrointestinal symptoms such as rectal bleeding and abdominal pain. The physical examination should be completed with a specific focus on the abdominal and perineal examination. If hypothyroidism is considered as the cause of constipation, the patient's skin should be examined for myxedema, the neck for goiters, and the heart rate for bradycardia. The abdomen must be examined to assess for bowel sounds and palpable masses, and a careful perineal examination must be performed with a particular focus on the rectal examination. The perineal area should be examined for scars, fissures, fistulas, and external hemorrhoids. The rectum should be viewed both with the patient relaxed and with the patient bearing down to examine the extent of pelvic descent. Decreased descent may indicate the presence of pelvic floor dysfunction, whereas excessive descent may indicate laxity of the perineum as a result of years of excessive straining during defecation. Continued straining may result in injury to the sacral nerves, which can lead to a decrease in rectal sensation and to incontinence. Digital examination of the rectum should be performed to evaluate rectal sphincter tone and consistency of the stool and check for the presence of anal fissures and strictures, fecal impaction, and rectal masses. Loss of sphincter tone may indicate a neurological disorder or spinal cord lesion. Inability to examine the rectum may related to the presence of a stricture or spasm of the anal sphincter.

Initial laboratory assessment should include a complete blood count, stool guaiac smear test, thyroid function tests, and measurement of serum electrolytes, glucose, and calcium levels. If occult blood is found, the patient should be referred to a gastroenterologist for further evaluation. If slow-transit constipation is suspected, a sitz marker study is recommended. The patient should discontinue taking any medications that slow colonic transit and should be placed on a high-fiber diet. The patient swallows the sitz marker (a gelatin capsule that includes 24 radio-opaque agents) and returns 5 days later for an abdominal X ray. Normal colonic transit time is 72 hours. If 20% of the markers are present after 5 days, the patient has slow-transit constipation (Wald et al. 2002).

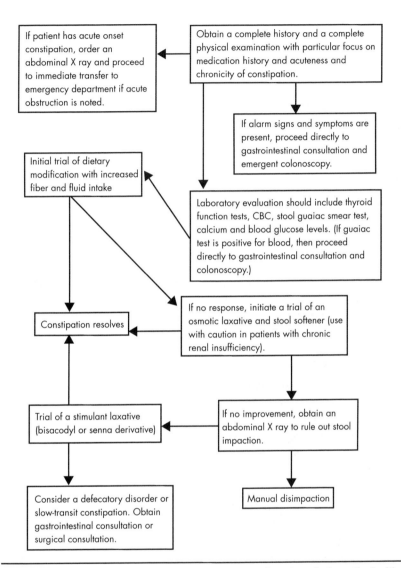

**FIGURE 26–1.** Algorithm for the assessment and treatment of a patient with constipation.

*Note.* CBC=complete blood count.

All patients who complain of constipation should have a trial of increased dietary fiber and liquid consumption. An osmotic laxative and an emollient stool softener should be prescribed. The dose of the laxative can be titrated until the constipation resolves or until symptoms of diarrhea or bloating occur.

If further testing is needed, the tests should be focused on more specific causes of constipation. If fecal impaction is considered, an abdominal X ray should be done. Patients for whom fecal impaction is suspected can be given a water-soluble enema, which can be both diagnostic and therapeutic, as it softens the stool in the distal colon. If no improvement results from the initial trial of dietary fiber and liquids along with the use of a stool softener, then additional medications must be used.

Osmotic laxatives are poorly absorbed substances that cause intestinal secretion of water, thus loosening stool. They take a few days to work and require adequate intake of water to work correctly. Osmotic laxatives should be used with extreme caution in patients with renal insufficiency or cardiac disease because of the risk of fluid overload states and electrolyte imbalance. Common side effects include bloating, flatulence, and muscle cramps. Enemas or suppositories work by stimulating distal colonic contractions and mechanically softening the stool.

Nonabsorbable sugars are intact when they reach the colon, where they are fermented by colonic bacteria. This process produces smaller unabsorbed sugars, resulting in an osmotic gradient in the colon and an increase in the fluid and stool volume within the colonic lumen (Thompson and Longstreth 2000). Common side effects include bloating, flatulence, and abdominal pain. Examples of these agents include lactulose, mannitol, and polyethylene glycol.

Stimulant laxatives, such as senna, cascara, bisacodyl, and mineral oil, stimulate secretion and colonic contractions, resulting in a bowel movement within 6–12 hours.

Biofeedback has been used in cases of constipation caused by defecatory disorders (Lembo and Camilleri 2003). In refractory cases of slow-transit constipation, biofeedback has been used to train patients to relax their pelvic floor muscles during defecation (Wald 2002). Women with constipation related to irritable bowel syndrome may be treated with tegaserod (Lembo and Camilleri 2003). Cholinergic medications can be used for the treatment of constipation. Manual disimpaction is needed in patients with fecal impaction. If this procedure is attempted, local or general anesthesia may be needed. Once the hard stool has been removed, a stool softener and osmotic laxatives are given to facilitate defecation (see Table 26–1).

Special care must be taken with bedridden or wheelchair-bound patients. Fecal incontinence may occur with excessive laxative use. Enemas (with tap water) may be used to prevent fecal impaction.

**TABLE 26-1.** Medications used in treatment of constipation

| Medication | Dosage | Trade name |
|---|---|---|
| Fiber | | |
|   Dietary fiber | 10–20 g/day | |
|   Psyllium | 3.4 g 1–3 times/day prn | Metamucil |
|   Methylcellulose | 2 g 1–3 times/day prn | Citrucel |
|   Polycarbophil | 1 g 1–3 times/day prn | FiberCon |
| Osmotic laxatives | | |
|   Magnesium hydroxide | 15–30 mL 1–2 times/day | Milk of Magnesia |
|   Magnesium citrate | 150–300 mL prn | |
|   Sodium phosphate (liquid) | 10–25 mL with water (12 oz) | Fleets Phospho-soda |
|   Sodium phosphate (enema) | 120 mL per rectum prn | |
| Emollients | | |
|   Docusate sodium | 100 mg 1–3 times/day | Colace |
| Nonabsorbable sugars | | |
|   Lactulose | 15–30 mL 1–2 times/day | |
|   Sorbitol | 15–30 mL 1–2 times/day | |
|   Mannitol | 15–30 mL 1–2 times/day | |
|   Polyethylene glycol | 17–36 g 1–2 times/day | MiraLax, GoLYTELY |
| Stimulant laxatives | | |
|   Senna | 187 mg/day | Senokot, Ex-Lax |
|   Cascara | 325 mg/day or 5 mL/day or prn | |
|   Bisacodyl (tablet and enema) | 5–10 mg qhs | Dulcolax |
|   Mineral oil | 5–15 mL qhs | |
| Cholinergic agents | | |
|   Bethanechol | 10 mg/day | Urecholine |
| Prokinetic agent | | |
|   Tegaserod | 10–20 mg qid | Zelnorm |

# References

Camilleri M, Thompson WG, Fleshman JW, et al: Clinical management of intractable constipation. Ann Intern Med 121:520–528, 1994

Chengappa KN, Pollock BG, Parepally H, et al: Anti-cholinergic differences among patients receiving standard doses of olanzapine or clozapine. J Clin Psychopharmacology 20:311–316, 2000

Emmanuel AV, Mason HJ, Kamm MA: Relationship between psychological state and level of activity of extrinsic gut innervation in patients with functional gut disorder. Gut 49:165–166, 2001

Garvey M, Noyes R Jr, Yates N: Frequency of constipation in major depression: relationship to other clinical variables. Psychosomatics 31:204–206, 1990

Lembo A, Camilleri M: Chronic constipation. N Engl J Med 349:1360–1368, 2003

Levin TT, Bennett J, Mendolwitz A: Death from clozapine-induced constipation: a case report and literature review. Psychosomatics 43:71–73, 2002

Pare P, Ferrazzi S, Thompson WG, et al: An epidemiologic survey of constipation in Canada: definitions, rates, demographics, and predictors of health care seeking. Am J Gastroenterology 96:3130–3137, 2001

Thompson WG, Longstreth GF: Function bowel disorders, in Rome II: The Functional Gastrointestinal Disorders, 2nd Edition. Edited by Drossman DA, Corazziari E, Talley NJ, et al. McLean, VA, Degnon Associates, 2000, pp 351–3966

Wald A: Slow transit constipation. Curr Treat Options Gastroenterol 5:279–283, 2002

# CHAPTER 27

# Gastrointestinal Bleeding

## Angelo M. O. Fernandes, M.D.

## Clinical Presentation

Gastrointestinal bleeding is classified as upper, when it originates from a location proximal to Treitz's ligament, or lower, when it is distal to Treitz's ligament. Gastrointestinal bleeding can be overt, when blood or modified blood is readily visible in gastric contents or in the stool, or occult, when blood is detected by stool testing or suggested by iron-deficiency anemia. Acute hemorrhage can be further classified as major, when it is accompanied by hemodynamic instability, or minor, when hemodynamic instability is absent.

Occult bleeding is by far the most common form of gastrointestinal hemorrhage. Iron-deficiency anemia is the principal metabolic manifestation of chronic blood loss (Ahlquist 2003). The most widely used test to detect blood in the stool is the modified guaiac smear test (Hemoccult fecal blood test), which relies on the peroxidase activity of hemoglobin and reflects the amount of hemoglobin present in the stool. A positive finding on the test for occult blood may be due to an insignificant lesion, but the cause may also be life-threatening; the challenge is to find and possibly treat the culprit lesion. Iron supplementation or ingestion of bismuth-containing preparations (e.g., Pepto-Bismol) can lead to black stools that are heme-negative and nonmalodorous. The consumption of peroxidase-rich foods, such as uncooked broccoli, turnips, or cauliflower, or rare red meat may lead to a false-positive fecal blood test. The presence of blood in the stool or in the upper gastrointestinal tract is always a significant finding that warrants further investigation. Although massive hemorrhage invariably requires immediate hospitalization and emergency diagnostic assessment, most evaluations of gastrointestinal bleeding can be performed in the outpatient setting.

**TABLE 27–1.**   Differential diagnosis of acute upper gastrointestinal bleeding

**Common causes**
Duodenal ulcer
Gastric ulcer
Esophageal varices
Mallory-Weiss tear

**Less common causes**
Dieulafoy vascular malformation (abnormally large submucosal artery)
Angiodysplasia
Portal hypertensive gastropathy
Gastric antral vascular ectasia (watermelon stomach)
Gastric varices
Neoplasia
Esophagitis
Gastric erosions

**Rare causes**
Esophageal ulcer
Erosive duodenitis
Aortoenteric fistula
Stomal ulcer
Hemobilia
Pancreatic source
Crohn's disease
No lesion identified

*Source.*   Adapted from Rockey 2002 and Elta 2003.

## Differential Diagnosis

### Organic Disorders

Upper gastrointestinal bleeding accounts for 75%–80% of all cases of
acute digestive blood loss (Wilcox 2002). The most common causes are
gastric ulcers, duodenal ulcers, gastric erosions, esophageal varices, and
Mallory-Weiss tears (see Table 27–1).

The most common causes of acute lower digestive tract bleeding are
diverticula and angiodysplasia. Less common causes include cancer,
inflammatory bowel disease, colitis (ischemic, infectious, or radiation-
related), and hemorrhoids (see Table 27–2).

| **TABLE 27-2.** | Differential diagnosis of acute lower gastrointestinal bleeding |
|---|---|

**Common causes**
Diverticulosis
Angiodysplasia

**Less common causes**
Cancer
Polyp
Postpolypectomy hemorrhage
Inflammatory bowel disease
Colitis
    Ischemic
    Radiation
    Infectious
    Nonspecific
Anorectal disease (hemorrhoids, anal fissures)
Small bowel source
Upper gastrointestinal source
Vasculitis
No lesion identified
Aortocolonic fistula
Trauma from fecal impaction
Anastomotic bleeding

**Rare causes**
Dieulafoy vascular malformation (abnormally large submucosal artery)
Colonic ulcerations
Rectal varices

*Source.*   Adapted from Rockey 2002 and Elta 2003.

In the United States the most common causes of chronic gastrointestinal blood loss are ulcers, malignancies, and angiodysplasia, which can be present anywhere in the gastrointestinal tract. Erosive esophagitis is another important cause of chronic gastrointestinal bleeding (see Table 27–3).

## Drug Effects, Toxicities, and Withdrawal

Laxative drugs are known to increase the rate of positive guaiac smear tests, probably as a result of an irritant effect on the colonic mucosa. Aspirin and nonsteroidal anti-inflammatory drugs (NSAIDs) can have a

**TABLE 27–3.**   Differential diagnosis of occult gastrointestinal bleeding

**Tumors/Neoplasms**
Carcinoma at any site
Large polyp at any site
Lymphoma
Lipoma
Metastases to the gut
Leiomyoma
Leiomyosarcoma

**Inflammatory**
Erosive esophagitis
Ulcer at any site
Cameron lesions (erosions in a hiatal hernia)
Erosive gastritis
Celiac disease
Inflammatory bowel disease
Meckel's diverticulum
Solitary colonic ulcer

**Vascular**
Angiodysplasia at any site
Portal hypertensive gastropathy
Gastroesophageal varices
Gastric antral vascular ectasia (watermelon stomach)
Hemangioma
Dieulafoy vascular malformation (abnormally large submucosal artery)

**Infectious**
Hookworm
Strongyloidiasis
Whipworm
Ascariasis
Tuberculous enterocolitis
Amebiasis

**Miscellaneous**
Hemoptysis
Oropharyngeal bleeding
Long distance running
Factitious bleeding

*Source.*   Adapted from Ahlquist 2003 and Rockey 2002.

toxic effect on the gastrointestinal mucosa and lead to occult or overt gastrointestinal bleeding. Certain drugs are known to worsen these toxic effects, notably alcohol, corticosteroids, and bisphosphonates (Wilcox 2002). The use of anticoagulants such as warfarin or antiplatelet agents does not lead to gastrointestinal bleeding per se, but it may exacerbate bleeding from a minor lesion (Ahlquist 2003; Wilcox 2002).

A population-based case-control study in the United Kingdom found that patients taking selective serotonin reuptake inhibitors (SSRIs) were at increased risk for upper gastrointestinal hemorrhage; this risk was magnified by the concomitant use of SSRIs and NSAIDs, suggesting a synergistic effect between the two drug classes (de Abajo et al. 1999). The postulated mechanism was a decreased uptake of serotonin by platelets, which adversely affected hemostasis. The chronic use of alcohol may lead to liver disease and portal hypertension, which may cause bleeding problems. Alcohol is also an independent risk factor for the development of peptic ulcers and erosive mucosal disease.

## Risk Stratification

Some historical factors that place patients at high risk for gastrointestinal bleeding are age >60 years, the presence of more than one comorbid illness, cardiac disease (acute coronary syndrome, congestive heart failure), bleeding diathesis or use of anticoagulants, neurological disorder (encephalopathy, delirium, recent stroke), liver disease (cirrhosis, alcoholic hepatitis), recent major surgery, renal disease (acute renal failure, treatment with dialysis), and pulmonary disease (respiratory failure, pneumonia, symptomatic chronic obstructive pulmonary disease) (Elta 2003). In the clinical course, tachycardia, orthostatic changes in vital signs, and shock place patients at high risk for an unfavorable outcome (see Figure 27–1).

## Assessment and Management in Psychiatric Settings

Rapid assessment of hemodynamic parameters allows the physician to implement resuscitation where appropriate, with the goal of replacing lost intravascular volume and improving tissue perfusion. A blood sample should be sent for a complete blood count, routine chemistry panel, coagulation studies, and typing in case a transfusion is required (Wilcox 2002).

A careful history and physical examination should follow resuscitation and stabilization of the patient in the management of acute gas-

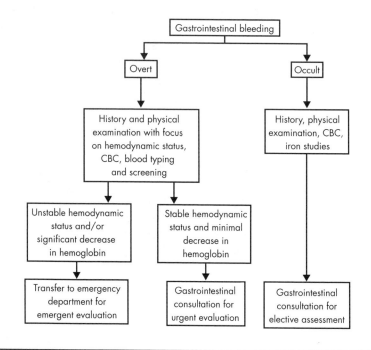

**FIGURE 27–1.**    Algorithm for the management of gastrointestinal bleeding.
*Note.*    CBC=complete blood count.

trointestinal bleeding. Hematemesis, or vomiting of blood, invariably reflects upper gastrointestinal bleeding (i.e., originating from the esophagus, stomach, or duodenum); if blood is altered by gastric secretions, it may have the appearance of coffee grounds. In the case of upper gastrointestinal bleeding, the stool commonly appears foul-smelling and tar-like (melena), but a briskly bleeding upper gastrointestinal lesion can also present as bright red blood per rectum (hematochezia). Hematochezia from an upper gastrointestinal source, with red blood in the nasogastric aspirate, is evidence of severe bleeding and is associated with a high mortality rate; it is almost always accompanied by hemodynamic instability. Lower gastrointestinal bleeding most often presents as hematochezia, but sometimes a lesion in the right side of the colon can manifest as melanotic stool. When hematochezia is seen only in the toilet paper or in the surface of solid stool it suggests perianal disease, such as hemorrhoids or anal fissures; the presence of tenesmus suggests rectal disease, such as proctitis.

In addition to monitoring the patient's vital signs, it is often helpful to perform a nasogastric aspirate in order to assess the rapidity of bleeding. The stool examination can also provide useful information, as patients with brown stool and infrequent bowel movements are less likely to have severe bleeding. On the other hand, patients passing red, maroon, or melanotic stools frequently are more likely to have significant bleeding (Wilcox 2002).

As the extravascular fluid moves into the vascular space to compensate for the loss of blood, the patient's hematocrit will decrease. This process, however, may take up to 72 hours to be completed; because of this interval, the hematocrit is less helpful in the initial evaluation of acute gastrointestinal bleeding than the assessment of the patient's hemodynamic parameters. Similarly, after bleeding has ceased, the hematocrit may continue to decrease for a few days, although this decrease does not constitute evidence of recurrent hemorrhage without clinical evidence of ongoing blood loss (Wilcox 2002).

The therapy for upper gastrointestinal bleeding depends on the underlying lesion. Upper endoscopy is usually the procedure of choice because it can be both a diagnostic and a therapeutic procedure. Peptic ulcers that bleed can be injected with saline or epinephrine, which tamponades the bleeding vessel, or they can be coagulated with a heating probe. If endoscopic therapy fails, angiographic embolization or surgery may be required. Intravenous proton pump inhibitors are used in the setting of endoscopic therapy for bleeding peptic ulcer to improve clot stabilization (Rockall et al. 1996). Patients taking NSAIDs or aspirin should stop taking them, if possible. The prophylactic use of misoprostol has been shown to reduce the incidence of ulcers in patients taking NSAIDs, but it is associated with a significant side effect profile. *Helicobacter pylori* infection should be eradicated in patients with upper gastrointestinal bleeding. Histamine type 2 ($H_2$) receptor blockers and sucralfate have been shown to reduce the incidence of gastritis related to acute illness (Cook et al. 1994). Patients at high risk for these lesions are those with respiratory failure who are receiving mechanical ventilation and those who have coagulopathy, head trauma, or burn injuries (Cook et al. 1996). Esophageal variceal bleeding occurs in the setting of portal hypertension, and its most common cause is liver cirrhosis. Control of active bleeding is best achieved through endoscopic means, ideally through variceal band ligation. Octreotide is a synthetic somatostatin analogue that reduces blood circulation to the splanchnic bed; it is used as an adjuvant therapy after endoscopic treatment to reduce the risk of rebleeding. Mallory-Weiss syndrome results from tears of the mucosa at the gastroesophageal junction that are usually associated with severe retching. Endoscopic therapy with injection or coagulation may be necessary in the 10%–20% of cases of Mallory-Weiss syndrome in which bleeding does not stop spontaneously (Wilcox 2002).

Because the most common causes of acute lower gastrointestinal bleeding are diverticula and angiodysplasia, angiography is usually performed to locate a bleeding vessel. If the patient is deemed at high risk for recurrent bleeding and if comorbid conditions coexist, surgery may be a preferable approach. Some authors advocate early colonoscopy with endoscopic injection or coagulation when there is evidence of recent diverticular bleeding; this procedure is becoming an acceptable alternative to angiography and surgery (Jensen et al. 2000).

Tests for fecal occult blood are routinely used as part of colorectal cancer screening. In this setting a colonoscopic examination is the gold standard, although a flexible sigmoidoscopy coupled with a barium enema is an acceptable alternative. If the colon is normal, an upper gastrointestinal investigation is warranted if there is significant anemia or if gastrointestinal symptoms are present. In asymptomatic patients without anemia, it is controversial whether any additional evaluation is needed; in patients with a family history of upper gastrointestinal tract malignancy, an esophagogastroduodenoscopy (EGD) should be obtained to rule out a tumor in the proximal gut (Ahlquist 2003; Wilcox 2002).

Patients with active gastrointestinal bleeding and negative findings from an endoscopic evaluation may need a bleeding scan or angiography to localize the source of bleeding. A bleeding scan can detect a bleeding rate of 0.1 mL of blood per minute; angiography is more accurate than a bleeding scan, but a bleeding rate of 0.5 mL/minute is required for detection. Angiography can also be used to embolize the bleeding vessel or to inject vasopressin intra-arterially. Patients with chronic obscure gastrointestinal bleeding with negative findings on an EGD and colonoscopy may need a push enteroscopy or a video capsule study to evaluate the small intestine (Ahlquist 2003; Wilcox 2002).

The risk of rebleeding after acute peptic ulcer bleeding is approximately 30% in 3 years if no treatment is pursued. Strategies to prevent rebleeding from peptic ulcers include long-term acid suppression, *H. pylori* eradication, and the avoidance of NSAIDs (Khuroo et al. 1997). There are no proven strategies for the prevention of rebleeding after lower gastrointestinal bleeding. Tumors that bleed should be resected if possible, and medical treatment of infectious or inflammatory colitides should reduce the likelihood of bleeding.

# References

Ahlquist DA: Approach to the patient with occult gastrointestinal bleeding, in Textbook of Gastroenterology, 4th Edition. Edited by Yamada T, Alpers DH, Laine L, et al. Philadelphia, PA, Lippincott Williams & Wilkins, 2003, pp 724–738

Cook DJ, Fuller HD, Guyatt GH, et al: Risk factors for gastrointestinal bleeding in critically ill patients. N Engl J Med 330:377–381, 1994

de Abajo FJ, Rodriguez LA, Montero D: Association between selective serotonin reuptake inhibitors and upper gastrointestinal bleeding: population based case-control study. BMJ 319:1106–1109, 1999

Elta GH: Approach to the patient with gross gastrointestinal bleeding, in Textbook of Gastroenterology, 4th Edition. Edited by Yamada T, Alpers DH, Laine L, et al. Philadelphia, PA, Lippincott Williams & Wilkins, 2003, pp 698–723

Jensen DM, Machiacado GA, Jutabha R, et al: Urgent colonoscopy for the diagnosis and treatment of severe diverticular hemorrhage. N Engl J Med 342:78–82, 2000

Khuroo MS, Yattoo GN, Javid G, et al: A comparison of omeprazole and placebo for bleeding peptic ulcer. N Engl J Med 336:1054–1058, 1997

Rockall TA, Logan RF, Devlin HB, et al: Risk assessment after acute upper gastrointestinal haemorrhage. Gut 38:316–321, 1996

Rockey DC: Gastrointestinal bleeding, in Sleisenger and Fordtran's Gastrointestinal and Liver Disease, 7th Edition. Edited by Feldman M, Friedman LS, Sleisenger MH. Philadelphia, PA, WB Saunders, 2002, pp 211–248

Wilcox CM: Acute gastrointestinal hemorrhage, in Digestive Diseases Self-Education Program III. Edited by Wilcox CM. Dubuque, IA, Kendall/Hunt, 2002, pp 123–145

# CHAPTER 28

# Abnormal Liver Function

Nakechand Pooran, M.D.

## Clinical Presentation

Liver function tests consist of serum measurement of aspartate aminotransferase (AST), alanine aminotransferase (ALT), bilirubin (direct and indirect), alkaline phosphatase, and γ-glutamyltransferase (GGT). The term "liver function test" has been criticized by some experts, because tests in this category reflect liver cell injury and do not give any information about the overall function of the liver. Serum albumin concentration and prothrombin time are used as surrogate markers for hepatic function.

Liver function tests are used to detect the presence and severity of liver disease, to distinguish among various types of liver disease, to follow the course of the disease, and occasionally to predict outcome and evaluate the response to treatment. When the results of all the individual tests are normal, the likelihood of liver disease is low (Green and Flamm 2002; Pratt and Kaplan 1999).

## Differential Diagnosis

Certain characteristic patterns of results for the individual liver function tests are useful in limiting the differential diagnosis. The general pattern of test results may suggest either hepatocellular necrosis or cholestasis. However, not all patients with liver disease fit into these two broad categories, and many present with a mixed biochemical pattern. The hallmark of hepatocellular necrosis is elevation in aminotransferase levels (AST/ALT). Cholestasis, impairment in bile flow, is characterized by elevation of alkaline phosphatase and bilirubin values. In patients with a mixed pattern, focus is placed on the predominant pattern (Davern and Scharschmidt 2002). For example, in patients in whom all the biochemical test values are elevated but the rise in AST/ALT is greater than the rise in alkaline phosphatase and bilirubin, hepatocellular necrosis is considered to predominate. If the rise in alkaline phosphatase and bilirubin is greater than the AST/ALT elevation, a cholestatic pattern dominates.

Striking elevations (>2,000 U/L) of the transaminase levels are seen predominantly in patients with ischemia, acute viral hepatitis, or a reaction to a toxin/medication (Davern and Scharschmidt 2002; Green and Flamm 2002). These patients should have a medical evaluation immediately to assess for liver failure. Milder elevations of AST/ALT levels have a broader range of differential diagnosis. One of the common causes is medication (Green and Flamm 2002). A careful history of all medications taken by the patient, including prescription, over-the-counter, illicit, and herbal preparations, should be obtained. Most medications can cause an elevation of liver enzyme values that usually occurs within 1–2 months of initiation of the medication (Green and Flamm 2002). Medications that can cause elevation of liver enzyme values include analgesics (e.g., nonsteroidal anti-inflammatory drugs, acetaminophen), antibiotics (e.g., penicillin derivatives, sulfonamides), antifungals (e.g., ketoconazole, fluconazole), lipid-lowering agents (e.g., 3-hydroxy-3-methylglutaryl coenzyme A [HMG-CoA] reductase inhibitors), antituberculosis medications (e.g., isoniazid), HIV medication (e.g., protease inhibitors), psychotherapeutic drugs (e.g., carbamazepine, phenytoin, trazodone, valproic acid), herb and alternative remedies (ephedra, gentian, germander, shark cartilage), and illicit drugs (anabolic steroids, cocaine, 3,4-methylenedioxymethamphetamine [Ecstasy], phencyclidine hydrochloride). If medication is essential in the patient's treatment, an alternative to the medication known to cause elevation in liver enzyme values should be sought. If no alternative medication is available, a gastroenterologist should be consulted. In many cases, the patient can continue taking the medication associated with elevated liver enzyme values, but the patient must be monitored closely with liver function tests. If the liver enzyme values continue to rise, the medication should be stopped to avoid liver failure. If medications have been eliminated as the etiology, other common causes of elevated transaminase levels include chronic viral hepatitis (hepatitis B and C), alcoholic hepatitis, nonalcoholic steatohepatitis, autoimmune hepatitis, hemochromatosis, Wilson's disease, $\alpha$1-antitrypsin deficiency, celiac disease, and cirrhosis (Green and Flamm 2002; Limdi and Myde 2003).

The patient with a cholestatic pattern of elevation in liver enzyme levels comes to medical attention either because he or she has developed jaundice or because the patient's liver function tests have shown an elevation of bilirubin or alkaline phospatase levels or both. The most common cause of a cholestatic pattern is obstruction of the bile duct, which is most commonly related to gallstones. Other etiologies of bile duct obstruction include benign strictures, papillary stenosis, cholangiocarcinoma, or pancreatic carcinoma. Evidence of bile duct obstruction can be found with an ultrasound or computed tomography scan of the abdomen, which will show dilated bile ducts proximal to the obstruction. If bile duct obstruction has been ruled out, other etiologies are sought. Medications that can induce cholestatic injury should be eliminated. Other causes of a cholestatic pattern include Gilbert syndrome, hemolysis, Dubin-Johnson syndrome, Rotor's syndrome, primary biliary cirrhosis, primary sclerosing cholangitis, benign recurrent cholestasis, vanishing bile duct syndrome, and infiltrating diseases of the liver (sarcoidosis, tuberculosis, amyloidosis, lymphoma).

## Risk Stratification

If the elevation in liver enzyme values is chronic, the assessment can be elective unless the values show a rising trend. If the onset of elevation in liver enzyme values is acute, the patient may require immediate medical evaluation. In a patient with elevated transaminase levels, transaminase values >2,000 U/L and/or an accompanying change in mental status, rising serum creatinine level, or prolonged prothrombin time signal the need for an emergent evaluation for possible liver failure (Hoofnagle et al. 1995).

Patients with a cholestatic pattern of elevation in liver enzyme values that is caused by bile duct obstruction should have an urgent evaluation if there is clinical evidence for ascending cholangitis, including the presence of right upper quadrant pain, fever, or leukocytosis. Patients with ascending cholangitis need biliary decompression, by means of either endoscopic retrograde cholangiopancreatography or percutaneous transhepatic cholangiography, and intravenous antibiotics. These patients should be transferred to a medical unit without delay.

## Assessment and Management in Psychiatric Settings

Medications are a common cause of abnormal liver enzyme values and should be evaluated as a potential etiology (see Table 28–1). As men-

**TABLE 28-1.**    Medications that cause abnormalities in liver enzyme tests

| Anesthetics | Antituberculosis drugs | Cardiovascular drugs |
|---|---|---|
| Halothane | Isoniazid | Angiotensin-converting |
| Methoxyflurane | Rifampin | enzyme inhibitors |
| Enflurane | Pyrazinamide | Methyldopa |
| **Analgesics** | **Antifungal** | Hydralazine |
| Acetaminophen | Ketoconazole | Amiodarone |
| Aspirin | Fluconazole | Quinidine |
| Sulindac | Itraconazole | **Hormones** |
| Diclofenac | Terbinafine | Anabolic steroids |
| **Anticonvulsants** | **Antineoplastic/** | Androgens |
| Phenytoin | **immunosuppressive** | Estrogens |
| Carbamazepine | **drugs** | **Psychoactive medications** |
| Valproic acid | Methotrexate | Neuroleptics |
| **Antibiotics** | Azathioprine | Monoamine oxidase |
| Amoxicillin/clavulanic | 6-Mercaptopurine | inhibitors |
| acid | 5-Fluorouracil | Tricyclic antidepressants |
| Fluoroquinolones | Cyclophosphamide | Trazodone |
| Erythromycins | Cyclosporine | **Miscellaneous** |
| Tetracycline | Tacrolimus | Allopurinol |
| Sulfonamides | **Antiviral agents** | Disulfram |
| Nitrofurantoin | Zidovudine | Herbs |
|  | Didanosine (ddI) |  |
|  | Zalcitabine (ddC) |  |

tioned earlier, most medications can have an adverse effect on liver enzyme levels. Hepatotoxicity can occur at any time during therapy. Most medications used in treating patients with psychiatric disorders can have an adverse effect on the liver. Soffer et al. (1983) reported two cases of liver injury due to carbamazepine. Risperidone-induced liver injury has been reported (Kumra et al. 1997). In liver injury secondary to use of risperidone, the patient develops steatosis that progresses to steatohepatitis.

An elevation of transaminase levels >2,000 U/L usually indicates a tremendous insult to the liver and massive necrosis of hepatocytes. Patients with this pattern of findings are at risk for hepatic failure and should have an urgent gastroenterological evaluation. Such severe acute injury may be caused by an ischemic event, a toxin/medication, or acute viral hepatitis. A through history and physical examination can eliminate the first two causes. Acute viral hepatitis is caused by hepatitis A, B, C, D, or E virus; Epstein-Barr virus; or cytomegalovirus. The diagnosis of acute hepatitis A, D, or E is based on detection of virus-specific IgM antibodies in the serum. A diagnosis of acute hepatitis B is made by finding a positive assay for hepatitis B surface antigen (HBsAg) and hepatitis B core IgM antibodies. Acute hepatitis C is rare but can be diagnosed by testing for the presence of hepatitis C virus RNA and hepatitis C virus antibodies. A diagnosis of acute Epstein-Barr virus or cytomegalovirus infection is based on a pattern of rising values in serial serological antibody titers (Berenguer and Wright 2002).

Milder elevation of transaminase levels has a wider differential diagnosis, including chronic viral hepatitis caused by hepatitis B or hepatitis C virus. The prevalence of chronic viral hepatitis is high among psychiatric patients (Dinwiddle et al. 2003; Rosenberg et al. 2001). This higher prevalence may be a result of greater rates of illicit drug use and sexual exposure to infected individuals in the psychiatric patient population. The hepatitis C virus antibody test and the hepatitis B serology (HBsAg antibodies, hepatits B core antigen antibodies) are the initial tests to exclude chronic viral hepatitis. When a patient is found to have chronic viral hepatitis, use of hepatotoxic medications in these patients is a source of concern. Chronic viral hepatitis does not preclude the use of hepatotoxic medications, but close monitoring is required, and the medication must be stopped if the patient has rising liver function test values. For example, valproic acid is safe for use in patients with chronic hepatitis C as long as the patient's liver function tests are monitored closely (Felker et al. 2003).

Psychiatric patients have a high prevalence of alcohol use (Kessler 1995). Patients with chronic alcohol use can have elevated liver enzyme values as a result of alcohol-related hepatitis or alcohol-induced cirrhosis. Alcohol use should be suspected when the AST:ALT ratio is greater than 2 and the GGT level is above normal (Cohen and Kaplan 1979; Pratt and Kaplan 2000).

Wilson's disease, a disorder of copper metabolism, can present as either acute or chronic hepatitis (Gitlin 2002). Some patients with Wilson's disease may be brought to medical attention because of the neuropsychiatric component of the disease. This diagnosis should be suspected in a patient with a low serum ceruloplasmin level, especially if the patient is less than 40 years old.

Hereditary hemochromatosis is a common genetic disorder of iron metabolism. Values for serum iron and total iron-binding capacity (TIBC) tested in the fasting patient are used to calculate the transferrin saturation (iron/TIBC). If the transferrin saturation is >45%, hemochromatosis should be suspected. An elevation of the ferritin level is an acute-phase reaction in any inflammatory disorder and therefore is not a sensitive marker for hemochromatosis.

Autoimmune hepatitis is a disorder that affects women more commonly than men and can present with an asymptomatic elevation of transaminase levels (Manns and Strassburg 2001). The serological marker that indicates autoimmune disorder is a positive antinuclear antibody (ANA) test and/or antismooth muscle antibody test. Psychiatric patients are also at risk for nonalcoholic steatohepatitis because they have a high prevalence of obesity, diabetes, and hyperlipidemia (Reid 2001). The diagnosis is made on the basis of an ultrasound finding of a fatty liver and liver biopsy findings of steatosis and inflammation.

In the majority of patients who present with a cholestatic pattern of elevation in liver enzyme values, either a medication or obstruction of the bile duct is the etiology. Once the effects of medications have been eliminated, an ultrasound of the abdomen is warranted to check for bile duct obstruction. A finding of dilated intrahepatic bile ducts suggests an obstruction of the biliary tree (Mittelstaedt 1997). This obstruction may be caused by gallstones, benign stricture, papillary stenosis, cholangiocarcinoma, or pancreatic cancer. If the obstruction is acute, the bile duct may not be dilated immediately but may later become dilated. Patients with bile duct obstruction may have elective evaluation of the bile duct, but if clinical evidence of ascending cholangitis is present, the patient requires immediate intravenous antibiotics and gastroenterological or surgical evaluation. If no evidence of bile duct obstruction is found, an antimitochondrial antibody titer should be obtained to evaluate for primary biliary cirrhosis. Primary bilary cirrhosis commonly affects females and sometime has the symptom of intense pruritis (Kaplan 2002). A diagnosis of a rarer cause of cholestatic injury, such as Gilbert syndrome, Dubin-Johnson syndrome, benign recurrent cholestasis, and infiltrative disorder, should be made after a gastroenterology or hepatology evaluation (Green and Flamm 2002).

Before seeking a consultation, the patients' medications should be reviewed, and a screening for viral hepatitis, ANA test, serum iron studies, measurement of the ceruloplasmin level (in a patient age <40 years), and an ultrasound scan of the liver should be obtained (Limdi and Myde 2003).

Patients with an acute rise in liver enzyme values accompanied by evidence of liver failure are monitored in an intensive care setting or a transplant unit. Hepatotoxic drugs are limited, and supportive care is instituted. For a patient to be a candidate for liver transplantation, he or she is required to cease alcohol and illicit drug use for at least 6 months.

The liver transplant candidate is also required to have strong social support and to adhere to all follow-up treatment. These requirements may be more problematic for psychiatric patients than for the general population.

Most liver diseases are treated in an outpatient setting. Therapy is directed at the specific cause of the underlying liver disease. If no specific therapy is available, then slowing or preventing the progression to cirrhosis and end-stage liver disease becomes the focus in management of these patients. If the liver disease is related to an obstruction caused by a stricture of the bile duct, treatment may involve dilating the stricture, placing a stent across the stricture, or surgical resection of the stricture (Banerjee 1993).

# References

Banerjee B: Extrahepatic biliary tract obstruction: modern methods of management. Postgrad Med 93:113–117, 1993

Berenguer M, Wright TL: Viral hepatitis, in Sleisenger and Fordtran's Gastrointestinal and Liver Disease, 7th Edition. Edited by Feldman M, Friedman LS, Sleisenger MH. Philadelphia, PA, WB Saunders, 2002, pp 1278–1341

Cohen JA, Kaplan MM: The SGOT/SGPT ratio: an indicator of alcoholic liver disease. Dig Dis Sci 24:835–838, 1979

Davern TJ, Scharschmidt BF: Biochemical liver tests, in Sleisenger and Fordtran's Gastrointestinal and Liver Disease, 7th Edition. Edited by Feldman M, Friedman LS, Sleisenger MH. Philadelphia, PA, WB Saunders, 2002, pp 1227–1239

Dinwiddie SH, Shicker L, Newman T: Prevalence of hepatitis C among psychiatric patients in the public sector. Am J Psychiatry 160:172–174, 2003

Felker B, Sloan K, Dominitz J, et al: The safety of valproic acid use for patients with hepatitis C infection. Am J Psychiatry 160:174–178, 2003

Gitlin JD: Wilson disease. Gastroenterology 125:1868–1877, 2002

Green RM, Flamm S: AGA technical review on the elevation of liver chemistry tests. Gastroenterology 123:1367–1384, 2002

Hoofnagle JH, Carithers RL, Shapiro C, et al: Fulminant hepatic failure: summary of a workshop. Hepatology 21:240–252, 1995

Kaplan MM: Primary biliary cirrhosis: past, present, and future. Gastroenterology 123:1392–1394, 2002

Kessler R: The National Comorbidity Survey: preliminary results and future directions. Int J Methods Psychiatr Res 5:139–151, 1995

Kumra S, Herion D, Jacobsen L, et al: Case study: risperidone-induced hepatotoxicity in pediatric patients. J Am Acad Child Adol Psychiatry 36:701–705, 1997

Limdi JK, Myde GM: Evaluation of abnormal liver function tests. Postgrad Med J 79:307–312, 2003

Manns MP, Strassburg CP: Autoimmune hepatitis: clinical challenges. Gastroenterology 120:1502–1517, 2001

Mittelstaedt CA: Ultrasound of the bile ducts. Semin Roentgenol 32:161–171, 1997

Pratt DS Kaplan MM: Laboratory tests, in Schiff's Diseases of the Liver. Edited by Schiff ER, Sorrell MF, Maddery WC. Philadelphia, PA, Lippincott-Raven, 1999, pp 205–244

Pratt DS, Kaplan MM: Evaluation of abnormal liver enzymes results in asymptomatic patients. N Engl J Med 342:1266–1271, 2000

Reid AE: Non-alcoholic steatohepatitis. Gastroenterology 121:710–723, 2001

Rosenberg SD, Goodman LA, Oscher FC, et al: Prevalence of HIV, hepatitis B, and hepatitis C in people with severe mental illness. Am J Public Health 91:31–37, 2001

Soffer E, Taylor R, Bertam P, et al: Carbamazepine-induced liver injury. Southern Med J 76:681–683, 1983

# PART VII

# Signs of
# Common Infections

Section Editor:

Barbara J. Barnett, M.D.

# CHAPTER 29

# Red Eye

## Dawne Kort, M.D.

## Clinical Presentation

To understand the common condition of red eye, one must be familiar with the anatomy of the eye. The conjunctiva, cornea, anterior chamber, iris, and ciliary body make up the anterior segment of the eye. This portion of the eye can be viewed by using the slit lamp. The posterior segment of the eye, which is collectively referred to as the fundus, includes the optic nerve, macula, and retina. These structures are visualized with the aid of a direct ophthalmoscope. Patients may or may not experience pain with their red eye. Some may complain of a discharge, pruritus, or visual change.

## Differential Diagnosis

Although the differential diagnosis of red eye is quite vast, certain signs are useful in differentiating one disease process from another. The portion of the eye involved (eyelid, conjunctiva, anterior chamber, etc.) often suggests the proper diagnosis. The nature of the onset of symptoms can help distinguish an acute and perhaps life-threatening condition from a chronic condition. Other factors that can help to narrow the differential diagnosis include the presence of visual changes, photophobia, pain, discharge (clear or colored), trauma, prior episodes, unilateral versus bilateral location, contact lens use, comorbid conditions (hypertension, diabetes, atrial fibrillation, cerebral events, collagen vascular diseases, etc.), and previous ophthalmological history.

The physical examination should begin with an assessment of visual acuity and visual fields. Each eye should be tested individually. If the patient uses glasses or contact lenses that are not present at the time of the examination, pinhole testing can be performed to obtain an estimate of corrected visual acuity. If the patient is unable to read the vision chart, visual acuity can be estimated by having the patient count fingers, detect hand motion, or even perceive light in a dark environment. Testing the visual field of each eye is important to distinguish intracranial conditions from ocular disease processes. After the visual assessment has been completed, the external eye is examined, including inspection of the periorbital skin and lids for trauma, infection, dysfunction, or deformity. Asymmetry should be noted. Palpation of the area may reveal subcutaneous emphysema or point tenderness over the orbital bone, which can be associated with orbital wall fractures. The eyelids must be everted to check for foreign bodies that may be trapped behind the lid. The conjunctiva should also be inspected for foreign bodies, evidence of trauma, inflammation, hemorrhages, and discharge. Pupil evaluation (size, reactivity, defect, etc.) and extraocular movements should be assessed next. Abnormalities found in this part of the examination may indicate that the etiology is an infectious process related to cerebral events, endocrine disorder, malignancy, aneurysm, neuromuscular disease, or trauma.

The most common cause of red eye is an infection. An external *hordeolum* (sty) is an acute infection (usually staphylococcal) of an oil gland associated with an eyelash. It is located at the lash line and has the appearance of a small pustule. Signs and symptoms include pain, erythema, focal swelling, and tenderness of the affected eyelid. Warm compresses and an antistaphylococcal antibiotic ointment constitute the recommended treatment (Farina and Mazarin 2001). An internal hordeolum (*chalazion*) is an acute or chronic inflammation of the eyelid due to blockage of the meibomian oil glands. An internal hordeolum often evolves from an incompletely resolved external hordeolum and manifests as a reddened, tender lump in the lid or at the lid margin. Treatment consists of warm compresses and an antistaphylococcal antibiotic ointment, along with ophthalmology follow-up. For chronic and recurrent infections, a 3-week course of doxycycline is recommended (Farina and Mazarin 2001).

*Anterior blepharitis* is a chronic and frequently bilateral inflammation of the lid margins. Common causes include staphylococcal species and/or seborrheic dermatitis. Examination of the eyes reveals greasy, scaly lid margins that may be erythematous and slightly swollen. Management includes gentle scrubbing of the eyelids and lashes with baby shampoo to remove debris, followed by application of a topical antibiotic ointment to the eyelid margins. If seborrheic dermatitis of the scalp and eyebrows is present, selenium sulfide shampoo should be used (Lowery and Roy 2001).

*Dacryocystitis* is an inflammation of the lacrimal sac that is caused by obstruction of the nasolacrimal duct. It is characterized by localized pain, edema, and erythema over the lacrimal sac at the medial canthus of the eye. Dacryocystitis is usually unilateral, and there is often purulent drainage from the punctum. In infants, this condition results from failure of canalization that normally occurs by the end of the first month. However, in adults, acute forms are caused by *Staphylococcus aureus* or β-hemolytic streptococcus. Treatment includes broad-spectrum oral antibiotics, warm compresses, gentle massage of the lacrimal sac, and ophthalmological referral (Gilliland 2001).

*Corneal abrasions, inflammations, or infections* are other known causes of red eye. These conditions are usually associated with decreased visual acuity, photophobia, severe pain, a sensation of a foreign body in the eye, and purulent discharge. Examination of the eye reveals conjunctival hyperemia, lid edema, and a localized whitish corneal infiltrate that may be associated with a hypopyon (an accumulation of white exudates in the anterior chamber). These disease entities can be diagnosed with fluorescein staining. An area of increased fluorescein uptake is diagnostic. Common pathogens include *Staphylococcus* and *Streptococcus* species. However, in patients who use extended-wear soft contact lenses, a common pathogen is *Pseudomonas*. Treatment consists of antibiotic drops and ophthalmological follow-up. For corneal abrasions, tetanus prophylaxis is also recommended (Farina and Mazarin 2001).

Inflammation of the iris is known as *iritis*. In this condition, the eye develops a "perilimbal flush" (dilated blood vessels in the conjunctiva adjacent to the cornea). White blood cells are present in the anterior chamber and can be seen under high magnification with the slit lamp. Signs and symptoms include decreased visual acuity, direct and consensual photophobia, and keratic precipitates on the endothelium. Iritis is usually unilateral. Common causes of this disease process include trauma, seronegative arthritides (idiopathic ankylosing spondylitis, Reiter's syndrome, etc.), inflammatory bowel diseases, chronic granulomatous conditions (tuberculosis, sarcoidosis, etc), local infection, sexually transmitted diseases, corneal abrasions, foreign bodies, and idiopathic conditions. Iritis can be differentiated from a corneal irritation by the placement of a topical anesthetic agent. Topical anesthetic agents will not relieve the pain of iritis, although they will relieve the pain of corneal abrasion. Treatment for iritis includes a long-acting topical cycloplegic, a topical steroid, and ophthalmological follow-up within 24 hours

(Gordon 2001). The topical cycloplegic is used to provide comfort by eliminating ciliary spasm and to prevent formation of posterior adhesions between the iris and the lens. The topical steroid is used to relieve inflammation.

*Keratoconjunctivitis sicca,* also known as dry eye, may result from any disease that is associated with deficiency of tear film components and lid surface or epithelial abnormalities. In most cases the eye appears normal. Common causes include rheumatoid arthritis, Sjögren's syndrome, and other autoimmune diseases. Management involves treating the underlying disorder (Farina and Mazarin 2001).

*Acute angle glaucoma,* which is a true ocular emergency, occurs in people with shallow (narrow) anterior chambers. Narrowing of this angle results in closer contact between the iris and the lens and produces resistance to flow of aqueous humor from the posterior to the anterior chamber. Complete closure of the angle blocks aqueous flow and causes an abrupt rise in the intraocular pressure. In an examination of the eye, the patient will have decreased visual acuity, a shallow anterior chamber, a red, congested-appearing eye with a fixed, mid-dilated pupil, a hazy cornea, and ciliary injection. The intraocular pressure will also be elevated. Treatment includes topical miotics (to reopen the angle and allow flow of the aqueous humor), carbonic anhydrase inhibitors (to decrease the secretion of the aqueous humor), topical β-adrenergic antagonists (to decrease the secretion of the aqueous humor), hyperosmotic agents (to decrease the volume of the fluid in the eye), analgesics as needed, and immediate ophthalmological consultation. Definitive therapy is surgical (Webb 1995).

Several different drugs have the potential to cause elevation of intraocular pressure, which can induce acute closed angle glaucoma (Table 29–1). These medications will incite an attack only in those individuals with occludable angles. The offending agents produce acute closed angle glaucoma by causing pupillary dilation, which elevates the intraocular pressure.

Patients with *conjunctivitis* complain of eyelids sticking together, pruritus, burning, or the sensation of a gritty foreign body in the eye. A thick purulent discharge may distort vision, although visual acuity is normal. Photophobia, if present, is usually minimal. Although conjunctivitis usually begins in one eye, spread to the other eye is quite common because of the infectious nature of the disease process (Kanski 1999).

Conjunctivitis can be a bacterial, viral, allergic, and even chemical process. Bacterial conjunctivitis is usually characterized by acute onset, minimal pain, occasional pruritus, and sometimes an exposure history.

**TABLE 29–1.**   Common drugs that can cause acute closed angle glaucoma

- Anticholinergic eye drops
- Antihistamines
- Antiparkinsonian drugs
- Antipsychotic agents
- Antispasmolytic agents
- Monoamine oxidase inhibitors
- Selective serotonin reuptake inhibitors
- Sulfa-containing agents
- Sympathomimetic eye drops
- Tricyclic antidepressants

Symptoms include eye pain, swelling, redness, and a moderate to large amount of discharge, usually yellow or greenish in color. Staphylococcal, streptococcal, and pneumococcal species are the most common pathogens. Treatment involves keeping the area clean and dry, avoiding direct contact, avoiding the use of contact lenses, and use of antibiotic ointment or drops against staphylococcal, streptococcal, and pneumococcal species. Chlamydia conjunctivitis is less common but can be a devastating condition. It should be suspected in anyone with a history of a sexually transmitted disease. Treatment typically includes systemic and topical antibiotics (oral erythromycin, doxycycline, or tetracycline plus topical erythromycin or tetracycline), as well as evaluation and treatment of all sexual partners (Silverman and Bessman 2003).

Viruses are the most common cause of conjunctivitis. Viral conjunctivitis is characterized by acute or subacute onset, minimal pain level, and pruritus. It is usually preceded by an upper respiratory illness or other viral prodrome. A clear, watery discharge is typical. Lymphoid follicles on the undersurface of the eyelid and enlarged, tender preauricular nodes can often be found. This infection is usually unilateral initially but spreads quickly through autoinoculation to involve both eyes. Adenovirus is the most common pathogen. Although this form of conjunctivitis is highly contagious, it is a self-limiting illness that requires only supportive care (Farina and Mazarin 2001). This form of conjunctivitis is highly contagious, especially in the healthcare arena. Outbreaks within hospital units are not uncommon and can be prevented by strict contact precautions.

Allergic conjunctivitis can be acute or subacute and is not associated with pain. This form of conjunctivitis is usually accompanied by intense itching, tearing, and swelling of the eye membranes. A clear, watery discharge with a moderate amount of mucus production is commonly seen with allergic conjunctivitis. Frequent causes include pollens, animal dander, and dust. Allergic conjunctivitis is frequently seasonal and is found with other typical "allergy" symptoms such as sneezing, itching nose, or scratchy throat. A cold moist washcloth applied to the eyes and over-the-counter decongestant eye drops give some relief.

Chemical conjunctivitis can result when any irritating substance enters the eye. Common offending irritants are household cleaners, sprays of any kind, smoke, smog, and industrial pollutants. Immediate thorough washing of the eyes with large amounts of water is essential. The local poison control center should be contacted at once to identify potentially damaging toxins and to ensure proper management.

*Herpes simplex keratitis* may be the result of primary or recurrent infection with the herpes simplex virus (usually type 1). Skin and mucocutaneous lesions are more common in primary infections, whereas corneal involvement (keratitis) is more common in recurrent infections. Herpes simplex keratitis can present with ocular pain, a sensation of a foreign body in the eye, photophobia, and tearing. Visual acuity may be decreased. Further examination may reveal a diffusely reddened eye, decreased corneal sensation, and preauricular adenopathy. Treatment includes prompt ophthalmological consultation, a topical antiviral agent, and a topical cycloplegic (Farina and Mazarin 2001).

*Herpes zoster ophthalmicus* results from reactivation of latent varicella zoster virus in the trigeminal ganglion. Clinical presentations include pain, paresthesias, tearing, and unilateral vesicular eruption in the trigeminal dermatomal distribution. If there is a lesion on the tip of the nose, possible ocular involvement is a concern. Ocular involvement can range from conjunctivitis to iritis, keratitis, corneal anesthesia, or ocular muscle palsies. Therapy consists of immediate ophthalmological consultation, an oral antiviral, a topical broad-spectrum antibiotic to prevent secondary infection, a topical cycloplegic, and oral analgesics as needed (Bessman and Mickel 2002).

*Orbital cellulitis* is an infection deep in the orbital septum. It is a serious ocular infection that can be life-threatening. Orbital cellulitis occurs because of an extension of a paranasal sinus infection. Patients with orbital cellulitis typically present with the same clinical findings seen in preseptal cellulitis, but they also have chemosis, ocular pain, pain with extraocular movements, limitation of extraocular function, papillary paralysis, and proptosis. Decreased visual acuity, increased intraocular pressure, and loss of sensation in the ophthalmic and max-

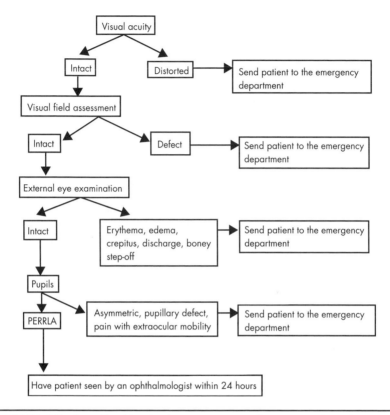

**FIGURE 29–1.**   Algorithm for the assessment and treatment of a patient with red eye.

*Note.*   PERRLA=pupils equal, round, and reactive to light and accommodation.

illary branches of the trigeminal nerve may also be seen. The management includes blood cultures, soft-tissue aspirates for Gram stain and culture, a computed tomography (CT) scan of the orbit, and hospital admission for administration of broad-spectrum intravenous antibiotics (Mitchell 2000).

*Preseptal cellulitis* is a periocular superficial cellulitis that has not breached the orbital septum. It is caused by hematogenous spread or direct extension from ethmoid sinusitis, skin infections, or trauma. Patients with preseptal cellulitis typically present with erythema, edema, warmth, and tenderness of the eyelid, conjunctival injection, and occasionally fever. Visual acuity, eye movements, and papillary findings are all normal in patients with preseptal cellulites. Additional testing includes blood cultures, soft-tissue aspirates for Gram stain and culture, and a CT scan of the orbits. Intravenous broad-spectrum antibiotics to cover *Streptococcus*, *Staphylococcus*, and *Haemophilus* species should be administered without delay on a medical unit (Mitchell 2000).

## Risk Stratification

Certain medical and environmental situations can predispose patients to ophthalmological conditions. For example, patients with diabetes, hypertension, connective tissue diseases, and rheumatologic illnesses are at an increased risk for having ophthalmological pathology. These patients should have eye examinations more frequently. Poor hygiene is another factor that can contribute to ophthalmological pathology. Patients with poor hygiene are at higher risk for ophthalmological infections, such as conjunctivitis, blepharitis, hordeolums, and chalazions. Patients who use contact lenses are also at greater risk for eye infections. These patients should also have routine eye examinations and should be instructed in proper lens wear, storage, and manipulation.

## Assessment and Management in Psychiatric Settings

Figure 29–1 shows steps for the evaluation and treatment of red eye.

## References

Bessman E, Mickel H: Herpes zoster ophthalmicus. 2002. Available at: http://www.emedicine.com/emerg/topic249.htm. Accessed March 1, 2004.

Farina GA, Mazarin G: Red eye evaluation. 2001. Available at: http://www.emedicine.com/oph/topic267.htm. Accessed April 1, 2004.

Gilliland GG: Dacryocystitis. 2001. Available at: http://www.emedicine.com/oph/topic708.htm. Accessed April 1, 2004.

Gordon K: Iritis and uveitis. 2001. Available at: http://www.emedicine.com/emerg/topic284.htm. Accessed April 1, 2004.

Kanski JJ: Clinical Ophthalmology: A Systemic Approach. Boston, MA, Butterworth-Heinemann, 1999, pp 94–156

Lowery RS, Roy H Sr: Blepharitis, adult. 2001. Available at: http://www.emedicine.com/oph/topic81.htm. Accessed April 1, 2004.

Mitchell JD: Ocular emergencies, in Emergency Medicine: A Comprehensive Study Guide, 5th Edition. Edited by Tintinalli JE, Kelen GD, Stapczynski JS. New York, McGraw-Hill, 2000, pp 1507–1508.

Silverman MA, Bessman E: Conjunctivitis, 2003. Available at http://www.emedicine.com/emerg/topic110.htm. Accessed March 1, 2004.

Webb LA: Eye Emergencies: Diagnosis and Management. Boston, MA, Butter-worth-Heinemann, 1995, pp 11–63

# Sore Throat, Earache, and Upper Respiratory Infections

## Grace Chen, M.D.

## Sore Throat

### Clinical Presentation

Pharyngitis, or inflammation of the pharynx, can be caused by viruses (most common), bacteria, fungi, or parasites. Infections caused by group A β-hemolytic streptococci (GABHS) are common and should be promptly diagnosed and treated. Clinical findings that increase the likelihood of GABHS include tonsillar exudates, tender anterior cervical lymphadenopathy, history of fever, and no cough. A patient with three or four of these signs is likely to have GABHS pharyngitis (75% sensitivity and specificity) (Centor et al. 1981). Other possible symptoms include throat pain, odynophagia, chills, malaise, headache, mild neck stiffness, nausea, vomiting, or abdominal pain. Examination may reveal pharyngeal swelling and erythema, tonsillar swelling, and foul breath. The patient may have a scarlatiniform rash (fine red papules, coarse to touch and blanching to pressure, that begin on the trunk and spread to the extremities, sparing palms and soles). A "white strawberry tongue" (enlarged papillae on a yellowish-white–coated tongue) may accompany the rash. The rash fades in 6–9 days and the palms and soles may desquamate afterward (Ebell et al. 2000).

### Differential Diagnosis

*Gonococcal pharyngitis* is another important variety of pharyngitis with a bacterial cause. The presumptive diagnosis of gonococcal pharyngitis can be made in a patient who complains of sore throat as well as ure-thritis or vaginitis.

*Viral pharyngitis* may be caused by infectious mononucleosis (Ep-stein-Barr virus), which occurs most commonly in the 15–24-year age group. The classic triad includes sore throat, fever, and lymphadenopa-thy. Hepatomegaly, splenomegaly, rarely jaundice, and maculopapular skin rash distinguish the disease from streptococcal infection. The ton-sils are enlarged, the pharynx may have exudates, and palatal petechiae may be present. Patients may have relative or absolute lymphocytosis and thrombocytopenia (Bisno 2001). *Primary herpes simplex virus type 1* infection often presents as exudative pharyngitis in adults. Patients have symptoms of fever, malaise, myalgia, cervical lymphadenopathy, pharyngitis, and painful vesicular lesions of the soft palate, buccal mu-cosa, tongue, and floor of the mouth, making it difficult to tolerate food.

Pharyngitis may also be the first manifestation of *agranulocytosis*. Agranulocytosis, defined as an absolute neutrophil count <500 µL) is very rare and occurs more commonly in female and elderly patients (Berliner et al. 2004). The antipsychotic clozapine has been associated with a risk of agranulocytosis of 0.8%–1.5% per year. Most cases oc-curred within the first 3 months of use (Alvir et al. 1993). Several case reports have also linked olanzapine to agranulocytosis. A complete blood count should be obtained in patients who are taking these medi-cations.

## Risk Stratification

It is important to separate those patients with GABHS pharyngitis, who require antibiotics, from those with viral pharyngitis, who do not re-quire antibiotics. Patients with GABHS pharyngitis receive antibiotics to prevent acute rheumatic fever, suppurative complications, and con-tagious spread. Suppurative complications of GABHS are rare and in-clude peritonsillar and retropharyngeal abscess. A complication that deserves mention but is not preventable by antibiotic treatment is acute poststreptococcal glomerulonephritis.

## Assessment and Management in Psychiatric Settings

To confirm GABHS pharyngitis, one may use rapid antigen tests to de-tect GABHS carbohydrate products. These tests have a sensitivity of 76%–87% and a specificity of 90%–96% (Gerber and Shulman 2004). The throat culture, however, with a sensitivity of 90% or greater, is still the gold standard for diagnosis of GABHS (Gerber and Shulman 2004). If clinical suspicion is high for gonococcal pharyngitis, genital, rectal, and oral cultures should be obtained to increase the likelihood of yielding the organism.

The treatment of choice for GABHS is either 1.2 million units of parenteral benzathine penicillin given intramuscularly (which eliminates the problem of nonadherence to treatment) or 500 mg of oral penicillin V two times daily for 10 days. For patients who are allergic to penicillin, 500 mg of oral erythromycin four times a day for 10 days is recommended (Fiebach and Rastegar 2003).

Patients with gonococcal pharyngitis should be treated for possible *Chlamydia* infection as well. Patients can be treated for gonorrhea with a single 125-mg dose of ceftriaxone intramuscularly or a single dose of an oral quinolone (50 mg of ciprofloxacin or 400 mg of ofloxacin) and treated for *Chlamydia* with either a single 1-g dose of azithromycin or 100 mg of doxycycline two times daily for 10 days (Fiebach and Rastegar 2003).

Treatment of viral pharyngitis, including infectious mononucleosis, is usually supportive. Splenic rupture is a rare, life-threatening complication. However, it has been reported to occur between the fourth and twenty-first day of symptomatic illness, so patients should be counseled to avoid contact sports during this time frame (Ebell 2004). Standard treatment for herpes simplex virus infection is 200 mg of acyclovir orally five times daily for 7 days (Bisno 2001).

In patients with pharyngitis associated with agranulocytosis, the contributing drug should be discontinued. The patient usually recovers after cessation of the contributing drug (Berliner 2004).

Patients without complete resolution of symptoms should seek further medical care. Complications of pharyngitis include peritonsillar abscess or other deep neck infections.

Chronic pharyngitis or tonsillitis is a diagnosis made in patients with more than six sore throats in 1 year or three or more episodes with enlarged tonsils in 2 or more years. In patients with chronic episodes, other noninfectious etiologies of sore throat, such as postnasal drip or reflux disease, should be excluded before pursuing further treatment (such as tonsillectomy) (Fiebach and Rastegar 2003).

## The Common Cold (Upper Respiratory Infection)

### Clinical Presentation

Coryza, otherwise known as the common cold, is a self-limited syndrome caused by viral infection of the upper respiratory mucosa. Patients have varying experiences, but the common cold may start with rhinorrhea, congestion, and sneezing or a sore throat. Cough may be present later in the illness, after nasal symptoms subside (Turner 2005). Patients with the common cold usually do not have fever. The incubation period is usually 48–72 hours. Patients usually have cold symptoms for a week, but a cold may last up to 2 weeks in 25% of cases (Fiebach and Rastegar 2003).

## Asessment and Management in Psychiatric Settings

Gonzales et al. (2001) listed principles to guide the physician in treating upper respiratory infections. First, it is necessary to separate coryza (viral in origin and without localizing features) from lower respiratory infection, sinusitis, and GABHS pharyngitis or other pharyngeal symptoms that require treatment. Second, antibiotic treatment of adults with the common cold is not recommended, because it does not speed illness resolution and increases antibiotic resistance. Finally, purulent nasal discharge or sputum alone does not predict bacterial infection or benefit from antibiotic treatment. However, purulent nasal discharge in addition to other symptoms or signs of sinusitis may indicate a need for treatment.

Treatment for the common cold is symptomatic. Analgesics, such as nonsteroidal anti-inflammatory drugs and acetaminophen, relieve fever, headache, and myalgias. Topical over-the-counter analgesics may provide relief for a sore throat. Nasal congestion can be treated with over-the-counter topical decongestants, such as phenylephrine and oxymetazoline sprays. Patients must be warned not to use these sprays for more than 3–5 days in order to avoid rebound effects or rhinitis medicamentosa (reflex vasoconstriction or increased nasal congestion occurring after decongestant medication.

# Epiglottitis

## Clinical Presentation

Epiglottitis is inflammation of the epliglottis or supraglottic area and is potentially fatal if not treated. Symptoms of epiglottitis include sore throat, dysphagia, fever, and stridor. In a physical examination, the patient is often drooling (thick secretions) and leaning forward, or the patient may be sitting up, panting, with the mouth open and head extended. Movement of the thyroid cartilage elicits pain (Herr and

Joyce 1997). The differential diagnosis includes pharyngitis, deep neck infections, and foreign body ingestion. Children who have not received the *Haemophilus influenzae* type B (Hib) vaccine are at risk for epiglottitis. The Hib vaccine has decreased the incidence of epiglottitis in children, and it is essentially nonexistent in this population, but the incidence in adults is increasing.

### Assessment and Management in Psychiatric Settings

In treating the patient with epiglottitis, securing an airway is the priority. An otolaryngology consultation should be obtained immediately, and the patient should be observed closely in the event that an artificial airway becomes necessary. On a lateral cervical X ray, the epiglottis appears enlarged and shaped like a thumb ("the thumbprint sign") (Hackeling and Triana 2000). Indirect laryngoscopy, performed with an emergency intubation kit by the bedside, demonstrates edema of the supraglottic and epiglottic area (Fiebach and Rastegar 2003).

Treatment includes supplemental humidified oxygen, intravenous fluids, and antibiotics. Steroids may be given to decrease inflammation. The patient should be admitted to an intensive care unit (Felter 2003).

## Otitis Externa

### Clinical Presentation

Acute diffuse external otitis, or "swimmer's ear," is an inflammation of the external ear canal or auricle. It presents with symptoms of pain, pruritis, and tenderness of the external ear. Hearing loss may occur if the disease becomes severe. The external auditory canal may be edematous and erythematous, and otorrhea may be present (Tintinalli and Lucchesi 2000).

### Differential Diagnosis

The differential diagnosis include trauma, infection, foreign bodies, cerumen impaction, cholesteatoma, neoplasms, referred pain from other areas (dental, retropharyngeal, oropharyngeal, nasal cavity, throat, and neck sources), trigeminal neuralgia, herpetic geniculate (Ramsay Hunt syndrome), and the infectious etiologies described in subsequent sections of this chapter (Tintinalli and Lucchesi 2000).

## Risk Stratification

Otitis externa should be differentiated from malignant external otitis, which is immediately life-threatening (see "Malignant Otitis Externa" on this page).

## Assessment and Management in Psychiatric Settings

Analgesia, cleansing, and decreasing the inflammation are vital to fighting the infection. Cerumen should be removed with a cotton swab or wire loop (Rutka 2004).

Agents that have been used to treat otitis externa include acidifying solutions, antiseptics that act as bacteriostatic agents, topical corticosteroids to decrease inflammation, and topical antibiotics (Rutka 2004). Examples of multidrug topical suspensions include the combination of ciprofloxacin and hydrocortisone and the combination of neomycin, polymyxin B, and hydrocortisone. Otomycosis should be treated with antifungal agents, such as clotrimazole. Medication should be instilled into the ear four times a day for at least 10 days (Tintinalli and Lucchesi 2000). Oral and intravenous antibiotics recommended for severe disease include β-lactams, cephalosporins, and fluoroquinolones (Rutka 2004).

Patients with mild disease should receive a topical agent and follow-up in 14 days. Patients with moderate disease may need an oral antibiotic and follow-up in 7 days. Patients with severe disease need to be referred to an otolaryngologist for cotton wick placement to allow topical medications to reach the ear canal (Rutka 2004).

# Malignant Otitis Externa

## Clinical Presentation

Malignant otitis externa is an invasive infection of the external auditory canal (necrotizing external otitis) or skull base (skull-base osteomyelitis) that begins as otitis externa and spreads to deeper tissues through clefts in the external auditory canal. Elderly diabetic patients and immunocompromised patients are most likely to be affected by malignant otitis externa (Kristiansen 1999). Malignant otitis externa should be differentiated from otitis externa. The symptoms of malignant otitis externa are similar to those of diffuse otitis externa, but are more intense.

## Assessment and Management in Psychiatric Settings

An otolaryngology consultation should be obtained for debridement. Additional tests should include a computed tomography scan to assess bone erosion. In routine laboratory tests, the only abnormality associated with malignant otitis externa may be an elevated erythrocyte sedimentation rate (Kristiansen 1999). Patients with malignant otitis externa are unresponsive to topical treatment and require intravenous antibiotics that also address *Pseudomonas aeruginosa*.

# Otitis Media

## Clinical Presentation

Acute otitis media is inflammation of the middle ear associated with middle ear effusion, often preceded by a viral upper respiratory tract infection (Berman 1995). Patients with acute otitis media have inflammation of the tympanic membrane, fever, irritability (in children), otorrhea, otalgia (or ear pulling), and nonspecific symptoms, such as nausea, vomiting, and anorexia. In a literature review, ear pain was found to be the most useful symptom for making the diagnosis (Rothman et al. 2003). Otoscopic findings include opacification of the tympanic membrane with bulging due to middle ear secretions and erythema of the tympanic membrane; immobility of the tympanic membrane may be found with pneumatic otoscopy (Tintinalli and Lucchesi 2000). The incidence of acute otitis media peaks in the preschool years and decreases with age. With growth, the increasing angle and length of the eustachian tube enhances drainage of the middle ear, preventing migration of bacteria from the nasopharynx (Tintinalli and Lucchesi 2000).

## Assessment and Management in Psychiatric Settings

Amoxicillin is the first-line antibiotic for acute otitis media, and a dosage of 90 mg/kg/day for 7–10 days is recommended to extinguish drug-resistant *Streptococcus pneumoniae* (McCracken 2002). For patients who are allergic to penicillin, other options are erythromycin, clindamycin, and trimethoprim-sulfamethoxazole (Niparko and Francis 2003). If 3 days of treatment fails, treatment with high-dose amoxicillin-clavulanate (Augmentin 250/125 or 500/125), cefuroxime axetil (Ceftin, available in 250–500-mg tablets), or ceftriaxone is recommended. The advantage of ceftriaxone is that it can be given as a single-dose injection

(McCracken 2002). Aspirin, acetaminophen, or ibuprofen can be given every 4–6 hours for pain (Niparko and Francis 2003). The follow-up should be directed at the response to treatment (McCracken 2002) and the diagnosis of complications, which may include tympanic perforation, acute serous labyrinthitis, facial nerve paralysis, mastoiditis, meningitis, extradural abscess, subdural empyema, lateral sinus thrombosis, cholesteatoma, and brain abscess (Niparko and Francis 2003).

# References

Alvir JM, Lieberman JA, Safferman AZ, et al: Clozapine-induced agranulocytosis: incidence and risk factors in the United States. N Engl J Med 329:162–167, 1993

Berliner N, Horwitz M, Loughran TP Jr: Congenital and acquired neutropania, in Hematology. Edited by Broudy VC, Berliner N, Larson RA, et al. Washington, DC, American Society of Hematology, 2004, pp 63–79

Berman S: Otitis media in children. N Engl J Med 332:1560–1565, 1995

Bisno AL: Acute pharyngitis. N Engl J Med 344:205–211, 2001

Centor RM, Witherspoon JM, Dalton HP, et al: The diagnosis of strep throat in adults in the emergency room. Med Decis Making 1:236–246, 1981

Ebell MH: Epstein-Barr virus infectious mononucleosis. Am Fam Physician 70:1279–1287, 2004

Ebell MH, Smith MA, Barry HC, et al: Does this patient have strep throat? JAMA 284:2912–2918, 2000

Felter R: Pediatrics, epiglottitis [Emedicine Web site]. 2003. Available at: http://www.emedicine.com/emerg/topic375.htm. Accessed December 16, 2003.

Fiebach NH, Rastegar DA: Respiratory tract infections, in Principles of Ambulatory Medicine, 6th Edition. Edited by Barker LR, Burton JR, Zieve PD, et al. Philadelphia, PA, Lippincott Williams & Wilkins, 2003, pp 421–444

Gerber MA, Shulman ST: Rapid diagnosis of pharyngitis caused by group A streptococci. Clin Microbiol Rev 17:571–580, 2004

Gonzales R, Bartlett JG, Besser RE, et al: Priniciples of appropriate antibiotic use for treatment of nonspecific upper respiratory tract infections in adults: background. Ann Emerg Med 37:698–702, 2001

Hackeling TA, Triana RJ: Disorders of the neck and upper airway, in Emergency Medicine: A Comprehensive Study Guide, 5th Edition. Edited by Tintinalli JE, Kelen GD, Stapczynski JS. New York, McGraw-Hill, 2000, pp 1556–1564

Herr RD, Joyce SM: Upper respiratory tract infections, in Infectious Disease in Emergency Medicine. Edited by Brillman JC, Quenzer RW. Philadelphia, PA, Lippincott-Raven, 1997, pp 479–494

Kristiansen P: The diagnosis and management of malignant (necrotizing) otitis externa. J Am Acad Nurse Pract 11:297–300, 1999

McCracken GH: Diagnosis and management of acute otitis media in the urgent care setting. Ann Emerg Med 39:413–421, 2002

Niparko JK, Francis HW: Hearing loss and associated problems, in Principles of Ambulatory Medicine, 6th Edition. Edited by Barker LR, Burton JR, Zieve PD, et al. Philadelphia, PA, Lippincott Williams & Wilkins, 2003, pp 1685–1697

Rothman R, Owens T, Dimel DL: Does this child have acute otitis media? JAMA 290:1633–1640, 2003

Rutka J: Acute otitis externa: treatment and perspectives. Ear Nose Throat 83:20–21, 2004

Tintinalli A, Lucchesi M: Common disorders of the external, middle, and inner ear, in Emergency Medicine: A Comprehensive Study Guide, 5th Edition. Edited by Tintinalli JE, Kelen GD, Stapczynski JS. New York, McGraw-Hill, 2000, pp 1518–1526

Turner RB: New considerations in the treatment and prevention of rhinovirus infections. Pediatr Ann 34:53–57, 2005

# CHAPTER 31

# Dysuria and Pyuria

## Vicki Figen, M.D.

## Clinical Presentation

Dysuria is the sensation of painful burning with urination. It is important to rule out external dysuria that is caused by the passage of urine over irritated vaginal mucosa, most likely caused by a vaginal discharge or vaginal irritation (Kurowski 1998). Pyuria is the presence of white blood cells (WBCs) in the urine. Pyuria alone does not indicate a urinary tract infection (UTI). UTI is the symptomatic presence of bacteria anywhere in the urinary tract, with pyuria (more than 3–5 WBC/mm$^3$ of urine).

## Differential Diagnosis

The presumptive diagnosis of an uncomplicated lower UTI can be made, if necessary, on the basis of symptoms alone, which include dysuria, frequency, urgency, and bladder fullness. A urinalysis should show bacteria and WBCs. Hematuria may be present. A lower UTI may progress to acute pyelonephritis with the development of fever, nausea, vomiting, flank pain, or costovertebral angle tenderness (Orenstein and Wong 1999).

## Risk Stratification

The distinction between complicated and uncomplicated UTI is important because it has implications for the duration of the antimicrobial regimen and possible follow-up (Hooton and Stamm 1997).

## Uncomplicated UTI

Uncomplicated UTI occurs in nonpregnant patients with no history of functional or anatomical abnormalities in the genitourinary tract. These infections are caused by a predictable group of organisms and affect otherwise healthy women. Uncomplicated UTIs are treated with a 3-day course of antibiotics (Fihn 2003; Hooton and Stamm 1997). A urine culture is not necessary. Uncomplicated UTIs become complicated if the patient develops fever, chills, vomiting, or flank pain; if these symptoms begin after instrumentation or catheterization; or if the symptoms have persisted for more than 7–10 days before the patient sought treatment (Fihn 2003).

## Complicated UTI

Complicated UTIs are those that occur in the presence of factors that predispose the patient to persistent infection, recurrent infection, or treatment failure. Asymptomatic bacteriuria should not be treated, except in patients who are pregnant, immunosuppressed, or scheduled for a urological procedure and in patients with a change in behavior or mental status without other identifiable cause who are unable to relate symptoms (e.g., patients with dementia or catatonia). In cases of complicated UTI, a urine culture should be done, and the patient should be treated with a 10–14-day course of antibiotics. If the patient's UTI was recently treated with an antibiotic, another suitable agent should be used (Anderson 1999).

UTIs in men should always be considered complicated and should be treated for 7–14 days with a suitable agent after urine has been obtained for culture and sensitivity testing. UTIs most commonly occur in older men with prostatic disease or outlet obstruction or who have undergone urinary tract instrumentation (Orenstein and Wong 1999).

# Assessment and Management in Psychiatric Settings

Trimethoprim-sulfamethoxazole is the drug of choice for patients who are not allergic to the two antibiotics and in settings where the prevalence of resistant organisms is less than 15%. The fluoroquinolones ciprofloxacin and levofloxacin are equally effective, but they are more expensive and may promote multidrug resistance. Both of these types of treatment provide excellent coverage for infections with *Escherichia coli* and *Staphylococcus saprophyticus* but inadequate coverage for *Enterococcus faecalis* (Anderson 1999) (see Figure 31–1).

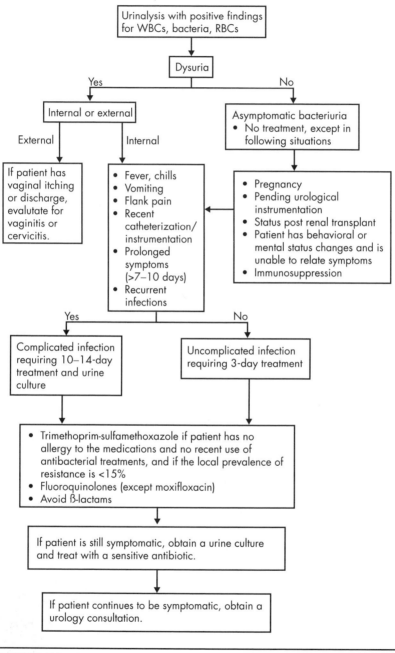

**FIGURE 31–1.** Algorithm for evaluation of urinary tract infection.

*Note.* RBC=red blood cell; WBC=white blood cell.

These therapies may lead to Q–Tc prolongation and should be used cautiously in patients who are taking second-generation antipsychotic drugs (Anderson 1999). The β-lactam antibiotics ampicillin and amoxicillin are best avoided because of frequent resistance and low cure rates (McCarty et al. 1999). In female patients with an uncomplicated UTI, a 3-day course of antibiotics should be prescribed. A urine culture is not necessary. For patients with complicated infections, a urine culture must be done, and the correct antibiotic should be given for a total of 7–10 days in female patients and 14 days in male patients (Harding et al. 2002). Routine posttreatment cultures in asymptomatic patients are not indicated. If symptoms do not resolve by the end of treatment or recur within 2 weeks, a urine culture and sensitivity testing should be performed. In this case, one should assume that the infecting organism is not susceptible to the agent originally used, and the patient should be re-treated with a 7–10-day regimen of a different suitable agent (McCarty et al. 1999).

Patient education strategies help prevent recurrent infection. If UTIs are clearly correlated with sexual intercourse in young sexually active women, the patient should be instructed to urinate immediately after intercourse and to avoid the use of spermicidal creams or jelly (Kurowski 1998). Postmenopausal women with frequent UTIs must be referred for gynecological consultation, as they may benefit from topical estrogen treatment of atrophic vaginitis.

## References

Anderson RU: Management of lower urinary tract infections and cystitis. Urol Clin N Am 26:729–735, 1999

Fihn SD: Acute uncomplicated urinary tract infection in women. N Engl J Med 349:259–266, 2003

Harding G, Zhanel G, Nicole LE, et al: Antimicrobial treatment in diabetic women with asymptomatic bacteriuria. N Engl J Med 347:1576–1583, 2002

Hooton TM, Stamm WE: Diagnosis and treatment of uncomplicated urinary tract infection. Infect Dis Clin N Am 11:551–581, 1997

Kurowski K: The women with dysuria. Am Fam Physician 57:2155–2164, 2169–2170, 1998

McCarty JM, Richard G, Huck W, et al: A randomized trial of short-course ciprofloxacin, ofloxacin, or trimethoprim/sulfamethoxazole for the treatment of acute urinary tract infection in women. Am J Med 106: 292–299, 1999

Orenstein R, Wong ES: Urinary tract infections in adults. Am Fam Physician 59:1225–1234, 1999

# CHAPTER 32

# Cough

## Gnanaraj Joseph, M.D.

## Clinical Presentation

Cough is the most common reason for which patients seek medical care, accounting for 38% of outpatient pulmonary care visits. Cough can be caused by many disorders and by any condition that stimulates cough receptors. Categorization is according to the duration of symptoms, which is described as acute (<3 weeks), subacute (3–8 weeks), or chronic (>8 weeks). Acute and subacute coughs are usually transient and have minor consequences; however, they can be associated with life-threatening events such as pulmonary embolism, congestive heart failure, or pneumonia.

## Diferential Diagnosis

### Acute Cough

In diagnosing acute cough, a clinical approach based on empirical therapies is recommended. Clinically, upper respiratory tract infections are the leading cause of acute transient cough (see Table 32–1).

*Upper respiratory tract viral infection* is diagnosed when the patient presents with rhinorrhea, sneezing, nasal obstruction, postnasal drip, fever, lacrimation, and pharyngitis and no abnormal findings in the chest examination (Diehr et al. 1984). Cough comes from the stimulation of the cough reflex in the upper respiratory tract by postnasal drip, clearing of the throat, or both.

**TABLE 32–1.**  Causes and treatment of acute cough

| Cause | Therapeutic options |
| --- | --- |
| Common cold (viral rhinosinusitis) | First-generation antihistamines, ipratropium bromide nasal spray |
| Allergic rhinitis | Avoidance of allergens; use of antihistamines, nasal corticosteroids, nasal cromolyn |
| Acute bacterial sinusitis | Dexbrompheniramine, oxymetazoline, antibiotics against common pathogens such as *Streptococcus pneumoniae* and *Haemophilus influenzae* |
| Exacerbation of chronic obstructive pulmonary disease | Ipratropium, oxygen (if $PaO_2 \leq 55$ mm Hg or if $SaO_2 \leq 88\%$), corticosteroids, antibiotics if indicated, cessation of smoking |

*Note.*  $PaO_2$=partial pressure of oxygen in arterial blood; $SaO_2$=oxygen saturation.

*Allergic rhinitis* can also produce acute cough. Avoidance of allergen is key to controlling symptoms. Nasal corticosteroids may be of some benefit. Also, nonsedating antihistamine therapy can be useful. Antibiotic therapy should be avoided unless there is suspicion of bacterial superinfection (Madison and Irwin 1998).

*Exacerbations of chronic obstructive pulmonary disease* can present with worsening cough with sputum production and dyspnea. In the physical examination, wheezing or diminished breath sounds may be present.

In evaluating a patient with acute cough, it is important to rule out lower respiratory tract infection (i.e., pneumonia). The patient should be asked about smoking, sputum secretion, travel, and gastrointestinal symptoms. A complete physical examination should be performed, and consultation should be sought for a complete examination of the chest. If there are abnormal findings in the lung examination and the patient is a nonsmoker with a history consistent with community-acquired pneumonia, the patient should be empirically treated with antibiotics.

*Bacterial sinusitis* is often difficult to distinguish from viral rhinosinusitis (common cold) (Madison and Irwin 1998). It should be suspected if the patient fails to improve when treated with antihistamines and decongestants or if the patient has at least two of the following symptoms: maxillary pain, toothache; purulent nasal secretions; abnormal findings on transillumination of any sinus; and a history of discolored nasal discharge. Imaging studies of the sinuses are not usually necessary, but antibiotics are recommended (Williams et al. 1992).

**TABLE 32–2.** Causes and treatment of subacute cough

| Cause | Therapeutic options |
|---|---|
| Previous infection | First-generation antihistamines with decongestants, ipratropium bromide, central antitussives, systemic corticosteroids if cough persists |
| *Bordetella pertussis* infection | Erythromycin or trimethoprim-sulfamethoxazole for 14 days |
| Subacute bacterial sinusitis | Treatment is similar to that for acute bacterial sinusitis (see Table 32–1), except for a 3-week course of an antihistamine-decongestant combination and antibiotics. |
| Asthma | β-Agonists, inhaled corticosteroids, leukotriene inhibitors, oral steroids |

## Subacute Cough

Patients with subacute cough should receive the same evaluation given to patients with chronic cough (see the next section, "Chronic Cough"). When subacute cough follows respiratory infection, conditions such as postinfectious cough, bacterial sinusitis, and asthma should be considered (see Table 32–2).

Postinfectious cough begins with an acute respiratory tract infection (Irwin et al. 1998) and is caused by postnasal drip, rhinitis, or tracheobronchitis. It is sometimes associated with transient bronchial hyperresponsiveness. If the patient has postnasal drip and frequent clearing of the throat or if mucus is seen in the oropharynx, a course of treatment similar to that for the common cold is recommended.

Should the cough persist beyond 1 week of treatment, imaging studies of the sinuses should be obtained to rule out bacterial sinusitis. If there are abnormal findings in the chest examination, a chest radiograph should be obtained. If the findings of the chest examination are normal, a short course of inhaled bronchodilators and corticosteroids is recommended. However, cough may be the sole presenting manifestation of asthma (as in cough-variant asthma).

## Chronic Cough

Although cough that lasts longer than 8 weeks can be caused by many different diseases, most cases are attributable to a few diagnoses (see Table 32–3). The most common causes include postnasal drip syndrome,

**TABLE 32-3.**   Causes and treatment of chronic cough

| Cause | Therapeutic options |
| --- | --- |
| Postnasal drip syndromes (nonallergic rhinitis, allergic rhinitis, vasomotor rhinitis) | Antihistamine-decongestant, ipratropium bromide, nasal corticosteroids, avoidance of allergens |
| Chronic bacterial sinusitis | Antibiotics for 6 weeks, nasal decongestant with antihistamines |
| Asthma | β-Agonists, inhaled corticosteroids, leukotriene inhibitors (Cough may take 6–8 weeks to resolve.) |
| Gastroesophageal reflux disease | Diet restriction, lifestyle modification, elevation of head end of bed, histamine type 2 agonist or proton pump inhibitor, prokinetic agents, surgery (Nissen fundoplication) |
| Chronic bronchitis | Elimination of irritants (smoking cessation), ipratropium bromide |
| Effect of angiotensin-converting enzyme inhibitors | Discontinuation of drug (Cough usually improves in 4 weeks. If this class of drugs is necessary, switch to angiotensin II receptor antagonist.) |
| Eosinophilic bronchitis | Inhaled corticosteroids (oral steroids may sometimes be required), avoidance of irritants (acrylates) |
| Others: Interstitial lung disease, bronchogenic carcinoma, left ventricular failure, pharyngeal dysfunction, sarcoidosis | Individual therapeutic options vary |

asthma, and gastroesophageal reflux disease (GERD) (Irwin et al. 1990, 1998). It is interesting to note that a single cause is responsible for chronic cough in 39%–75% of patients, and more than one cause is responsible in the remaining proportion of patients (Irwin et al. 1990; Mello et al. 1996).

*Postnasal drip* is the most common cause of persistent cough (Irwin et al. 1990). Underlying reasons for postnasal drip include acute nasopharyngitis, sinusitis, and allergic, perennial nonallergic, and vasomotor rhinitis. However, postnasal drip may also be "silent," and the absence of these symptoms does not necessarily exclude the diagnosis (Pratter et al. 1993). Clues in the physical examination are a cobblestone appearance to the nasopharyngeal mucosa and the presence of secretions in the nasopharynx. When a specific cause for cough is not apparent, empirical therapy for postnasal drip should be attempted before starting an extensive diagnostic evaluation for other etiologies (Irwin et al. 1998).

Cough can be the only symptom of *asthma* (Mello et al. 1996; O'Connell et al. 1991). However, wheezing and dyspnea commonly accompany cough in asthma. Atopy or a family history of asthma helps in the differential diagnosis. Spirometry is necessary to confirm the diagnosis of asthma. In some patients with asthma for whom spirometry results are normal, airway hyperreactivity can be demonstrated by broncho-provocation testing (Corrao et al. 1979). The best way to confirm asthma as a cause of cough is to demonstrate improvement with appropriate therapy, such as inhaled β-agonist therapy, inhaled corticosteroids, or a short trial of oral steroids (Irwin et al. 1997). The maximum symptom benefit of the inhaled corticosteroids may not be seen for 6–8 weeks.

*GERD* is the third most common cause of persistent cough (Irwin et al. 1990, 1998), occurring in 30%–40% of patients with chronic cough (Mello et al. 1996). These patients may also have symptoms such as heartburn; however, gastrointestinal symptoms are absent in more than 75% of patients in whom cough is due to reflux. Possible mechanisms responsible for the cough associated with GERD are stimulation of receptors in the upper respiratory tract by aspiration of gastric contents and esophageal-tracheobronchial cough reflex induced by reflux of acid into the distal esophagus.

Cough that occurs after a viral or other *upper respiratory tract infection* can persist for more than 8 weeks after the acute infection. A viral etiology is usually presumed to be the initial trigger. However, *Bordetella pertussis* is one of the common causes of persistent cough (Wright et al. 1995). Some patients may have unsuspected bacterial suppurative disease of the large airways (Schaefer and Irwin 2003). Most patients with bronchiectasis chronically produce sputum. The lung examination may reveal rhonchi or wheezes. The chest X ray may be suggestive, but examination of the chest with computed tomography with high-resolution imaging is the optimal method of diagnosis.

Cough is one of the main diagnostic features in *chronic bronchitis*. Almost all patients with chronic bronchitis are smokers, except for a small number who have airway inflammation because of exposure to other irritants such as fumes or dusts. However, most smokers do not seek medical attention for their cough, and in most case series of patients with chronic cough, chronic bronchitis accounts for at most 5% of the cases (Irwin et al. 1990). Treatment should be targeted at reduction of sputum production and airway inflammation by removing environmental irritants, particularly through smoking cessation. Treatment may consist of antibiotics, bronchodilators, inhaled steroids, or mucolytics, depending on the severity of the airway obstruction and symptoms (Irwin et al. 1998).

*Bronchogenic carcinoma,* an uncommon cause of chronic cough, is found in only about 2% of cases (Irwin et al. 1998). Most cases that manifest with cough involve neoplasms that originate in the large central airways, where cough receptors are common. Pulmonary lymphangitic carcinomatosis from extrapulmonary malignancies can also present as cough, generally accompanied by dyspnea. A history suggestive of a new cough or a recent change in chronic "smoker's cough," cough that persists more than 1 month after smoking cessation, and/or hemoptysis should raise concern for lung cancer. Chest X ray, sputum cytologies, and flexible bronchoscopy are useful diagnostic procedures in evaluation of possible lung cancer.

A *drug-induced cough* is a well-recognized complication of treatment with angiotensin-converting enzyme (ACE) inhibitors in 3%–20% of patients who take these medications (Israili and Hall 1992). The cough is an effect of this class of drugs and is not dose related. One hypothesis for this effect is that accumulation of bradykinin, which is normally degraded in part by ACE, may stimulate afferent C-fibers in the airway. Drug-induced cough caused by ACE inhibitors usually begins within 1 week of instituting ACE therapy, but it can be delayed up to 6 months (Lacourciere et al. 1994). Treatment consists of discontinuing the ACE inhibitor. The cough usually ends within 1–4 days after discontinuation of the drug, but it can take as long as 4 weeks to resolve (Lacourciere et al. 1994). Sulindac, indomethacin, nifedipine, and inhaled sodium cromoglicate may provide symptomatic relief.

*Psychogenic cough* is a diagnosis of exclusion. Short of observing the results of a therapeutic trial, it is hard to distinguish habit cough from cough caused by postnasal drip syndrome (Irwin et al. 1998).

## Risk Stratification

Pneumonias acquired in the community or hospital are often due to oropharyngeal aspiration and must be promptly treated to avoid serious morbidity and mortality in the elderly, patients with degenerative

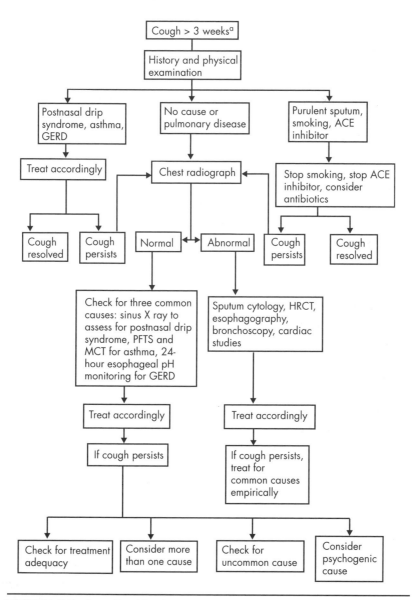

**FIGURE 32–1.** Algorithm for evaluation of cough.

*Note.* ACE=angiotensin-converting enzyme; GERD=gastroesophageal reflux disorder; HRCT=high-resolution computed tomography; MCT=methacholine challenge test; PFTS=pulmonary function test.

aA clinical approach is recommended in evaluation of cough lasting <3 weeks (acute cough), depending on the cause (see Table 32–1).

neurological disorders, and patients with neuroleptic-induced dysphagia (Marik and Kaplan 2004). At high risk for severe complications are also patients with the increasingly common pertussis infection, a prolonged cough illness associated with pharyngeal discomfort, hoarseness, headaches, episodic diaphoresis, sleep disturbance and weight loss that may lead to pneumonia, seizures, pneumothorax, and rib fractures (Rothstein and Edwards 2005). Clinicians need also be aware that dry cough is the most common symptom of the severe acute respiratory syndrome, a coronavirus infection that leads to pneumonia, respiratory failure, and death in about 10% of patients (Tsang and Seto 2004). Finally, cough with acute onset may be the presenting symptom in patients with pulmonary embolism (Laack and Goyal 2004).

## Assessment and Management in Psychiatric Settings

The following stepwise approach is recommended for evaluation and treatment of cough:

- The patient's history should be reviewed, and a physical examination performed with a focus on common causes of cough.
- A chest X ray should be ordered.
- No additional tests are required in current smokers, patients who are taking ACE inhibitors, and patients with a recent upper respiratory tract infection at the onset of the cough.
- A stepwise diagnostic approach (see Figure 32–1) helps the physician to stratify the risk and proceed from simple and less invasive tests (sinus and chest radiography and methacholine challenge) to more invasive studies (esophageal pH monitoring and bronchoscopy).
- The causes of cough may be determined by observing which specific therapy eliminates the cough as a complaint. If the evaluation suggests more than one possible cause, therapies should be initiated in the same sequence in which the abnormalities were discovered.
- The role of empirical therapy in diagnosis of the cause of chronic cough has not been rigorously studied. A detailed history and a physical examination with empirical treatment are sometimes more cost-effective than rigorous testing in the management of cough.

## References

Corrao WM, Braman SS, Irwin RS: Chronic cough as the sole presenting manifestation of bronchial asthma. N Engl J Med 300:633–637, 1979

Diehr P, Wood RW, Bushyhead JB, et al: Prediction of pneumonia in outpatients with acute cough—a statistical approach. J Chronic Dis 37:215–225, 1984

Irwin RS, Curley FJ, French CL: Chronic cough: the spectrum and frequency of causes, key components of the diagnostic evaluation, and outcome of specific therapy. Am Rev Respir Dis 141:640–647, 1990

Irwin RS, French CT, Smyrnios NA, et al: Interpretation of positive results of a methacholine inhalation challenge and 1 week of inhaled bronchodilator use in diagnosing and treating cough-variant asthma. Arch Intern Med 157:1981–1987, 1997

Irwin RS, Boulet L-P, Cloutier MM, et al: Managing cough as a defense mechanism and as a symptom: a consensus panel report of the American College of Chest Physicians. Chest 114(suppl):133S–181S, 1998

Israili ZH, Hall WD: Cough and angioneurotic edema associated with angiotensin-converting enzyme inhibitor therapy: a review of the literature and pathophysiology. Ann Intern Med 117:234–242, 1992

Laack TA, Goyal DG: Pulmonary embolism: an unsuspected killer. Emerg Med Clin North Am 22:961–963, 2004

Lacourciere Y, Brunner H, Irwin R, et al: Effects of modulators of the renin-angiotensin-aldosterone system on cough. J Hypertens 12:1387–1393, 1994

Madison JM, Irwin RS: Chronic obstructive pulmonary disease. Lancet 352:467–473, 1998

Marik PE, Kaplan D: Aspiration pneumonia and dysphagia in the elderly. Chest 124:328–336, 2003

Mello CJ, Irwin RS, Curley FJ: Predictive values of the character, timing, and complications of chronic cough in diagnosing its cause. Arch Intern Med 156:997–1003, 1996

O'Connell EJ, Rojas AR, Sachs MI: Cough-type asthma: a review. Ann Allergy 66:278–282, 285, 1991

Pratter MR, Bartter T, Akers S, et al: An algorithmic approach to chronic cough. Ann Intern Med 119:977–983, 1993

Rothstein E, Edwards K: Health burden of pertussis in adolescents and adults. Pediatr Infect Dis J 24(suppl):S44–47, 2005

Schaefer OP, Irwin RS: Unsuspected bacterial suppurative disease of the airways presenting as chronic cough. Am J Med 114:602–606, 2003

Tsang K, Seto WH: Severe acute respiratory syndrome: scientific and anecdotal evidence for drug treatment. Curr Opin Investig Drugs 5:179–185, 2004

Williams JW Jr, Simel DL, Roberts L, et al: Clinical evaluation for sinusitis: making the diagnosis by history and physical examination. Ann Intern Med 117:705–710, 1992

Wright SW, Edwards KM, Decker MD, et al: Pertussis infection in adults with persistent cough. JAMA 273:1044–1046, 1995

# PART VIII

# Skin and Soft Tissue Abnormalities

Section Editor:

Barbara J. Barnett, M.D.

# CHAPTER 33

# Dermatological Disorders

## Steven A. Valassis, M.D.

## Common Bacterial Skin Infections

### Clinical Presentation

#### Impetigo

Impetigo is a highly contagious superficial skin infection that generally involves the face and is more commonly seen in the pediatric population. It is commonly caused by *Staphylococcus* or *Streptococcus* species. Impetigo has two forms: bullous and nonbullous. In the bullous form, the lesions coalesce to form large bullae with clear fluid. The vesicles mature and collapse, leaving the pathognomonic honey-colored crusts overlying erythematous, nonulcerated skin (Brown et al. 2003).

#### Ecthyma

Ecthyma is a bacterial skin infection that is very similar to impetigo. In some individuals, it is a chronic form of impetigo. Patients with ecthyma have vesicles similar to those seen in impetigo that lead to crusts. The crusts in ecthyma are thicker than those in impetigo and appear "punched out." Group A β-hemolytic streptococci are responsible for the initial infection, although the lesions are usually coinfected with staphylococci.

#### Cellulitis

Cellulitis is an infection involving the skin and underlying subcutaneous tissue. The offending pathogen, usually *Staphylococcus aureus* or *Streptococcus pyogenes*, often gains entrance to the body through breakdowns in the skin but can also spread through lymphatic or hematogenous dissemination. Cellulitis presents with painful, erythematous skin that is warm and exhibits localized swelling. The erythema blanches with pressure and has indistinct borders. The infection can occur anywhere on the body, although it has a predilection for the extremities (Brady et al. 2004).

### Erysipelas

Erysipelas is a more superficial cellulitis traditionally thought to be caused by group A β-hemolytic streptococci. Although historically known to involve the face, it is also commonly seen in the lower extremities and in patients with chronic lymphedema. The pathogen invades the skin and then spreads through the lymphatic system. Patients exhibit an acute onset with high fever, chills, malaise, and nausea, followed by painful "burning," erythematous skin within 24–48 hours of the constitutional symptoms. Red, shiny, warm plaques that are well demarcated from the surrounding tissue occur.

### Fasciitis

Fasciitis refers to an infection that has spread from a simple cellulitis to one involving the fascial layers deep to the subcutaneous tissue. This condition is a medical emergency and requires immediate medical and surgical care. Patients with fasciitis appear toxic and manifest a febrile response and derangements in their vital signs from mere tachycardia to frank shock. These patients appear sicker than expected on the basis of the cutaneous involvement and may describe pain out of proportion to the physical findings. Severe edema and necrotic tissue may be seen (Green et al. 1996).

## Risk Stratification

Fasciitis should always be suspected in patients with abnormal vital signs and quickly spreading infection. This condition constitute a medical emergency.

Patients with cellulitis and erysipelas may require hospital admission if they have abnormal vital signs, lymphangitis, and premorbid conditions such as immunocompromised states and diabetes.

## Assessment and Management in Psychiatric Settings

A systematic approach should be taken in dealing with patients with cutaneous findings (see Figure 33–1). The patient's complete set of vital signs should be measured, and the patient should be completely un-

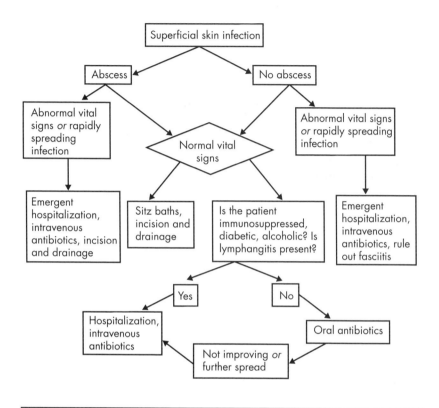

**FIGURE 33-1.**    Algorithm for assessment and treatment of superficial skin infections.

dressed so that the entire body can be examined. In the history, any recent changes in medication or past skin eruptions should be noted, and the presence of immunocompromised states, including alcohol abuse and diabetes, should be determined.

Careful attention should be taken in measuring vital signs and in assessing the overall appearance of the patient and any recent changes in the patient's appearance. It may be prudent to check the patient's rectal temperature, because this measurement has been shown to be more sensitive than the traditional oral temperature. Patients with a fever and those who are lethargic or are toxic-appearing require immediate referral to an emergency department.

The margins of the infection should be marked on the skin with a pen so that the rate of spread of the infection can be noted. An X ray should be taken of the area involved to check for the presence of foreign bodies and for subcutaneous emphysema, which is seen in gas gangrene. Tetanus immunization status should be assessed, and the standard dose of tetanus toxoid should be administered if needed (Brady et al. 2004).

Impetigo is treated with the topical antibiotic mupirocin (2% ointment). Studies have shown that this regimen is as efficacious as oral antibiotics (Stulberg et al. 2002). In addition, washing the skin with antimicrobial soaps and removing crusts by soaking them with warm compresses to facilitate topical antibiotic absorption hastens healing. Patients with ecthyma can be treated similarly to those with impetigo, although patients with ecthyma require oral antibiotics in addition to topical antibiotics.

Cellulitis should be treated with an antistaphylococcal, antistreptococcal antibiotic such as a first-generation cephalosporin or a macrolide. Patients with diabetes, immunosuppressed states, or a limb-threatening infection should receive a broader-spectrum antibiotic such as ampicillin-sulbactam. Patients in whom cellulitis is superimposed on lymphedema or who have a high fever have a higher prevalence of bacteremia, and a blood culture is indicated (Swartz 2004). Parenteral antibiotics are recommended in patients with infections that involve large portions of the extremities, face, neck, and perineum; in patients with any immunosuppressed state, including diabetes and alcoholism; and in patients with lymphangitis (Trubo et al. 1997).

Erysipelas, unlike simple cases of cellulitis, requires parenteral antibiotics, for example, penicillin G. Extended-spectrum antibiotics are warranted in patients with severe cases of erysipelas and in diabetic patients.

If fasciitis is suspected, immediate medical and surgical consultation is paramount. The patient requires aggressive fluid resuscitation, careful monitoring of electrolyte abnormalities, and parenteral broad-spectrum antibiotics (Brady et al. 2004).

Patients who are beginning oral antibiotic therapy for simple cellulitis should have medical follow-up within 24–48 hours. If the erythema does not diminish, if it spreads beyond the demarcated area, or if the patient develops a fever, immediate medical evaluation is indicated.

Patients with impetigo should be observed for the development of signs of renal insufficiency with nephritis about 10 days after the skin infection. Signs of renal insufficiency include hematuria and proteinuria seen in a urinary analysis, and this test can be used to screen patients. The overall incidence of acute nephritis with impetigo is 5% and can be as high as 15% with certain strains of *Streptococcus*.

## Cutaneous Abscesses

### Clinical Presentation

An abscess is a collection of pus within the soft tissue secondary to infection that is localized and surrounded by a wall of indurated granulation tissue. The area is tender, has a fluctuant center, and may have surrounding erythema and lymphangitis. Abscesses can occur anywhere on the body but most often occur in the neck, axillae, extremities, and inguinal and perirectal areas.

### Differential Diagnosis

#### Folliculitis

Folliculitis is the invasion of a hair follicle by skin flora, which causes inflammation and erythema and results in formation of a small pustule surrounding the hair.

#### Furuncles and Carbuncles

Furuncles and carbuncles are infections that spread from a simple folliculitis. A furuncle is the extension of a superficial folliculitis to the deeper and surrounding tissue, where a small abscess is formed. A carbuncle is a collection of furuncles that have developed interconnected sinuses below the skin. The offending organism is generally a *Staphylococcus* or *Streptococcus* species (Rhody 2002).

#### Hidradenitis Suppurativa

Hidradenitis suppurativa is a disease of repeated abscess formation in infected apocrine sweat glands. It is seen more often in women, and it is believed that obesity, poor hygiene, excessive perspiration, and shaving further exacerbate the condition. These abscesses may drain spontaneously and have scant pus. They often occur in the axillae but are also commonly seen in the inguinal and perianal areas. Analogous to carbuncle formation, these abscesses may also become interconnected and form extensive sinus tracts below the skin (Meislin and Guisto 2002).

#### Pilonidal Abscess

Pilonidal abscesses occur in the superior portion of the gluteal fold overlying the coccyx. The natural history of a pilonidal abscess is minor trauma resulting in disruption of the skin's protective barrier. A small cavity lined by squamous epithelium is created at the site of trauma. The resulting cavity may become blocked by hair or keratin and act as a nidus for bacterial invasion and abscess formation (Meislin and Guisto 2002).

### Bartholin Cyst Abscess

Bartholin cyst abscesses occur in sexually active women with obstruct-ed Bartholin ducts. These ducts are located on the inferior-lateral mar-gin of the vaginal vestibule at the 5- and 7-o'clock positions. The ducts are secretory and can become obstructed and invaded by normal vagi-nal flora or, in approximately 10% of cases, by *Neisseria gonorrhoeae* or *Chlamydia trachomatis*.

### Perianal and Perirectal Abscesses

Perianal and perirectal abscesses involve the crypts surrounding the anus. These abscesses tend to be caused by fecal flora and have mixed aerobic and anaerobic pathogens. The condition may spread to involve the deeper tissue below. These abscesses are most often seen in adult men (Meislin and Guisto 2002).

## Risk Stratification

The cutaneous abscesses, although painful and unpleasant, do not often constitute a medical emergency. Patients with a cutaneous abscess should have normal vital signs and be afebrile. If the patient is febrile or the infection has spread beyond the confines of the abscess, immedi-ate medical care must be obtained. Patients who are immunocompro-mised need more aggressive management. Perirectal abscesses that have spread into deeper tissue planes may require surgical debride-ment.

## Assessment and Management in Psychiatric Settings

The definitive treatment for abscesses is incision and drainage (see Fig-ure 33–1). During the incision and drainage, loculate collections of pus and debris must be disrupted and drained for resolution to occur. The resulting cavity can then be loosely packed with gauze to facilitate drainage. Antibiotics are indicated only if there is surrounding cellulitis. The patient requires a follow-up medical visit for a wound check and dressing change 24–48 hours after the incision and drainage. If the pa-tient develops a fever or worsening erythema, prompt medical attention is required.

Hidradenitis suppurativa, pilonidal abscess, and Bartholin cyst abscess may have high recurrence rates. It is therefore recommended that patients with recurring abscesses be referred for surgical consultation. In patients with a Bartholin cyst abscess, a cervical culture for gonorrhea and chlamydia should be performed at the time of incision and drainage.

## Erythema Multiforme

### Clinical Presentation

*Erythema multiforme* consists of three separate clinical syndromes caused by drug hypersensitivity reactions that lead to lymphocytic infiltrates and keratinocyte necrosis of the skin and mucous membranes. Although erythema multiforme can affect persons of any age, it is most often seen in young adults and is seen twice as often in male patients as in female patients. Erythema multiforme has severe systemic complications and is associated with a high mortality rate.

### Differential Diagnosis

Stevens-Johnson syndrome (SJS), also known as *erythema multiforme major*, begins as an erythematous rash 1–3 weeks after a drug administration. This eruption spreads symmetrically over the body in 3–4 days. The erythema is tender and is often described as "burning." Blisters develop over the erythematous areas, and necrosis of the skin occurs. There is involvement of mucous membranes, including painful eruptions in the oral, ocular, and genital areas that may result in great morbidity. Patients with SJS have flu-like symptoms such as fever and malaise, develop hypotension, and have detachment of the epidermis on both skin and mucous membranes (Habif 1996).

*Toxic epidermal necrolysis* (TEN) has a presentation similar to that of SJS. Patients with TEN have skin eruptions similar to those in SJS but do not exhibit target lesions. Unlike SJS, which occurs weeks after administration of an offending drug, TEN may develop within a few days after such a drug is taken.

*Erythema multiforme minor* is a disease in the same spectrum as SJS and TEN, but it has few systemic complications. Target and bullous lesions are seen mostly in the extremities, and mucous membrane involvement can be seen.

## Risk Stratification

SJS and TEN are potentially lethal diseases and require aggressive and emergent medical intervention. Regardless of treatment, mortality rates approach 30%. Although erythema multiforme minor has a more benign course that SJS and TEN, patients with a new rash and mucosal involvement associated with drug administration require expedited medical evaluation to rule out the more serious conditions.

## Assessment and Management in Psychiatric Settings

A systematic approach should be taken in dealing with patients with cutaneous findings. The patient's vital signs should be measured, and the patient should be completely undressed so that the entire body can be examined. In the history, any recent changes in medication and history of past skin eruptions should be noted. Patients exhibiting a fever, lethargy, hypotension, or difficulty breathing or controlling their oral secretions and those with any mucosal involvement require immediate medical care to rule out an anaphylactic-type reaction or erythema multiforme. Other patients may be seen by an internal medicine or dermatology consultant. Patients who require immediate medical care should be transferred to the nearest emergency department, preferably one that is a burn treatment center.

The manufacturers' reports indicate that many common psychiatric drugs have caused either SJS or TEN (Physicians' Desk Reference 2004). The list includes the antipsychotics fluphenazine, chlorpromazine, and clozapine; the antidepressant mirtazapine; and the mood stabilizers lamotrigine, gabapentin, carbamazepine, and valproic acid.

Whether the patient has SJS or TEN, the basic approach to treatment is similar. The patient requires immediate medical evaluation and admission to an intensive care or burn unit. The offending drug should be discontinued. Aggressive intravenous fluid administration and careful electrolyte monitoring are paramount. The patient's airway should be carefully monitored. Prophylactic antibiotics are not indicated. There is a role for intravenous immunoglobulin early in the course of the disease, and trials of intravenous steroids have been used with various levels of success. Patients with minimal symptoms may be treated on an outpatient basis with close medical and dermatological follow-up. These patients may benefit from topical corticosteroids and oral antihistamines.

# Common Drug Reactions

## Clinical Presentation

### Maculopapular Rash

The most common drug reaction is maculopapular rash. It consists of erythematous macules and papules that occur symmetrically and are often pruritic. The lesions become confluent, may occur on mucous membranes, and can be seen on the palms and soles. The rash tends to occur 7–10 days after a new medication is started, and it is indistinguishable from viral exanthems (Habif 1996). The following common psychiatric medications have been known to cause maculopapular rashes: haloperidol, olanzapine, carbamazepine, lamotrigine, gabapentin, and lithium (Physicians' Desk Reference 2004).

### Urticaria

Urticaria is a pruritic rash that consists of red wheals that can be small papules or large plaques. The wheals fade within 1 day, after which new ones emerge in other locations. Urticaria may involve the mucous membranes. Angioedema, a localized nonpitting edema, may occur and can be life-threatening if it involves the oral airway. Drug-induced urticaria can occur through three distinct mechanisms: anaphylactic reaction (which is IgE-mediated and occurs within minutes to hours after drug ingestion), serum sickness (which is mediated by circulating immune complexes and occurs 4–21 days after drug ingestion), and nonimmunologic reaction (a mast cell reaction, which occurs minutes after drug ingestion). Anaphylaxis can lead to systemic shock because of increased permeability and dilation of blood vessels and because of arrested breathing related to airway constriction, airway angioedema, and development of pulmonary edema. The following common psychiatric medications have been known to cause urticaria: phenothiazines, risperidone, tricyclic antidepressants, and mirtazapine (Physicians' Desk Reference 2004).

### Eczematous Eruptions

Eczematous eruptions consist of epidermal inflammation that occurs on the flexural surfaces. In the acute phase, vesicles are present. When they resolve, the affected area shows red, dry, flaky patches of skin that appear "scaly." The following common psychiatric medications have been known to cause eczematous eruptions: fluphenazine, clozapine, and gabapentin (Physicians' Desk Reference 2004).

### Photosensitivity

Photosensitivity reactions are commonly seen with antibiotic use, but they also occur with use of psychiatric medications. Patients exhibit signs of exaggerated sunburn with dry, painful skin within 24 hours of sun exposure. Blistering may occur in severe cases. The rash encompasses only sun-exposed skin, and darker pigmentation occurs upon resolution. Onycholysis can occur with photosensitivity reactions (Habif 1996). The following common psychiatric medications have been associated with photosensitivity: haloperidol, fluphenazine, risperidone, sertraline, and mirtazapine (Physicians' Desk Reference 2004).

### Lichenoid Reaction

Lichenoid reactions present as hyperpigmented papules and plaques. There is involvement of the buccal mucosa, and reticulated, lacelike changes are noted (Habif 1996). Risperidone and carbamazepine have been reported to cause lichenoid reactions (Physicians' Desk Reference 2004).

### Fixed Drug Reaction

A fixed drug reaction appears as single or multiple round, dusky-red plaques or blisters. These plaques are sharply demarcated and can occur anywhere on the body but commonly occur in the perineal area. The reaction tends to occur within a few hours after ingestion of a new drug and to recur in the same area each time the drug is taken. Repeated exacerbations may be milder and may manifest as only a pruritic or burning sensation (Habif 1996). Chlorpromazine and fluphenazine have been reported to cause fixed drug eruptions (Physicians' Desk Reference 2004).

### Cutaneous Vasculitis

Cutaneous vasculitis presents as areas of purpura or petechiae, especially on the lower extremities. In addition, various skin eruptions can occur, including urticarial, bullous, or ulcerative lesions (Habif 1996). Clozapine and lamotrigine have been reported to cause cutaneous vasculitis (Physicians' Desk Reference 2004).

## Risk Stratification

Erythema multiforme and anaphylactic-type reactions are severe drug reactions with cutaneous manifestations than must be quickly identi-

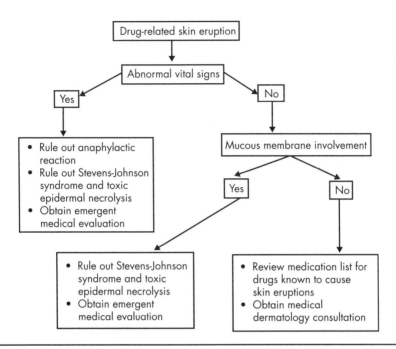

**FIGURE 33–2.** Algorithm for assessment of drug-related skin eruptions.

fied because of the associated high mortality rate. Other drug reactions with cutaneous manifestations, including maculopapular rash, urticaria, eczematous eruptions, photosensitivity, lichenoid reactions, fixed drug reactions, and cutaneous vasculitis, are not life-threatening.

## Assessment and Management in Psychiatric Settings

A systematic approach should be taken in dealing with patients with cutaneous findings (see Figure 33–2). The patient's complete set of vital signs should be measured, and the patient should be completely undressed so that the entire body can be examined. In the history, any recent changes in medication and history of past skin eruptions should be noted. Patients who exhibit a fever, lethargy, hypotension, wheezing, or difficulty breathing or controlling their oral secretions and those with any mucosal involvement require immediate medical care to rule out an anaphylactic-type reaction or erythema multiforme.

Patients who have urticaria with evidence of angioedema, dyspnea, hypotension, or other signs of an impending anaphylactic reaction require immediate subcutaneous epinephrine and acute emergency medical care. The remainder of the cutaneous reactions can be treated by discontinuing the offending medication and administering oral antihistamines as needed. Patients with photosensitivity reaction should limit their sun exposure and should use sunscreen. Topical corticosteroids may be helpful in relieving maculopapular eruption and lichenoid reactions. Systemic corticosteroids and colchicine are often necessary in treatment of severe cases of drug-induced cutaneous vasculitis (Habif 1996).

Patients with nonemergent skin eruptions may be seen within 1–2 days by a dermatologist or an internist who is comfortable treating dermatological conditions.

## References

Brady WJ, Perron AD, Martin ML: Approach to the dermatologic patient in the emergency department, in Emergency Medicine: A Comprehensive Study Guide, 65th Edition. Edited by Tintinalli JE, Kelen GD, Stapczynski JS. New York, McGraw-Hill, 2004, pp 1507–1512

Brown J, Shriner DL, Schwartz RA, et al: Impetigo: an update. Int J Dermatol 42:251–255, 2003

Green RJ, Dafoe DC, Raffin TA: Necrotizing fasciitis. Chest 110:219–229, 1996

Habif TP: Clinical Dermatology: A Color Guide to Diagnosis and Therapy, 3rd Edition. St. Louis, MO, Mosby, 1996, pp 409–442

Meislin HW, Guisto JA: Soft tissue infections, in Rosen's Emergency Medicine: Concepts and Clinical Practice, 5th Edition. Edited by Marx JA, Hockberger RS, Walls RM, et al. St. Louis, MO, Mosby, 2002, pp 1944–1957

Physicians' Desk Reference, 57th Edition. Montvale, NJ, Medical Economics, 2003

Rhody C: Bacterial infections of the skin. Prim Care 27:459–473, 2002

Stulberg DL, Penrod MA, Blatny RA: Caring for common skin conditions. Am Fam Physician 66:119–124, 2002

Swartz MN: Cellulitis. N Engl J Med 350:904–912, 2004

Trubo R, Bisno AL, Hacker SM, et al: Today's strategies for bacterial skin infections. Patient Care 31:78–94, 1997

# CHAPTER 34

# Edema

## Juliet Caldwell, M.D.

## Clinical Presentation

Edema is palpable swelling produced by excess accumulation of fluid in the body's interstitial space. Its causes are numerous and range in severity from benign to life-threatening, making careful clinical decision making paramount. Astute clinicians consider factors such as edema location, rapidity of onset, associated symptoms, and medical history in order to safely triage patients to their respective levels of care; some patients require urgent emergency department assessment, and others benefit more from outpatient evaluation.

Edema can be a global phenomenon, reflecting an increase in total body fluid caused by renal retention of salt and water. Alternatively, it can be a local phenomenon that reflects trauma to, inflammation of, or incompetent venous return from a particular part of the body. Edema is most often pitting, that is, the fluid shifts to other local areas when the edematous area is pressed, leaving an indentation in the skin and soft tissue. Nonpitting edema is usually seen when the fluid is protein rich, such as in lymphatic incompetence (Braunwald 1998); it may otherwise reflect skin changes from long-standing disease or an infiltrative process such as myxedema or lipedema, an unusual phenomenon sometimes seen in young women (Ciocon et al. 1993; Powell and Armstrong 1997).

## Differential Diagnosis

### Bilateral Edema

Systemic processes that increase total body fluid manifest as generalized edema. This condition is often first noted as bilateral leg edema because fluid collection is most prominent in dependent areas of the body.

In bedridden patients edema may first collect in the presacral area (Braunwald 1998). Most patients with generalized edema have advanced cardiac, renal, hepatic, or nutritional deficiencies.

*Congestive heart failure, valvulopathies, and restrictive and constrictive heart diseases* lead to decreased cardiac output and a reduction in the glomerular filtration rate; these reductions result in the subsequent upregulation of aldosterone and the accumulation of excess total body salt and water (Braunwald 1998). In the physical examination, patients with these conditions might exhibit high jugular venous pressure. In left heart failure, patients may also complain of orthopnea and paroxysmal nocturnal dyspnea; the physical examination can reveal bilateral crackles, and a chest X ray may show evidence of pulmonary edema. In *pulmonary hypertension* high pulmonary pressures result in congestion of the right heart and a subsequent elevation in venous pressures (Blankfield et al. 1998). Echocardiography, the single most useful test for pulmonary hypertension, should be performed without delay. If respiratory symptoms or signs (dyspnea, tachypnea, or decreased oxygen saturation) accompany the bilateral edema, if the patient's history is suggestive of a recent cardiac event (chest pain, nausea, diaphoresis), or if the patient presents with acute onset or worsening of edema, the patient should be transferred immediately to a medical unit to rule out an acute cardiac event such as a myocardial infarction.

Decreased oncotic pressure also leads to generalized or bilateral leg edema. The decreased oncotic pressure may be secondary to decreased intake and absorption of protein, impaired albumen synthesis, or increased loss of protein (O'Brien et al. 2005). *Renal disease* is a fairly common cause of outpatient hypoproteinic edema. The *nephrotic syndrome* is a clinical entity characterized by hypoalbuminemia, pronounced proteinuria, edema, hyperlipidemia, and hypercoagulability (Braunwald 1998; Cho and Atwood 2002). Bedside urinalysis to check for proteinuria is an easy test that can help suggest nephrotic syndrome. Hematuria and hypertension coupled with new-onset edema might signal acute *glomerulonephritis. Chronic renal insufficiency* can also cause edema as a result of inadequate salt and water excretion.

*Cirrhosis* causes hypoalbuminemic edema because of decreased protein synthesis in the diseased liver. The clinician can attempt to elicit a history of alcohol abuse or hepatitis and can search for supporting evidence of ascites, caput medusae, jaundice, abnormal liver function tests, and prolonged prothrombin time (Braunwald 1998). Patients with edema secondary to cirrhosis require referral for treatment of the underlying disease. Hypoalbuminemia secondary to *malnutrition* is a common cause of generalized edema in the chronically ill patient with poor feeding. The clinician can usually elicit a history of anorexia, and the physical examination reveals a cachectic yet edematous patient. *Malabsorption* can be suggested by a history of intestinal surgery or a complaint of chronic diarrhea. These disease states generally require close outpatient evaluation.

Generalized or bilateral leg edema occurs in 80% of *pregnancies*. The edema is caused by a number of factors, most obviously by uterine compression of the iliac vessels, which results in elevated hydrostatic pressure and extravasation of fluid. The normal edema of pregnancy forms gradually and does not require any particular intervention. However, it is critical to understand that pregnancy itself predisposes the pregnant woman to thrombosis. A high level of clinical suspicion for deep vein thrombosis must prevail when a pregnant patient is being evaluated for new-onset or asymmetric leg edema. In addition, sudden onset of non-pitting edema—particularly of the hands and face—in a *hypertensive* pregnant patient beyond her first trimester signals the need for emergency department evaluation for likely *preeclampsia* (Castro 1998). Proteinuria further supports this diagnosis. A potentially fatal disease, preeclampsia requires aggressive inpatient blood pressure control and seizure prophylaxis and may ultimately necessitate emergent delivery of the fetus (Castro 1998).

Pretibial myxedema is caused by *hyperthyroidism* and *hypothyroidism*, although it is more commonly seen in the latter (Braunwald 1998; Cho and Atwood 2002). Pretibial myxedema is a nonpitting, rubbery edema over the tibia and is thought to be secondary to the accumulation of mucopolysaccharides (Braunwald 1998; Cho and Atwood 2002). Edema of the hands and eyelids is often observed as well (Cho and Atwood 2002). The clinician can search for historical evidence such as heat/cold intolerance, depression, agitation, psychosis, weight change, and altered bowel habits. The physical examination may reveal tachycardia, bradycardia, exophthalmos, or goiter.

Bulky *pelvic* or *intra-abdominal tumors* can cause bilateral leg edema by compression of the iliac vessels or inferior vena cava. The edema is of gradual onset and often develops in the context of anemia, weight loss, and fatigue. Tumors and masses in the thorax or mediastinum can likewise cause the *superior vena cava (SVC) syndrome*. The tumor compresses the SVC, causing gradual venous congestion of the face, neck, arms, and brain. There is plethora and fullness of the face as well as mild edema of the arms and head. Headache can indicate increased cerebral pressure, and papilledema may be noted in the physical examination.

Any patient with suspected SVC syndrome should be transferred to the nearest emergency department so that decompressive treatment with steroids and diuretics can begin immediately (Schamban and Borenstein 2002).

*Lipedema* is a benign condition found in young women; it is characterized by fatty infiltration of the legs, resulting in nonpitting bilateral edema (Powell and Armstrong 1997). *Idiopathic edema* manifests as bilateral lower-extremity pitting edema of unknown etiology often found in young, menstruating women. It is a benign diagnosis of exclusion (Powell and Armstrong 1997).

*Drug-induced edema* is quite common and should be considered in every patient who presents with diffuse swelling (see Table 34–1) (Cho and Atwood 2002; Powell and Armstrong 1997; Wood 1998). Among the psychopharmacological agents, monoamine oxidase inhibitors are generally accepted to cause edema. Anecdotal reports have implicated the tricyclic antidepressants as possible culprits, but no clear evidence has surfaced. Evidence does exist to implicate risperidone in edema formation (Katz et al. 1999), and olanzapine and valproate have been loosely associated with edema (Ettinger et al. 1990). If dangerous causes of edema have been excluded, the clinician may choose to discontinue the potential offending agent and watch for edema resolution.

**TABLE 34-1.**    Drugs that can cause edema and angioedema

**Drugs that can cause edema**

| | |
|---|---|
| Psychotropic medications | Diabetes medications |
| Monoamine oxidase inhibitors | Pioglitazone |
| Olanzapine | Rosiglitazone |
| Risperidone | Troglitazone |
| Tricyclic antidepressants | Nonsteroidal anti-inflammatory drugs |
| Valproate | (including cyclooxygenase-2 [COX-2] |
| Antihypertensives | inhibitors) |
| β-Blockers | Hormones |
| Calcium channel blockers | Corticosteroids |
| Clonidine | Estrogen |
| Diazoxide | Progesterone |
| Guanethidine | Testosterone |
| Hydralazine | **Drugs that can cause angioedema** |
| Methyldopa | Angiotensin-converting enzyme |
| Minoxidil | inhibitors |
| Reserpine | Penicillin |

## Unilateral Edema

The most dangerous cause of unilateral leg (and occasionally arm) edema is *deep vein thrombosis*. Rapid deterioration and death may occur if the clot breaks off and lodges within the pulmonary vasculature. Risk factors for deep vein thrombosis include immobility, trauma, fractures, surgery, smoking while taking an oral contraceptive, recent air travel, hypercoagulability, and previous deep vein thrombosis. The symptoms include unilateral limb swelling that is usually accompanied by pain. The physical examination reveals a swollen, tender calf or leg with or without erythema; a tender cord may be palpated, and Homans' sign can often be elicited. If respiratory symptoms are present, the patient should be sent immediately to the emergency department for treatment of pulmonary embolism. Stable patients can either be sent to the emergency department for evaluation, or, if the clinician is confident of the diagnosis, the patient may be treated with immediate subcutaneous anticoagulation with low-molecular-weight heparin and scheduled for an urgent outpatient Doppler/ultrasound examination. Contraindications to anticoagulation must always be sought before administration.

*Cellulitis* is often difficult to differentiate from deep vein thrombosis. The limb is swollen, hot, and tender to the touch. Fever is often present. Many patients with cellulitis require a Doppler/ultrasound examination to rule out deep vein thrombosis. Treatment consists of intravenous or oral antibiotics.

*Venous stasis* can be unilateral or bilateral. It is a benign chronic condition of incompetent venous valves that is usually caused by trauma or recurrent deep vein thrombosis. Stasis dermatitis (thickening and hyperpigmentation of the involved skin) evolves from long-standing venous insufficiency (Ciocon et al. 1993). Venous stasis is always chronic; acute-onset edema merits thorough evaluation to rule out more dangerous causes of unilateral edema. The diagnosis of venous insufficiency should never be made without prior investigation. Treatment consists of leg elevation and use of compression stockings and diuretics.

*Lymphedema* manifests as chronic painless swelling in one or many extremities. It can be congenital or acquired. In the physical examination, the edema is slow to pit and is usually not associated with erythema, warmth, or tenderness (Ciocon et al. 1993). In the United States, the most common cause of lymphedema is axillary node dissection after breast surgery; the resulting lymphedema occurs in the arm where the node dissection was done.

*Reflex sympathetic dystrophy* is a rare cause of gradual unilateral painful edema. Patients with this condition complain of a painful limb, usually an arm, after some inciting insult, such as a stroke or myocardial infarction. Local trauma to a shoulder or nerve root can also result in reflex sympathetic dystrophy. Over time autonomic instability ensues and the limb becomes discolored, atrophic, and edematous.

*Factitious edema* may be produced by psychiatric patients by means of prolonged application of a tourniquet around a limb (Ciocon et al. 1993).

## Risk Stratification

Rather than pinning down the exact cause, the clinician may find it more important to categorize edema as a sign of an emergent, urgent, or nonurgent condition. The general categories shown in Table 34–2 are guidelines only, and exceptions always exist. Emergent causes require immediate action and usually need emergency evaluation by a physician. Urgent causes require close outpatient follow-up by an internist or specialist within 1–2 days. Nonurgent causes require routine follow-up within a week or two.

## Assessment and Management in Psychiatric Settings

The history should begin with determination of the time course of the edema formation (see Figure 34–1). Edema that has formed over a period of hours to days usually deserves immediate medical attention. Any history of difficulty breathing, chest discomfort, nausea, vomiting, or diaphoresis should be sought. If those symptoms are present, the patient should be evaluated in an emergency department, and the diagnoses of myocardial infarction, cardiac disease, and pulmonary embolism should be excluded. Urinary symptoms such as decreased volume or change in color should arouse suspicion of acute renal failure. In patients who are past 20 weeks of pregnancy, care should be taken to distinguish between the normal edema of pregnancy and the much more ominous diagnoses of deep vein thrombosis and preeclampsia. A history of a recent crush injury, bite, or burn should alert the clinician to the possibility of compartment syndrome (any condition in which a structure such as a nerve or tendon is being constricted in a space).

An increased respiratory rate or low oxygen saturation suggests congestive heart failure or an embolized deep vein thrombosis. Fever may indicate pulmonary embolus, deep vein thrombosis, myocardial

---

**TABLE 34−2.**    Risk stratification of conditions associated with edema

| Emergent | Nonurgent |
|---|---|
| Deep vein thrombosis | Medication-induced lymphedema |
| Compartment syndrome | Chronic venous insufficiency |
| New-onset congestive heart failure (myocardial infarction, valvulopathy, myocardial or pericardial disease, acute renal failure) | Factitious edema |
| | Idiopathic edema |
| | Lipedema |
| | Normal pregnancy |
| Abscess | Reflex sympathetic dystrophy |
| Cellulitis | Popliteal cyst |
| Superior vena cava syndrome | |
| Angioedema | |
| Preeclampsia | |

**Urgent**

Congestive heart failure (without
  pulmonary edema)
Nephrotic syndrome
Glomerulonephritis
Graves' disease (hyperthyroidism)
Hypothyroidism
Cirrhosis
Hypoproteinemia (malnutrition,
  malabsorption)
Venous compression (tumor)
Ruptured muscle or tendon

---

infarction, cellulitis, or abscess. Extremes in blood pressure obviously warrant emergency attention, but even mild hypertension in a woman beyond 20 weeks of pregnancy requires emergent evaluation for preeclampsia. Bilateral crackles on chest auscultation may indicate pulmonary edema. Facial swelling and oropharyngeal swelling are potential emergencies and should be evaluated by an emergency physician. A hoarse or muffled voice is an ominous examination finding and may harbinger airway compromise. Facial plethora with arm swelling suggests SVC syndrome. A patient with new-onset unilateral limb edema should usually be sent to the emergency department to be evaluated with a duplex sonogram to rule out deep vein thrombosis. Pain, warmth, and redness in the affected limb are consistent with cellulitis as well as deep vein thrombosis. The absence of a pulse and the presence

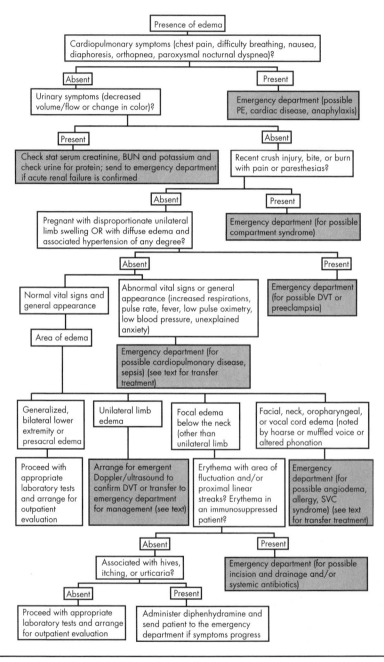

**FIGURE 34–1.** Algorithm for identification of emergency edema.

*Note.*   BUN=blood urea nitrogen; DVT=deep vein thrombosis; PE = pulmonary embolism; SVC=superior vena cava.

of pallor and paresthesias confirm the diagnosis of compartment syndrome, a surgical emergency.

Once these potential emergencies have been ruled out by the history and physical examination, the clinician may proceed with a more detailed assessment. Useful laboratory tests include measurement of blood urea nitrogen and serum creatinine to assess renal function; liver function tests, measurement of the albumin and cholesterol levels, and a coagulation profile to look for malnutrition, malabsorption, and liver failure; and urinalysis and measurement of serum thyroid-stimulating hormone concentration to diagnose proteinuria.

Patients with prominent respiratory symptoms (who may have heart failure, myocardial infarction, pulmonary embolism, or angioedema) should be administered high-flow oxygen and should be propped in an upright sitting position. The patient should be sent swiftly to the emergency department for definitive management.

Urgent and nonurgent causes of edema (see Table 34–2) can await definitive treatment by a medical doctor. Elevation of a swollen limb above the level of the heart can reduce swelling. Removal of any offending medicine is reasonable. It is not recommended that new-onset edema be treated with diuretics, because this strategy yields symptomatic relief only; the cause of the edema should be sought because edema is often the first sign of significant pathology. In general, it is most important to understand that benign causes of edema should never be presumed without definitive evaluation.

## References

Blankfield RP, Finkelhor RS, Alexander JJ, et al: Etiology and diagnosis of bilateral leg edema in primary care. Am J Med 105:192–197, 1998

Braunwald E: Edema, in Harrison's Principles of Internal Medicine, 14th Edition, Vol 1. Edited by Fauci A, Braunwald E, Isselbacher K, et al. New York, McGraw-Hill, 1998, pp 210–214

Castro L: Hypertensive disorders of pregnancy, in Essentials of Obstetrics and Gynecology, 3rd Edition. Edited by Hacker N, Moore J, Gambone J, et al. Philadelphia, PA, WB Saunders, 1998, pp 196–207

Cho S, Atwood JE: Peripheral edema. Am J Med 113:580–586, 2002

Ciocon JO, Fernandez BB, Ciocon DG: Leg edema: clinical clues to the differential diagnosis. Geriatrics 48:34–41, 1993

Ettinger A, Moshe S, Shinnar S: Edema associated with long-term valproate therapy. Epilepsia 31:211–213, 1990

Katz IR, Jeste DV, Mintzer JE, et al: Comparison of risperidone and placebo for psychosis and behavioral disturbances associated with dementia: a randomized, double-blind trial. J Clin Psychiatry 60:107–115, 1999

Powell AA, Armstrong MA: Peripheral edema. Am Fam Physician 55:1721–1726, 1997

O'Brien JG, Chennubhotla SA, Chennubhotla RV: Treatment of edema. Am Fam Physician 71:2111–2117, 2005

Schamban N, Borenstein M: Selected oncologic emergencies, in Rosen's Emergency Medicine: Concepts and Clinical Practice, 5th Edition. Edited by Marx JA, Hockberger RS, Walls RM, et al. St. Louis, MO, Mosby Inc., 2002, pp 1701–1705

Wood A: Adverse reactions to drugs, in Harrison's Principles of Internal Medicine, 14th Edition, Vol 1. Edited by Fauci A, Braunwald E, Isselbacher K, et al. New York, McGraw-Hill, 1998, pp 422–430

# PART IX

# Hematological Abnormalities

Section Editor:

Dilip Patel, M.D.

# CHAPTER 35

# Neutropenia

Rajasrre Roy, M.D.

Manish Sheth, M.D.

Dilip Patel, M.D.

## Clinical Presentation

Neutropenia refers to an absolute neutrophil count (ANC) that is less than two standard deviations below the normal mean value for a certain population. (ANC is calculated by multiplying the total white blood cell count [WBC/μL] by the percentage of neutrophils in the WBC count.) Because the neutrophil count varies by age, sex, race, and other factors, the lower limit for a normal neutrophil count is somewhat variable in different populations. In general, 1,500 neutrophils/μL is considered the lower limit of normal ANC for most children and adults. Blacks may demonstrate slightly lower normal neutrophil counts than whites. The incidence of neutropenia is higher in women and in elderly persons, perhaps reflecting more frequent medication use or other genetic or physiological traits in these populations.

Clinical features of neutropenia vary according to severity, duration of neutropenia, and the presence of other associated immune system deficiencies or comorbidities. Fever is the most common presentation. Underlying infection may manifest as earache, sinus pain or pressure, inflammation around a cut or wound in the skin, dysuria, or diarrhea. Patients may also present with life-threatening infections such as bacterial septicemia, pneumonia, urosepsis, or systemic fungal infections.

---

**TABLE 35-1.**   Causes of neutropenia

---

Pseudoneutropenia

**Acquired neutropenia**
Drugs and chemicals
Felty's syndrome
Immune system causes
Infections (viral, bacterial, protozoal, rickettsial, fungal)
Neutropenia associated with complement activation
Nutritional causes
Splenic sequestration

**Congenital or chronic neutropenia**
Cyclic neutropenia
Chronic benign neutropenia
Idiopathic chronic severe neutropenia
Neutropenia associated with congenital immune defects
Neutropenia associated with phenotypic abnormalities
   Shwachman syndrome
   Cartilage-hair hypoplasia
   Congenital dyskeratosis
   Barth syndrome
   Chédiak-Higashi syndrome
Myelokathexis
Severe congenital neutropenia (Kostmann's syndrome)
Lazy leukocyte syndrome
Metabolic disease

---

# Differential Diagnosis

The causes of neutropenia can be classified in three main groups: pseudoneutropenia, acquired neutropenia, and congenital neutropenia (Table 35–1). Neutropenia is also a common manifestation of bone marrow defects such as myelodysplastic syndrome, leukemia, or aplastic anemia.

## Pseudoneutropenia

Spurious neutropenia can occur in the presence of paraproteinemia and certain anticoagulants, which can cause neutrophil clumping. The neutrophil count can be spuriously low if the blood count is performed by an automated process long after the blood has been drawn. A final cause of pseudoneutropenia is the asymmetrical distribution of circulating neutrophils to the marginal granulocyte pool.

## Acquired Neutropenia

There are many causes of acquired neutropenia. Drug-induced neutropenia occurs with a relatively high frequency in patients who are receiving psychotropic medication or cancer chemotherapy. Infection is the most common cause overall. Other causes of acquired neutropenia include nutritional deficiencies, immune system causes, complement activation, and splenic sequestration.

### Drug-Induced Neutropenia

Several mechanisms for drug-induced neutropenia have been postulated and supported by experimental evidence (see Table 35–2). These mechanisms include immune-mediated destruction of neutrophils or neutrophilic precursors, dose-dependent inhibition of granulopoiesis, and direct toxic effect on the myeloid precursors or the bone marrow microenvironment. Drug-induced immune-mediated neutropenia can occur when the drug acts as a hapten that then induces antibody formation, complement fixation, and subsequent neutrophil destruction. A variant of this process is the formation of circulating immune complexes that bind to neutrophils and destroy them. Phenothiazines may produce neutropenia as a result of dose-dependent inhibition of granulopoiesis. Carbamazepine and valproic acid can cause inhibition of granulocyte-monocyte colony forming units in the bone marrow, and chlorpromazine can cause inhibition of nucleic acid synthesis in myeloid precursor cells. Genetics also plays a role in inducing drug-related neutropenia in certain populations. This role is probably related to inherent differences in drug metabolism and/or clearance, as suggested by the association between clozapine-induced agranulocytosis and the *HLA-B38, DR4,* and *DQw3* alleles in Ashkenazi Jews (Lieberman et al. 1990).

Initial monitoring data after *clozapine* became available for marketing in the United States in 1990 showed that the incidence of agranulocytosis with clozapine therapy was 0.8% at 1 year and 0.91% at 1.5 years (Alvir et al. 1993). The risk of agranulocytosis was higher in elderly and female patients. With weekly monitoring of patients' WBC counts (see Table 35–3), the incidence of agranulocytosis associated with clozapine decreased to 0.38% (versus 0.1% with typical antipsychotics) by the end of the 1990s (Alphs and Anand 1999). The period of highest risk for agran-

**TABLE 35-2.**   Drugs associated with neutropenia

| | |
|---|---|
| **Heavy metals (e.g., gold, mercury, arsenic compounds)** | Ranitidine |
| | Brompheniramine |
| **Analgesics and anti-inflammatory agents** | **Cardiovascular drugs** |
| | Procainamide |
| Aminopyrine | Captopril |
| Phenylbutazone | Propranolol |
| Indomethacin | Hydralazine |
| Ibuprofen | Methyldopa |
| Quinine | Quinidine |
| **Antipsychotics, antidepressants,** | Nifedipine |
| **neuropharmacological agents** | Ticlopidine |
| Phenothiazines (chlorpromazine, | **Antimicrobials** |
| methylpromazine, mepazine, | Penicillins |
| promazine, prochlorperazine, | Cephalosporins |
| thioridazine, trifluoperazine, | Vancomycin |
| trimeprazine) | Chloramphenicol |
| Clozapine | Gentamycin |
| Risperidone | Clindamycin |
| Olanzapine | Metronidazole |
| Imipramine, desipramine | Nitrofurantoin |
| Diazepam, chlordiazepoxide | Doxycycline |
| Meprobamate | Rifampin |
| Thiothixene | Isoniazid |
| Haloperidol | Sulfonamides |
| Riluzole | Antimalarials |
| **Anticonvulsants** | Antivirals (zidovudine, acyclovir, |
| Valproic acid | gancyclovir) |
| Phenytoin | **Miscellaneous** |
| Trimethadione | Allopurinol |
| Carbamazepine | Colchicine |
| Lamotrigine | Famotidine |
| Ethosuximide | Aminoglutethimide |
| Mesantoin | Ethanol |
| **Antithyroid drugs** | Flutamide |
| Thiouracil | Tamoxifen |
| Propylthiouracil | Retinoic acid |
| Methimazole | Omeprazole |
| Carbimazole | Levodopa |
| Potassium perchlorate | Diuretics (e.g., spironolactone, |
| Thiocyanate | acetazolamide, thiazide diuretics) |
| **Antihistamines** | Oral hypoglycemic agents (e.g., |
| Cimetidine | chlorpropamide, tolbutamide) |

ulocytosis is during the first 12–18 weeks after clozapine initiation. Various mechanisms of clozapine-induced agranulocytosis have been proposed. In one proposed mechanism, granulocytes oxidize clozapine to a reactive intermediate that irreversibly binds to the cells, causing agranulocytosis. In another contributory mechanism, clozapine-induced agranulocytosis does not result in a compensatory increase in the level of granulocyte colony stimulating factor (G-CSF) in the body. Researchers have tried to identify ways to predict clozapine-induced agranulocytosis. A WBC elevation of at least 15% above the previous measurement is a sensitive but nonspecific marker for developing agranulocytosis (Alvir et al. 1995). On the other hand, eosinophilia did not prove to be a predictor of neutropenia (Ames et al. 1996). As for the role of G-CSF or granulocyte-macrophage colony stimulating factor (GM-CSF), Chengappa et al. (1996) showed that the average duration of agranulocytosis was not significantly different in G-CSF-treated and -untreated patients, although the treated group had a significantly shorter average duration of hospitalization (8.2 days vs. 13.5 days). This finding was important because many patients experience acute, severe psychosis when clozapine is discontinued after clozapine-induced agranulocytosis is found. A shorter acute hospital stay would permit such patients to be returned rapidly to a psychiatric facility. Clozapine should be used with extreme caution and as the last resort in patients who have experienced drug-induced agranulocytosis and only after obtaining the agreement of hematology and psychopharmacology consultants (Honingfield et al. 1998). Reexposure may be associated with a shorter latency to development of agranulocytosis and a more severe agranulocytosis episode that could lead to death.

In early trials of *olanzapine,* there was no evidence of agranulocytosis or hematological toxicity. However, subsequent reports have included a few cases of prolonged agranulocytosis when olanzapine was used immediately after discontinuation of clozapine (Swartz et al. 1999). It is very rare for olanzapine to cause neutropenia by itself in the absence of exposure to clozapine. The structural similarity between clozapine and olanzapine metabolites could play a role in prolongation of clozapine-induced neutropenia. Another possible contributing factor may be that olanzapine affects the metabolism and clearance of clozapine from the serum. It is prudent to postpone olanzapine therapy in patients with clozapine-induced agranulocytosis until the patient's hematological status has normalized. Both olanzapine- and clozapine-related agranulocytosis respond well to lithium, which acts by stimulating G-CSF and elevating the serum cortisol level.

**TABLE 35–3.** Clinical management of clozapine-related neutropenia

| White blood cell (WBC) count or absolute neutrophil count (ANC) | Clinical findings | Treatment plans |
|---|---|---|
| WBC count 3,000–3,500 cells/µL<br><br><br><br><br><br>ANC ≥1,500 cells/µL | Advise patient to report immediately the appearance of lethargy, fever, sore throat, or weakness. | 1. Monitor patient closely.<br>2. Perform twice-weekly WBC count with differential.<br>3. Clozapine therapy may continue.<br>4. Treat infections appropriately. |
| WBC count 2,000–3,000 cells/µL<br><br><br><br><br><br>ANC 1,000–1,500 cells/µL | Advise patient to report immediately the appearance of lethargy, fever, sore throat, or weakness. | 1. Interrupt clozapine therapy at once, and notify the Clozaril National Registry (CNR).<br>2. Obtain WBC count with differential every day until WBC count is >3,000 cells/µL and ANC is >1,500 cells/µL, then perform twice-weekly WBC count with differential until WBC count >3,500 cells/µL. Treat infections appropriately.<br>3. Clozaril therapy may be reinstituted with twice weekly monitoring when WBC count is ≥3,000 cells/µL and ANC is ≥1,500 cells/µL and no symptoms of infection are present. |

**TABLE 35–3.** Clinical management of clozapine-related neutropenia *(continued)*

| White blood cell (WBC) count or absolute neutrophil count (ANC) | Clinical findings | Treatment plans |
| --- | --- | --- |
| WBC count <2,000 cells/µL<br><br>ANC 500–1,000 cells/µL | Advise patient to report immediately the appearance of lethargy, fever, sore throat, or weakness. | 1. Discontinue clozapine at once, and notify the CNR.<br>2. Obtain hematology consultation.<br>3. Treat infections aggressively.<br>4. Monitor patient daily until WBC and differential counts return to normal (WBC count >3,500 cells/µL and ANC >1,500 cells/µL).<br>5. Clozapine must not be restarted.<br>6. Obtain follow-up WBC counts for at least 4 weeks after discontinuation of clozapine. |

**TABLE 35-3.** Clinical management of clozapine-related neutropenia *(continued)*

| White blood cell (WBC) count or absolute neutrophil count (ANC) | Clinical findings | Treatment plans |
| --- | --- | --- |
| ANC <500 cells/μL | Signs and symptoms of local or systemic infections, with fever, lethargy, weakness, and malaise, may represent a medical emergency. | 1. Discontinue clozapine at once, and notify the CNR.<br>2. Obtain consultation with a hematologist and infectious disease specialist.<br>3. Consider hospital admission if the patient has a fever.<br>4. Consider starting granulocyte colony stimulating factor/granulocyte-macrophage colony stimulating factor within 48 hours of agranulocytosis; continue until ANC is >500 cells/μL.<br>5. Monitor patient daily until WBC count is >3,500 cells/μL and differential count returns to normal.<br>6. Clozapine must not be restarted.<br>7. Obtain follow-up WBC counts for at least 4 weeks after discontinuation of clozapine. |

Case reports have also associated *risperidone* and *quetiapine* with neutropenia in the absence of clozapine. The neutropenia resolved once the offending drug was discontinued (Croarkin and Rayner 2001).

Anticonvulsants used for mood stabilization are also associated with blood dyscrasias, but severe neutropenia is very infrequent. *Carbamazepine* is the more common offender, but neutropenia has also been reported with valproate, phenytoin, and lamotrigine. Careful monitoring of the WBC count is strongly recommended for at least 4 months after the first prescription of these medications (Blackburn et al. 1998; Lambert et al. 2002; Stubner et al. 2004; Tohen et al. 1995).

Tricyclic antidepressants, especially *clomipramine*, have reportedly been associated with severe neutropenia. The newer antidepressant *mirtazapine* is associated with a risk of neutropenia of approximately 1 in 1,000 patients (Gravener et al. 1986; Kasper et al. 1997).

### Infection

Infection is the most common cause of acquired neutropenia in the general population. Viral infection is the most common infectious etiology. Neutropenia caused by infection is usually short-lived. In most acute viral infections, the neutrophil count usually recovers in a few weeks. However, certain viral infections, such as hepatitis, Epstein-Barr virus, and HIV, cause protracted neutropenia. Bacterial septicemia, particularly if caused by a Gram-negative organism, is one of the most serious causes of acquired neutropenia.

### Nutritional Causes

Starvation, anorexia nervosa, marasmus, and cachexia, which can cause severe, generalized nutritional deficiencies, may produce pancytopenia or selective neutropenia. Vitamin $B_{12}$ and folic acid deficiency can cause megaloblastic pancytopenia.

### Immune System Causes

Neutropenia can be caused by antineutrophil antibodies that mediate destruction either by splenic sequestration of opsonized cells or by complement-mediated neutrophil lysis. Immune neutropenia can occur as an isolated condition involving only the neutrophils and/or cells of the myeloid series or can occur in association with other immune-mediated cytopenias. Immune neutropenia is more common in young females and may be associated with other autoimmune diseases such as systemic lupus erythematosus and rheumatoid arthritis. Felty's syndrome is an eponym used to describe the triad of rheumatoid arthritis, splenomegaly, and neutropenia.

### Complement Activation

The exposure of blood to artificial membranes used in medical procedures, including dialysis, cardiopulmonary bypass, apheresis, and extracorporal membrane oxygenation, may result in complement activation and neutrophil lysis in vivo.

### Splenic Sequestration

Enlargement of the spleen may result in neutropenia because of splenic trapping and destruction of neutrophils. Neutropenia caused by splenic sequestration is often accompanied by a similar degree of anemia and/ or thrombocytopenia.

## Congenital Neutropenia

### Kostmann's Syndrome

Kostmann's syndrome, also known as severe congenital neutropenia, is characterized by recurrent bacterial infections with onset in early infancy in association with persistent agranulocytosis. In a bone marrow examination, arrest of myeloid maturation at the promyelocyte-myelocyte stage is found in patients with Kostmann's syndrome.

### Cyclic Neutropenia

Cyclic neutropenia is characterized by a regular periodic oscillation in the circulating neutrophil count from normal to neutropenic levels as low as $\leq 200$ cells/$\mu$L. In about three-quarters of patients, the mean ($\pm$ standard deviation) periodicity of neutrophil cycling is $21 \pm 3$ days. During the periods of neutropenia, patients usually experience symptoms of malaise, fever, and skin and/or mucosal infections. During periods of normal neutrophil counts, patients are usually asymptomatic.

### Chronic Benign Neutropenia

Patients with chronic benign neutropenia exhibit moderate to severe chronic neutropenia without leukopenia and with relative monocytosis, lymphocytosis, and variable eosinophilia. In contrast to patients with cyclic neutropenia, patients with chronic benign neutropenia have no periodic oscillations in the neutrophil count and little if any increased risk of infection. Both familial and nonfamilial cases have been described. Familial cases are seen in Jewish Yemenite, African, and western European lineages.

### Idiopathic Chronic Severe Neutropenia

In some patients, chronic, symptomatic, severe neutropenia presents in later childhood or during adulthood. Patients with idiopathic chronic severe neutropenia tend to be more symptomatic than those with chronic benign neutropenia. Evidence of myeloid hypoplasia and maturation arrest or even normal morphology is found in bone marrow evaluation in patients with idiopathic chronic severe neutropenia.

## Risk Stratification

The risk of infection is strongly related to the severity and the duration of neutropenia. In general, individuals with an ANC of 1,000–1,500 cells/$\mu$L are at little risk, and those with an ANC of 500–1,000 cells/$\mu$L are at moderate risk. Individuals with an ANC of <500 cells/$\mu$L, who have agranulocytosis, are at high risk, but the frequency of infection varies substantially from patient to patient.

## Assessment and Management in Psychiatric Settings

The approach to the diagnostic evaluation of a patient with neutropenia can be largely guided by the clinical history and physical examination and does not always require an extensive laboratory evaluation at the onset. The laboratory evaluation at a minimum should include a complete blood count (CBC) with manual WBC differentiation and a thorough review of the peripheral smear. Medication assessment and abnormalities of other blood counts may help to narrow the list of differential diagnoses. If the patient is asymptomatic or has minimal symptoms, has mild to moderate neutropenia, and has no significant history or physical findings to warrant immediate further evaluation, clinical observation is the best approach. Patients who are taking a medication that is known to cause neutropenia should be monitored closely with frequent CBCs. Discontinuation of the offending drug usually results in the patient's recovery from neutropenia within a few days. Neutropenia with associated anemia and/or thrombocytopenia may suggest underlying bone marrow suppression. If the neutropenia is persistent and no obvious cause is identified by routine diagnostic measures, expert hematology consultation, bone marrow examination, marrow cytogenetic techniques, and a collagen vascular evaluation may be necessary.

Management of neutropenia is based on the etiology, chronicity, and severity of the disorder as well as on associated disease states. The major focus in treating neutropenic patients involves preventive measures to limit the number and severity of infections, as well as direct measures to rapidly identify and treat any evolving infection. Despite all efforts, infections do occur in patients with chronic severe forms of neutropenia. Fever may be the only sign, because these patients may not exhibit the inflammatory response to infection and may not show any radiological findings. The clinician must have a high index of suspicion for bacterial and fungal infections and initiate rapid diagnostic evaluation and appropriate antibiotic therapy.

In patients with severe neutropenia and fever, prompt evaluation, including a thorough physical examination followed by culture of all accessible body fluids and open wounds, is necessary. In the physical examination, sore throat and aphthous ulcers in the mouth may be found. The perineum and perirectal area should be examined because the rectum is a common location for mucosal irritation and infection. Growth failure or phenotypic abnormalities, especially bony defects, should be noted.

Severe neutropenia with fever should be considered a medical emergency, and prompt institution of management is of prime importance. Patients with an ANC of <500 cells/μL and fever above 100.4°F require hospitalization and prompt administration of parenteral broad-spectrum antibiotics until they recover from the neutropenia. Hospitalization is necessary to allow close monitoring for sepsis syndromes, which can be fatal within hours if not managed adequately in neutropenic patients.

Preventive measures begin with close attention to areas of high infection risk. Because chronic gingivitis and stomatitis can be major sources of morbidity, good oral hygiene is imperative, including cleaning and attention to and correction of dental problems. An antibiotic mouthwash such as chlorhexidine can be very helpful in preventing gingivitis. Any type of invasive dental work should be discouraged if the patient has a neutrophil count <1,000 cells/μL. The perirectal area is protected by avoidance of trauma, such as rectal temperature measurement or suppository insertion. If constipation is a concern, stool softeners are prescribed to reduce trauma and straining. Patients should be educated to report perirectal pain or irritation. The skin, another common site of bacterial entry in neutropenic patients, should be kept clean. Patients should be advised to use an electric shaving device instead of razor blades for shaving. For female patients, use of tampons should be discouraged. Most clinicians recommend that patients refrain from eating fresh fruit and vegetables at the time of critical neutropenia (ANC <500 cells/μL). Prophylactic antibiotics are used in some instances and may limit infectious risks in patients with severe chronic neutropenia.

The advent of recombinant human G-CSF and GM-CSF has revolutionized the management of neutropenic patients. Both G-CSF and GM-CSF are recombinant hematopoietic growth factors that stimulate proliferation of progenitor cells and differentiation of committed progenitor cells into mature granulocytes. In addition to stimulating proliferation of neutrophils, GM-CSF stimulates proliferation of monocytes and eosinophils. Most patients respond to G-CSF doses of 5–10 μg/kg/day, although response in individual patients varies. G-CSF is well tolerated by most patients. The most common side effect is bone pain, which can be managed with acetaminophen. G-CSF should be continued until an ANC of 500 cells/μL is reached. A rise in the monocyte count usually precedes neutrophil recovery.

## References

Alphs LD, Anand R: Clozapine: the commitment to patient safety. J Clin Psychiatry 60 (suppl 12):39–42, 1999

Alvir JM, Lieberman JA, Safferman AZ, et al: Clozapine-induced agranulocytosis: incidence and risk factors in the United States. N Engl J Med 329:162–167, 1993

Alvir JM, Lieberman JA, Safferman AZ:. Do white-cell count spikes predict agranulocytosis in clozapine recipients? Psychopharmacol Bull 31:311–314, 1995

Ames D, Wirshing WC, Baker RW, et al: Predictive value of eosinophilia for neutropenia during clozapine treatment. J Clin Psychiatry 57:579–581, 1996

Blackburn SC, Oliart AD, Garcia Rodriguez LA: Antiepileptics and blood dyscrasias: a cohort study. Pharmacotherapy18:1277–1283, 1998

Chengappa KN, Gopalani A, Haught MK, et al: The treatment of clozapine-associated agranulocytosis with granulocyte colony-stimulating factor (G-CSF). Psychopharmacol Bull 32:111–121, 1996

Croarkin P, Rayner T: Acute neutropenia in a patient treated with quetiapine. Psychosomatics 42:368, 2001

Gravenor DS, Leclerc JR, Blake G: Tricyclic antidepressant agranulocytosis. Can J Psychiatry 31:661, 1986

Honigfield G, Arellano F, Sethi J, et al: Reducing clozapine-related morbidity and mortality: 5 years of experience with the Clozaril National Registry. J Clin Psychiatry 59 (suppl 3): 3–7, 1998

Kasper S, Praschak-Rieder N, Tauscher J, et al: A risk-benefit assessment of mirtazapine in the treatment of depression. Drug Saf 17:251–264, 1997

Lambert O, Veyrac G, Armand C, et al: Lamotrigine-induced neutropenia following two attempts to increase dosage above 50 mg/day with recovery between episodes. Adverse Drug React Toxicol Rev 21:157–159, 2002

Lieberman JA, Yunis J, Egea E, et al: HLA-B38, DR4, DQw3 and clozapine-induced agranulocytosis in Jewish patients with schizophrenia. Arch Gen Psychiatry 47:945–948, 1990

Stubner S. Grohmann R, Engel R, et al: Blood dyscrasias induced by psychotropic drugs. Pharmacopsychiatry 37 (suppl 1):S70–S80, 2004

Swartz JR, Ananth J, Smith MW, et al: Olanzapine treatment after clozapine-induced granulocytopenia in 3 patients. J Clin Psychiatry 60:119–121, 1999

Tohen M, Castillo J, Baldessarini RJ, et al: Blood dyscrasias with carbamazepine and valproate: a pharmacoepidemiological study of 2,228 patients at risk. Am J Psychiatry 152(3):413-418, 1995

# CHAPTER 36

# Thrombocytopenia

Archana Bhargava, M.D.

Dilip Patel, M.D.

## Clinical Presentation

In healthy individuals, platelet production is approximately 35,000–50,000/μL of whole blood per day; this value can be increased up to eightfold during times of higher demand. Once having entered the circulation, the enucleate platelets survive for an average of 8–10 days, after which they are removed from the circulation by cells of the monocyte-macrophage system.

The normal platelet count in adults ranges from 150,000 to 450,000/μL. Thrombocytopenia is defined as a platelet count less than 150,000/μL ($150 \times 10^9$/L). Approximately 2.5% of the healthy population have a platelet count lower than 150,000/μL. If the count has recently fallen 50% or more from a prior value, an investigation is warranted. Clinical or spontaneous bleeding does not occur until the platelet count is less than 10,000–20,000/μL.

Patients with thrombocytopenia may be asymptomatic, and this abnormality may be first detected through a routine complete blood count. The most common symptomatic presentation of thrombocytopenia is bleeding, characteristically mucosal and cutaneous (Rutherford and Frenkel 1994). Mucosal bleeding may be manifest as epistaxis and gingival bleeding, and large bullous hemorrhages may appear on the oral mucosa. Bleeding into the skin is manifested as petechiae, purpura, or superficial ecchymoses. Petechiae are pinhead-sized, red, flat, discrete lesions that often occur in crops in dependent areas; they are most dense on the feet and ankles and fewer are present on the legs. Petechiae are not tender and do not blanch under pressure. Purpura is a purplish discoloration of the skin due to the presence of confluent petechiae. Patients with platelet abnormalities tend to bleed immediately after vascular trauma. Posttraumatic or postoperative surgical bleeding usually responds to local measures, but bleeding may persist for hours or days after small injuries. Bleeding into the central nervous system is the most common cause of death due to thrombocytopenia. Deep bleeding into joints, retroperitoneum, or muscles is not seen with thrombocytopenia and is seen more commonly with coagulopathies (Levine 2003).

## Differential Diagnosis

### Decreased Platelet Production

Platelet production by the bone marrow can be impaired when the marrow is suppressed or damaged after viral infections, such as rubella, mumps, varicella, parvovirus, hepatitis C, and Epstein-Barr virus. Certain infectious agents, such as HIV, are capable of damaging megakaryocytes directly. Thrombocytopenia is a common finding in individuals infected with HIV; approximately 40% of HIV-positive patients are affected during the course of their illness. Thrombocytopenia as the initial manifestation of HIV is not uncommon. A decrease in platelet count is expected after chemotherapy or radiation therapy to sites of platelet production and in cases of congenital or acquired bone marrow aplasia or hypoplasia. Aplastic anemia is a specific entity that reflects a primary deficiency of stem cells and results in aplasia and pancytopenia. In alcohol-induced thrombocytopenia, an enlarged spleen in the patient with alcoholic cirrhosis plays an important role, but alcohol also has a direct toxic effect on megakaryocytes, leading to decreased production. Vitamin $B_{12}$ and folic acid deficiency can also lead to thrombocytopenia.

### Increased Platelet Destruction

*Idiopathic thrombocytopenic purpura* (ITP) is an acquired disorder characterized by isolated thrombocytopenia with otherwise normal blood counts and no clinically apparent conditions known to cause thrombocytopenia. The pathogenesis of ITP is presumed to be related to platelet-specific autoantibodies. The onset may be acute and abrupt, or it may be insidious. A related condition is *alloimmune platelet destruction* after transfusion or organ transplantation. *Disseminated intravascular coagulation* is a consumptive coagulopathy that can result in either bleeding or thrombosis and may lead to multiorgan failure and death. Disseminated intravascular coagulation occurs secondary to another condition such as sepsis or advanced malignancy. *Thrombotic thrombocytopenic purpura–hemolytic uremic syndrome* (TTP-HUS) is an acute illness with abnormalities in multiple systems that is diagnosed in patients with fever, thrombocytopenia, microangiopathic hemolytic anemia, global neurological dysfunction, and azotemia (Tsai 2003).

*Antiphospholipid antibody syndrome* is characterized by the presence of antibodies to certain plasma proteins that are often bound to phospholipids. Patients with this syndrome may present with venous and/or arterial thrombosis and recurrent fetal losses. The *HELLP syndrome* (hemolytic anemia, elevated liver function tests, and low platelet count) develops in approximately 10%–20% of women with preeclampsia. Destructive thrombocytopenia can occur after certain infections, such as infectious mononucleosis and cytomegalovirus, and during cardiopulmonary bypass surgery.

## Drug-Related Thrombocytopenia

Drug toxicity is an important and reversible cause of thrombocytopenia. Certain drugs, most notably heparin, quinine, trimethoprim-sulfamethoxazole and other sulfonamides, quinidine, and valproic acid, are known to produce thrombocytopenia (George et al. 1998). The usual mechanism of thrombocytopenia caused by drugs is accelerated platelet destruction brought about by drug-dependent antibodies.

Thrombocytopenia is a well-recognized complication of heparin therapy, usually occurring within 4–10 days after heparin treatment has started (Warkentin et al. 1995). The mechanism of the thrombocytopenia caused by heparin is nonimmune and appears to be a direct effect of heparin on platelet activation. The more serious form (type II heparin-induced thrombocytopenia) is an immune-mediated disorder characterized by the formation of antibodies against the heparin-platelet factor 4 complex. A second form of heparin-related thrombocytopenia (called type I heparin-induced thrombocytopenia) is typically characterized by a lesser decrease in platelet count that occurs within the first 2 days after initiation of heparin therapy. This form of heparin-induced thrombocytopenia often resolves with continued heparin administration and is of no clinical consequence.

## Dilutional and Distributional Thrombocytopenia

Patients who have had massive blood loss and transfusional support with packed red blood cells (RBCs) develop dilutional thrombocytopenia due to the absence of viable platelets in packed RBC products.

Normally, about one-third of circulating platelets are sequestered in the spleen, where they are in equilibrium with circulating platelets that are not sequestered. Splenic sequestration of platelets can be increased to 90% in cases of extreme splenomegaly, although total platelet mass and overall platelet survival remain relatively normal. Thus, patients with cirrhosis, portal hypertension, and splenomegaly may have significant degrees of thrombocytopenia (with or without leukopenia and anemia).

### Pseudothrombocytopenia

The platelet count can be falsely low in two clinical situations. First, if anticoagulation of the blood sample is inadequate, the resulting platelet clumps can be counted as leukocytes by automated cell counters. Second, approximately 0.1% of normal subjects have ethylenediaminetetraacetic acid (EDTA)-dependent agglutinins that can lead to platelet clumping and to spurious thrombocytopenia and spurious leukocytosis.

## Risk Stratification

Many patients with drug-induced thrombocytopenia require no specific treatment, as their platelet counts will recover promptly after withdrawal of the offending agent. However, treatment is required for severe thrombocytopenia, such as in patients with a platelet count <10,000/µL or patients with bleeding symptoms. When bleeding is not severe, appropriate treatment is with 1 mg/kg of oral prednisone given once daily. For patients with major bleeding, treatment includes platelet transfusions, intravenous gamma globulin, and high doses of parenteral glucocorticoids. Median time to recovery after discontinuation of the suspected drug is 5–7 days. The first intervention in a patient with heparin-induced thrombocytopenia should be immediate cessation of all exposure to heparin, including heparin flushes. Avoidance of low-molecular-weight heparin is also recommended.

## Assessment and Management in Psychiatric Settings

An accurate history and physical examination are the most important parts of the initial evaluation. However, if the platelet count does not make sense within the context of the clinical findings, the platelet count should be repeated before extensive evaluation is undertaken.

In the history, conditions associated with thrombocytopenia are obvious and should be immediately recognized by the clinician, including recent viral or rickettsial infection; previously diagnosed hematological disease (such as acute or chronic leukemia, chronic myeloproliferative or myelodysplastic disease); nonhematological diseases known to decrease platelet counts (e.g., eclampsia, sepsis, disseminated intravascular coagulation, anaphylactic shock, hypothermia, massive transfusions); a family history of bleeding and/or thrombocytopenia; recent live virus vaccination; poor nutritional status, especially in elderly and alcoholic patients; medications, including over-the-counter and herbal products, quinine-containing beverages, and aspirin; and pregnancy, especially late in the third trimester or at onset of labor, but also with a prior history of ITP or TTP-HUS or with preeclampsia or eclampsia. Patients with a suspected bleeding disorder should be questioned about past bleeding problems, a history of iron-responsive anemia, bleeding outcomes with surgical procedures and tooth extractions, history of transfusion, character of menses, and dietary habits or antibiotic use.

In the physical evaluation, a number of critical areas must be examined. Examination of the skin and mucosa may reveal helpful findings. Purpura, petechiae, and ecchymoses are the most common findings in thrombocytopenia. Sites of bleeding, especially in the dependent parts of the body, should be noted. In ambulatory patients, this bleeding normally occurs in the feet and ankles, but it may occur in the presacral area in bedridden patients. Sites of indwelling catheters, areas of previous trauma, incision sites, and exit sites of venous access devices should be carefully examined. Examination of oral, nasal, and anal mucosa is important because clinical findings in these areas are evident with severe thrombocytopenia. The ocular fundus should be examined for evidence of bleeding, because central nervous system bleeding is the most common cause of death in the thrombocytopenic patient. It is important to examine the patient for lymphadenopathy and hepatosplenomegaly and to test the stool for occult blood.

An expert review of the peripheral smear is essential in diagnosing TTP-HUS and acute leukemia, and the review should be obtained as expeditiously as possible, because any delay in making these diagnoses and initiating appropriate treatment may prove fatal to the patient. A microangiopathic blood picture, with fragmented RBCs, hemolytic anemia, and increased serum concentration of lactate dehydrogenase, suggests the diagnosis of TTP-HUS.

Management of thrombocytopenia is guided by an understanding of its etiology and clinical course. The principal goal of treatment for patients with isolated thrombocytopenia is the prevention of bleeding and achievement of a safe platelet count (Zondor et al. 2002). In patients who have thrombocytopenia as part of a multisystem disorder (e.g., disseminated intravascular coagulation, acute myeloid leukemia, HIV infection), treatment of the primary disorder is the fundamental management principle. For TTP-HUS, prompt plasmapheresis is lifesaving. In case of pseudothrombocytopenia, the platelet count should be repeated with heparin or sodium citrate as an anticoagulant. If sodium citrate is used, the platelet count should be corrected for dilution caused by the amount of citrate solution used; no such correction is needed for heparin.

Platelet transfusions are generally recommended for patients with a platelet count <10,000/μL or bleeding that is directly related to the decreased count. Patients with ITP rarely require transfusions, and the efficacy is severely diminished because of the short half-life of the transfused platelets. Usual duration of response is 2–4 days. Platelets from a single donor are preferred to those from multiple or random donors, which are associated with an increased risk of alloimmunization (George et al. 1996).

# References

George JN, Woolf SH, Raskob GE: Idiopathic thrombocytopenic purpura: a practice guideline developed by explicit methods for the American Society of Hematology. Blood 88:3–40, 1996

George JN, Raskob GE, Shah SR, et al: Drug-induced thrombocytopenia: a systematic review of published case reports. Ann Intern Med 189:886–890, 1998

Levine SP: Thrombocytopenia: pathophysiology and classification, in Wintrobe's Clinical Hematology, 11th Edition. Edited by Greer JP, Foerster J, Lukens JN, et al. Philadelphia, PA, Lippincott Williams & Wilkins, 2003, pp 1579–1582

Rutherford CJ, Frenkel EP: Thrombocytopenia: issues of diagnosis and therapy. Med Clin North Am 78:555–575, 1994

Tsai HM: Advances in the pathogenesis, diagnosis, and treatment of thrombotic thrombocytopenic purpura. J Am Soc Nephrol 14:1072–1081, 2003

Warkentin TE, Levine MN, Hirsh J, et al: Heparin-induced thrombocytopenia in patients treated with low-molecular-weight heparin or unfractionated heparin. N Engl J Med 332:1330–1336, 1995

Zondor SD, George JN, Medina PJ: Treatment of drug-induced thrombocytopenia. Expert Opin Drug Saf 1:173–180, 2002

# CHAPTER 37

# Anemia

Simon Vinarsky, M.D.

Dilip Patel, M.D

## Clinical Presentation

Anemia is usually diagnosed when the patient's hemoglobin value is less than 12 g/dL or the hematocrit is less than 37%. The hemoglobin level is 10–12 g/dL in mild anemia, 7–9 g/dL in moderate anemia, and less than 7 g/dL in severe anemia (Tefferi et al. 2005). Some controversy still exists in defining normal values of hemoglobin and hematocrit for healthy elderly subjects, as some clinicians believe that older persons have slightly lower hemoglobin levels than younger adults. Our opinion is that elderly patients should not be presumed to have a lower "normal" range and that anemia in older patients is caused by disease rather than by aging and should always be investigated, even in the absence of an apparent clinical disease (Woodman et al. 2005).

The signs and symptoms induced by anemia are dependent on the degree of anemia as well as the rate at which the anemia has evolved. The severity of clinical symptoms is less related to the severity of the anemia than to the length of time over which the condition develops. Symptoms are much less likely with anemia that evolves slowly, because there is time for multiple homeostatic forces and compensatory mechanisms to adjust to a reduced oxygen-carrying capacity of blood. It is not uncommon in clinical practice to see a patient with more than a 70% loss of red blood cell (RBC) mass (hemoglobin level <4 g/dL) who is relatively asymptomatic or to see someone who lost as little as 20% of the total RBC mass as a consequence of an acute hemorrhagic event but who is severely symptomatic.

The symptoms related to anemia can result from decreased oxygen delivery to tissues and hypovolemia in patients with acute bleeding. The clinical signs and symptoms of a slowly developed anemia include pallor, tachycardia, systolic ejection murmur, exertional dyspnea, fatigue, and evidence of the hyperdynamic state, such as bounding pulses, palpitations, and "roaring in the ears." In rapidly developed anemia, such as anemia from hemorrhage and certain catastrophic hemolytic anemias, the symptoms include syncope on rising from a supine position, orthostatic hypotension, tachycardia, lethargy, confusion, heart failure, angina or myocardial infarction, persistent hypotension, shock, and death. Early in the clinical course of the acute bleeding, the hematocrit and hemoglobin levels will be normal, and the clinical signs and symptoms have higher diagnostic value than laboratory findings (Brugnara and Lux 1995).

## Differential Diagnosis

*Normochromic, normocytic anemia* (with normal mean corpuscular hemoglobin concentration [MCHC] and normal mean corpuscular volume [MCV]) includes anemias of chronic disease, hemolytic anemias, anemia of acute hemorrhage, and aplastic anemia. *Normochromic, macrocytic anemia* (normal MCHC, high MCV) is seen in patients with folic acid or vitamin $B_{12}$ deficiency. *Hypochromic, microcytic anemia* (low MCHC, low MCV) reflects iron deficiency or thalassemia (Clarke and Higgins 2000).

Aplastic anemia is a stemm cell disorder that leads to hypocellular bone marrow. Most cases are acquired and usually due to drug, viruses, and toxins (Brodsky and Jones 2005). Drugs that can cause aplastic anemia include antimicrobial drugs (chloramphenicol, dapsone, sulfonamide, β-lactams, amphotericin, chloroquine), nonsteroidal anti-inflammatory drugs (NSAIDs), anticonvulsants (carbamazepine, phenytoin), cancer chemotherapy agents, antihypertensives (angiotensin-converting enzyme inhibitors, methyldopa), antiplatelet agents (ticlopidine), antiarthritic drugs (colchicine, gold), and antipsychotics (clozapine, chlorpromazine). Hemolytic anemia may follow treatment with penicillin and its derivatives and with cephalosporins, levodopa, methyldopa, quinidine, and NSAIDs (Arndt and Garratty 2005).

## Risk Stratification

Patients with severe anemia (hemoglobin level <7 g/dL), hemodynamic instability, and myocardial ischemia or heart failure, as well as patients with a rapid decrease in the hemoglobin level, must be immediately transferred to a medical unit for evaluation and treatment.

## Assessment and Management in Psychiatric Settings

The initial evaluation of the patient should be directed toward assessing the evidence suggesting active bleeding (acute or chronic); vitamin $B_{12}$, folate, or iron deficiency; bone marrow suppression; and hemolysis.

A detailed history is very important because clues to the etiology may appear in any part of it, including the history of the present illness, past medical history, family history, and review of systems. It is helpful to determine the patient's ethnicity and country of origin, because sickle cell anemia, thalassemias, and other hemoglobinopathies are particularly common in African Americans and in patients from the Mediterranean region, the Middle East, and Southeast Asia. Family history can help in making a diagnosis of sickle cell disease, thalassemia, and other inherited hemoglobinopathies. Information regarding previous blood count measurements and blood transfusions can help to distinguish an acute problem from a chronic problem. Inquiry about nutritional habits, symptoms of malabsorption, substance abuse (alcohol), and use of various drugs (e.g., phenytoin, trimethoprim, methotrexate) will help in making a diagnosis of vitamin $B_{12}$ deficiency or folate deficiency. An assessment of nutritional status is especially important in elderly and alcoholic patients. Inquiry about past medical problems and comorbid conditions will help to establish a diagnosis of anemia related to chronic disease (e.g., infection, inflammation, malignancy) or anemia caused by chronic renal insufficiency.

The use of both prescribed and over-the-counter medications, as well as use of herbal supplements, should be examined in great detail. Specific questions should be asked about the use of alcohol, aspirin, and other NSAIDs because of their potential for causing multiple gastroduodenal toxicities, including chronic or acute gastrointestinal bleeding. Exposure to toxic chemicals and several medications, including a few psychiatric drugs (such as perhenazine valproate), has been linked to development of conditions of bone marrow failure such as aplastic anemia and pure RBC aplasia (Acharya and Bussel 2000; Oyewumi 1999).

The major aim in the physical examination is to find signs of organ or multisystem involvement and to assess the severity of the patient's condition. The physical examination of a patient with anemia should emphasize the evaluation of tissue oxygen delivery. With acute blood loss, signs of hypovolemia and tissue hypoxia are the most reliable indicators of anemia severity. The patient must be evaluated for the presence or absence of tachycardia, dyspnea, fever, and postural hypotension.

Evaluation for jaundice is also a standard part of the physical examination, but this sign can be misinterpreted and may be difficult to detect under artificial lighting conditions. Pallor of the skin and mucous membranes is another sign of severe anemia. This sign is less reliable in patients with subcutaneous edema or deeply pigmented skin. Therefore, the examination should focus on areas where vessels are close to the surface (e.g., nail beds, mucous membranes, and palmar creases of the hand). When the palmar creases are lighter in color than the surrounding skin, the hemoglobin level is usually <8 g/dL. Other items to search for in the physical examination include the presence or absence of lymphadenopathy, hepatosplenomegaly, and bone tenderness, especially over the sternum. Bone tenderness signifies expansion of the marrow space because of infiltrative disease (as in chronic myelogenous leukemia) or lytic lesions (as in multiple myeloma or metastatic cancer). Rectal examination and stool testing for the presence of occult blood have an important role in evaluating patients with suspected gastrointestinal bleeding.

Patients with suspected vitamin $B_{12}$ deficiency should receive a detailed neurological examination. It is also important to recognize the signs of other hematological abnormalities, including petechiae and ecchymoses caused by thrombocytopenia and other signs of bleeding related to abnormalities of coagulation.

Initial testing of the anemic patient is often based on the suspected diagnosis but should always include a complete blood count (CBC), a reticulocyte count, and examination of the peripheral smear. The CBC usually includes measurement of hemoglobin and hematocrit, RBC count, RBC indices, red cell distribution width, white blood cell count and differential, and platelet count. The reticulocyte count has great diagnostic value and helps to distinguish among the different types of anemia. Anemia with a high reticulocyte count is usually seen in the patient with hemolysis or blood loss and reflects an increased erythropoietic response in bone marrow. Hemolysis or blood loss can rarely be associated with a low reticulocyte count if a concurrent disorder, such as infection or effects of prior chemotherapy that impairs RBC production, is present. Anemia with a low reticulocyte count is strong evidence for deficient production of RBCs, a low reticulocyte count accompanied by pancytopenia is suggestive of aplastic anemia, and a reticulocyte percentage of zero with normal white blood cell and platelet counts suggests a diagnosis of pure red cell aplasia. Leukopenia with anemia can be seen in the patient with bone marrow suppression or replacement, hypersplenism, or deficiencies of vitamin $B_{12}$ or folate. Leukocytosis may reflect infection, inflammation, or a hematological malignancy. Thrombocytopenia in association with anemia can be seen in a variety of disorders, including hypersplenism, bone marrow involvement with malignancy, sepsis, and vitamin $B_{12}$ or folate deficiency. The presence of thrombocytosis suggests myeloproliferative disease, chronic iron deficiency, inflammation, infection, or neoplastic disorders.

Mild pancytopenia can be seen in patients with splenomegaly. In contrast, the presence of severe pancytopenia should trigger evaluation for aplastic anemia, severe folate or cobalamin deficiency, or acute leukemia.

When hemolysis is thought to be the cause of anemia, helpful laboratory findings will include elevated lactate dehydrogenase (LDH) level, indirect serum bilirubin level, and reticulocyte count, as well as a lowered serum haptoglobin level. The combination of an increased LDH level and reduced haptoglobin level is 90% specific for a diagnosis of hemolysis; the combination of a normal LDH level and a normal haptoglobin level is 90% sensitive for ruling out hemolysis.

Patients whose anemia is not readily explained must be evaluated by a hematology consultant, who will review the blood smear and consider direct bone marrow examination. The blood smear review will often lead to a correct diagnosis by identifying neutrophil hypersegmentation in vitamin $B_{12}$ or folate deficiency; nucleated RBCs in patients with hemolytic anemia, sickle cell anemia, thalassemia, or bone marrow infiltration; RBC fragmentations in various microangiopathic anemias; teardrop RBCs in myeloid metaplasia with bone marrow fibrosis; or parasites such as *Plasmodium* (in malaria) or *Babesia*. Bone marrow examination usually offers little additional diagnostic information in the more common forms of anemia, but it is of great value in identifying hypoproliferative anemia and disorders of erythroid maturation. Bone marrow examination should generally be reserved for patients with pancytopenia and with suspected bone marrow infiltration in leukemia, lympho- or myeloproliferative disease, and myelodysplasia.

Management of anemia often begins at the time of initial evaluation, especially if the anemia is so severe that the patient exhibits signs and symptoms of tissue hypoxia. Immediate management for patients with severe anemia or hypovolemia includes infusion of electrolyte and colloid solutions and blood transfusion, along with supplemental oxygen to ensure oxygen delivery to the tissues.

When anemia is less severe and does not immediately threaten the patient's survival, a careful history, physical examination, and appropriate laboratory tests often reveal the etiology. Until a diagnosis is made, blood transfusion along with simultaneous administration of vitamins and minerals is discouraged.

# References

Acharya S, Bussel JB: Hematologic toxicity of sodium valproate. J Pediatr Hematol Oncol 22:62–65, 2000

Arndt PA, Garratty G: The changing spectrum of drug-induced immune hemolytic anemia. Semin Hematol 42:137–144, 2005

Brodsky RA, Jones RJ: Aplastic anemia. Lancet 365:1647–1656, 2005

Brugnara C, Lux SE: Introduction to anemias, in Blood: Principles and Practice of Hematology. Edited by Handin RI, Lux SE, Stossel TP. Philadephia, PA, Lippincott, 1995, pp 1345–1360

Clarke GM, Higgins TN: Laboratory investigation of hemoglobinopathies and thalassemias: review and update. Clin Chem 46:1284–1290, 2000

Oyewumi LK: Acquired aplastic anemia secondary to perhpenazine. Can J Clin Pharmacol 6:169–171, 1999

Tefferi A, Hanson CA, Inwards DJ: How to interpret and pursue an abnormal complete blood cell count in adults. Mayo Clin Proc 80:923–936, 2005

Woodman R, Ferrucci L, Guralnik J: Anemia in older adults. Curr Opin Hematol 12:123–128, 2005

# PART X

# Renal and Electrolyte Abnormalities

Section Editor:

Hitesh Shah, M.D.

# CHAPTER 38

# Azotemia

### Sheron Latcha, M.D.

## Clinical Presentation

Azotemia, or acute renal failure, is a sharp decline in glomerular filtration rate (GFR) with a resulting accumulation of nitrogenous waste products. Blood urea nitrogen (BUN) and creatinine elevations are markers for a drop in GFR. A multitude of diseases and pathological mechanisms underlie acute renal failure. Understanding the etiology and managing the complications of acute renal failure require a systematic approach.

Traditionally, acute renal failure is divided into three categories according to the type of renal injury (see Table 38–1): prerenal, renal (intrinsic), and postrenal (postobstructive). Intrinsic acute renal failure is further classified according to tubular, interstitial, glomerular, or vascular injuries. Of course, the classification is an oversimplification, because the effects of different types of renal injury may overlap. For example, radiocontrast agents can produce both prerenal azotemia and ischemic acute tubular necrosis. In the psychiatric setting, prerenal factors account for the majority of cases of acute renal failure, followed by postrenal (postobstructive) and renal (intrinsic) factors. This chapter deals primarily with prerenal and intrinsic acute renal failure. Postobstructive acute renal failure is discussed in greater detail in Chapter 44, "Urinary Tract Obstruction."

## Differential Diagnosis

### Prerenal Azotemia

Prerenal azotemia results from an acute decline in renal perfusion. Renal hypoperfusion can occur in the setting of frank volume depletion

**TABLE 38–1.** Types of acute renal failure

Prerenal
    Renal hypoperfusion
Intrinsic
    Tubular injury
    Interstitial injury
    Glomerular insults (postinfectious glomerulonephritis, antiglomerular
        basement membrane disease, ANCA-mediated vasculitis,
        cryoglobulinemia, autoimmune disease such as systemic lupus
        erythematosus)
    Vascular (renal artery or renal vein thrombosis)
Postobstructive (bladder neck obstruction [benign prostatic hyperplasia],
    ureteral obstruction [stones, retroperitoneal fibrosis], bladder dysfunction
    [neurogenic bladder, effects of anticholinergic medications])

*Note.* ANCA=antineutrophil cytoplasmic antibody.

from hemorrhage, diarrhea, diuretic use, and fluid losses from the skin. Intravenous contrast can also result in renal hypoperfusion. Lithium causes many patterns of renal injury, including prerenal azotemia and nephrogenic diabetes insipidus.

Prerenal failure can also occur in states of apparent volume overload such as congestive heart failure. This phenomenon highlights the concept of effective intra-arterial volume. Diminished cardiac output in turn stimulates the kidney to retain salt and water in an attempt to maintain intravascular volume. This compensatory mechanism produces signs of apparent volume overload such as edema, ascites, and pleural effusions. Valvular heart disease, pericardial tamponade, and pulmonary hypertension cause acute renal failure by means of the same pathophysiological mechanisms.

The renal adaptive response to hypovolemia is to maintain GFR by dilating the afferent arteriole and constricting the efferent arteriole (see Table 38–2). Decreased perfusion pressures sensed in the juxtaglomerular apparatus activate the renin–angiotensin II–aldosterone pathway. These hormones constrict the efferent arteriole and stimulate tubular reabsorption of sodium.

The kidney's adaptive response to hypovolemic insults has limitations. Protracted prerenal compromise can result in ischemic acute tubular necrosis. Nonsteroidal anti-inflammatory drugs (NSAIDs) inhibit prostaglandin synthesis, and patients with prerenal acute renal function are dependent on the vasodilatory properties of prostaglandins to main-

**TABLE 38-2.** Hemodynamically mediated acute renal failure

| Hemodynamic change | Effect on afferent arteriole | Effect on efferent arteriole | Glomerular filtration rate |
|---|---|---|---|
| Prerenal azotemia | Dilates | Constricts | Maintained |
| Effects of nonsteroidal anti-inflammatory drugs | Constricts | No change | Decreases |
| Effects of angiotensin-converting enzyme inhibitors | No change | Dilates | Decreases |

tain GFR. NSAIDs effectively knock out this compensatory hormone (Table 38–3).

Similarly, angiotensin II maintains GFR in prerenal azotemia by constricting the efferent arteriole. The use of angiotensin-converting enzyme inhibitors and angiotensin II receptor blockers in the setting of prerenal azotemia knocks out this compensatory response.

## Intrinsic Renal Failure

### Acute Tubular Necrosis

In the hospital setting, acute tubular necrosis accounts for more than 50% of cases of acute renal failure. Direct toxicity to the tubular cells can result from drug exposure or from intratubular occlusion with pigments and crystals (see Table 38–4).

Acetaminophen is a renal toxin that can produce an acute tubular necrosis lesion (Bjorck et al. 1988). Cellular injury and death is mediated by a toxic intermediate, N-acetylimidoquinone, formed through the cytochrome P450 system. Patients who take anticonvulsants or other medications that stimulate the cytochrome P450 system are more susceptible to renal injury from this cause. N-Acetylimidoquinone is directly toxic to renal tubule epithelial cells, and it can cause acute tubular necrosis even in the absence of hepatic injury (Blakely and McDonald 1995; Cobden et al. 1982). Although some patients require acute dialysis during the acute phase of this disorder, the cellular injury is reversible, and restitution of baseline renal function usually occurs within 2–4 weeks.

---

**TABLE 38-3.**　Prerenal azotemia: etiologies of decreased effective intravascular volume

---

Volume loss
　　Hemorrhage
　　Gastrointestinal losses (diarrhea,vomiting, nasogastric tube suction)
　　Renal losses (diuretics, diabetes insipidus)
　　Excessive sweating
　　Third space lossses (pancreatitis, burns, crush injuries)
Diminished cardiac output (cardiogenic shock, congestive heart failure, pericardial tamponade)
Diminished venous return
　　Massive pulmonary embolism
　　Inferior vena cava thrombosis
Vasoconstriction
　　Effects of medications (vasopressors, calcineurin inhibitors)
Vasodilation
　　Peripheral (sepsis, anaphylaxis, effects of medications)
　　Splanchnic (hepatorenal syndrome)
Loss of renal autoregulation (effects of angiotensin-converting enzyme inhibitors, angiotensin II receptor blockers, nonsteroidal anti-inflammatory drugs)

---

**TABLE 38-4.**　Acute tubular necrosis

---

Ischemia from any cause listed in Table 38-1
　　Recreational drugs (cocaine, amphetamines)
　　Intravenous contrast
Direct tubular toxins
　　Endogenous (pigments, including hemoglobin and myoglobin; light chains)
　　Exogenous (drugs, including acetaminophen, aminoglycosides, foscarnet, amphotericin, cisplatin)
　　Intratubular obstruction (casts; crystals, including oxalate, uric acid, acyclovir, indinivar, methotrexate, sulfonamides)

---

　　Massive release of myoglobin pigments into the circulation following crush injuries, alcohol abuse, muscle ischemia, seizure activity, or direct drug toxicity can result in acute tubular necrosis. Myoglobin pigments produce acute tubular necrosis through three mechanisms: 1) obstructive uropathy as a result of pigment cast formation, 2) hypovolemia due to fluid sequestration in the injured muscles, and 3) direct intrarenal vaso-constriction caused by myoglobin itself. The end result is a nonoliguric acute renal failure associated with elevations in creatine kinase (usually above 10,000 U/mL), reddish-brown urine, and pigmented granular casts in the urine sediment. Myoglobin pigment will cause the orthotoli-dine test on the urine dipstick to show large red blood cells (RBCs), but no RBCs are seen in microscopic examination of the urine. Cocaine alone, or in combination with heroin, amphetamines, or phencyclidine hydro-chloride, can cause myonecrosis. Myonecrosis results primarily from an ischemic injury caused by arterial vasospasm. In addition, vasospasm can occur in the vessels to the kidney, brain, heart, skin, and bowels, produc-ing multiorgan ischemic injury (Parks et al. 1989; Zamora-Quezada et al. 1988). Heme pigment deposits released by cell lysis during sickle cell cri-sis, ABO-incompatible blood transfusion, tumor lysis syndrome, autoim-mune hemolytic disease, or drug exposure can produce intratubular ob-struction.

Management of pigment nephropathy includes discontinuation of any offending medications and establishment of a diuresis. Administra-tion of intravenous boluses of normal saline solution of up to 1 L/hour with close monitoring of urine output is recommended. If the patient is not responding to forced diuresis and renal function is worsening, then a nephrology consultant should be asked to evaluate the patient for he-modialysis. Hemodialysis does not remove the pigment from circula-tion. Rather, it facilitates fluid and electrolyte management.

Decreased urinary flow rate is the usual risk factor for crystal depo-sition in the renal tubules. Accidental or intentional ingestion of ethyl-ene glycol, contained in antifreeze, produces an oliguric renal failure associated with a high anion gap metabolic acidosis and a serum osmo-lar gap. Metabolism of ethylene glycol by alcohol dehydrogenase leads to glycolic acid and oxalic acid formation. Glycolic acid is a direct tubu-lar toxin, and oxalic acid causes an obstructive uropathy. Metabolic ac-idosis can result in respiratory failure and circulatory collapse.

Ethylene glycol intoxication should be managed in the intensive care unit in consultation with a nephrologist. Ethanol is administered to act as a competitor for alcohol dehydrogenase to prevent the metabolism of ethylene glycol to glycolic and oxalic acid. Fomepizole is a more specific inhibitor of alcohol dehydrogenase but is more expensive than ethanol (Barceloux et al. 1999). Hemodialysis is indicated for patients with an ethylene glycol level >20 mg/dL or a methanol level >50 mg/dL and for management of metabolic acidosis.

**TABLE 38-5.**   Drugs commonly implicated in acute interstitial nephritis

Anticonvulsants (valproic acid, phenytoin, phenobarbital, diazepam, carbamazepine)

Antimicrobials (penicillin, cephalosporins, sulfa-containing drugs, rifampin, isoniazid, ethambutol, interferon, ciprofloxacin)

Analgesics/anti-inflammatories (sulfasalazine, mesalamine, aspirin, nonsteroidal anti-inflammatory drugs)

Atypical antipsychotics (clozapine)

Diuretics (furosemide, thiazides, chlorthalidone)

## Acute Interstitial Nephritis

Acute interstitial nephritis accounts for a significant number of cases of drug-induced acute renal failure. Typically, there is a sudden decline in renal function within 2–3 weeks of initial exposure to the drug. Reexposure to a culprit medication can produce acute renal failure much more quickly (Table 38–5). Clozapine has been reported to cause a severe anuric acute interstitial nephritis that requires dialysis support (Elias et al. 1999). About 50% of patients with acute interstitial nephritis have a fever, rash, or eosinophilia. The classic triad of fever, rash, and acute renal failure occurs in only about 5% of cases. Negative findings of a gallium scan effectively rule out acute interstitial nephritis as the cause of acute renal failure.

Obviously, withdrawal of the offending agent is paramount in the treatment of drug-induced acute interstitial nephritis. Even so, complete recovery of renal function may not occur until 6–8 weeks after discontinuation of the drug. A significant portion of affected patients have chronic elevation of the serum creatinine level after drug withdrawal. The available data suggest that steroids may decrease the interval for recovery of renal function (Spital et al. 1987). A nephrology consultation should be obtained if the patient's creatinine level fails to show improvement within 7 days after discontinuation of the offending medication.

Lithium, a commonly prescribed medication in the psychiatric population, produces a chronic interstitial nephritis with a steady decline in creatinine clearance over decades. Neither antecedent acute interstitial nephritis nor lithium toxicity is a requisite predisposing factor for chronic interstitial nephritis. Although only a small percentage of patients progress to end-stage kidney failure that requires hemodialysis, patients who are taking lithium should have their creatinine clearance followed closely. It is recommended that any patient who shows a decline in renal function should stop taking lithium. In addition, if a patient manifests symptoms of polyuria and polydipsia while taking lithium, the medication should be discontinued. If the patient is unresponsive to alternative medications, then the patient should be advised about the small but real possibility of irreversible end-stage kidney disease if lithium is continued.

### Acute Glomerulonephritis

Acute glomerulonephritis is a rare cause of acute renal failure in the psychiatric patient. The clinical presentation ranges from that of an asymptomatic, normotensive patient with nonnephrotic-range proteinuria to that of a patient with rapidly progressing acute renal failure with nephrotic syndrome, hypertension, and active urine sediment.

### Vascular Insults

Renal artery occlusion is a rare cause of acute renal failure. Risk factors include an underlying hypercoagulable state, traumatic vascular injury, and embolic disease. Patients who are at risk for atheroembolic disease are those with diffuse atherosclerotic disease, especially after an invasive arterial procedure such as cardiac catheterization. The findings of the physical examination include livedo reticularis and painful purple toes. Acute renal artery occlusion presents with loin pain and hematuria. Malignant hypertension and microangiopathic hemolytic anemia produce a small-vessel vasculopathy.

Renal vein occlusion can occur in the setting of nephrotic syndrome, inferior vena cava occlusion, retroperitoneal fibrosis, or significant dehydration. With renal artery occlusion, a noncontrast computed tomography scan may show a wedge-shaped defect. Doppler ultrasonography of the renal vein and magnetic resonance imaging/magnetic resonance angiography can be used to evaluate venous and arterial abnormalities, respectively. Management usually includes anticoagulation and, rarely, interventional radiology or surgical intervention.

## Postobstructive Acute Renal Failure

Obstruction of the urinary tract can occur at the bladder neck, at the ureteropelvic junction, within the ureters, or at the level of the renal pelvis. Obstruction can occur from within the urinary system (from stones, blood clots, papillary necrosis) or because of extrinsic compression on any of its components. Obstructive uropathy will hinder normal urinary flow but does not always result in complete anuria. If the blockage

**TABLE 38-6.** Evaluation of acute renal failure

| Index | Prerenal azotemia | Acute tubular necrosis |
|---|---|---|
| Specific gravity | >1.018 | <1.015 |
| Fractional excretion of sodium | <1% | >1% |
| Urine osmolarity | >500 mOsm/kg | <300 mOsm/kg |
| Urine sodium | <10 mmol/L | >40 mmol/L |

is at the bladder neck, the patient may complain of urgency and frequency. Male patients with an enlarged prostate may complain of hesitancy. This topic is covered in greater depth in Chapter 44, "Urinary Tract Obstruction."

## Risk Stratification

It is important to realize that a doubling of the serum creatinine level represents a 50% loss of renal function. So, a change in serum creatinine level from 1 mg/dL to 2 mg/dL is equivalent to losing one kidney, assuming a baseline creatinine level of 1 mg/dL.

## Assessment and Management in Psychiatric Settings

Establishing the cause of acute renal failure is key to timely institution of the proper therapy. Most often, the diagnosis becomes apparent from a focused history and physical examination. Urinalysis, urine and serum chemistries, and imaging studies can be used to confirm the clinician's initial impression (see Table 38–6 and Table 38–7). Of key importance is an assessment of the patient's volume status.

The patient should be asked about the presence of specific symptoms of obstruction such as straining, hesitancy, and overflow incontinence. It is useful to remember that most patients with partial obstruction have normal or slightly increased urine outputs. Only in the setting of complete bilateral ureteral obstruction will the patient be anuric. Anticholinergic agents, opioid analgesics, and tricyclic antidepressants can worsen bladder dysfunction and obstruction in susceptible individuals. A distended bladder can be percussed in the physical examination. Insertion of a Foley catheter and measurement of a postvoid residual (PVR) can be both a diagnostic and a therapeutic intervention. A PVR of 200–300 mL or greater is suggestive of an obstructive process.

**TABLE 38–7.** Evaluation of acute renal failure

| Etiology | Clinical data | Urine sediment | Ultrasound findings |
|---|---|---|---|
| Prerenal azotemia | Decreased effective intravascular volume | Normal | Normal |
| Intrinsic acute renal failure | | | |
| Acute tubular necrosis | Nephrotoxin exposure or ischemia | Granular casts | Normal |
| Acute interstitial nephritis | Rash, drug exposure, fever | Leukocyturia and WBC casts, urine eosinophils | Increased echogenicity, normal size |
| Glomerulonephritis | Rash, fever, alopecia | Casts (RBC, WBC), dysmorphic RBC, nephritic syndrome | Increased echogenicity, normal size |
| Postobstructive acute renal failure | Frequency, urgency, hesitancy | Normal | Dilation in the collecting system or bladder |

*Note.* RBCs=red blood cell; WBCs=white blood cell.

The normal ratio of BUN to creatinine is 15:1. In prerenal azotemia, the ratio is typically >20:1. Other causes of an increased BUN-to-creatinine ratio include increased urea reabsorption from gastrointestinal bleeding or increased protein intake. Catabolic states and corticosteroid ingestion can also cause an elevated BUN-to-creatinine ratio.

The finding for specific gravity from the urinalysis can help to differentiate prerenal azotemia from acute tubular necrosis. In prerenal azotemia, the specific gravity is usually >1.018, as the kidney attempts to maximally concentrate the urine. Tubular damage in acute tubular necrosis results in isosthenuria and a specific gravity <1.015. For similar reasons, urine osmolality in prerenal azotemia is typically >500 mOsm/kg and is <300 mOsm/kg in acute tubular necrosis. Calculating the fractional excretion of sodium (FENa) can also help to differentiate prerenal azotemia from acute tubular necrosis. Decreased effective arterial volume causes a sodium-avid state at the proximal tubule, with FENa <1%. The FENa is measured by using simultaneous values of serum and urine electrolytes in the following equation: FENa = (urine $Na^+$ concentration / plasma $Na^+$ concentration) / (urine creatinine concentration / plasma creatinine concentration) × 100.

The FENa calculation is a reliably discriminating test for differentiating acute tubular necrosis from prerenal azotemia. Other clinical scenarios associated with a FENa <1% include acute glomerulonephritis, contrast nephropathy, sepsis, and early obstruction. On the other hand, a FENa ≥1% can also be seen with the use of diuretics, mannitol, and glycerol and in acute interstitial nephritis and postobstruction acute renal failure. In addition, if the patient has any underlying defect in urinary concentrating ability, the FENa is >1%, even if the patient has prerenal azotemia (Zarich et al. 1985).

The presence of hematuria or persistent proteinuria in the urinalysis can signal bladder or glomerular pathology. A nephrology consultation is advisable in this situation. Patients with nephritic urine sediment may need to be assessed with a kidney biopsy to determine further therapeutic interventions.

Imaging with a renal sonogram is helpful in ruling out an obstructive process. Bilateral hydronephrosis is consistent with a bladder neck obstruction. Unilateral ureteral or, less commonly, bilateral ureteral stenosis can be due to stones, masses, or retroperitoneal fibrosis. Renal sizes are an important clue to underlying kidney diseases. Large kidney sizes are seen with polycystic kidney disease, infiltrative diseases, amyloidosis, diabetes mellitus, and HIV disease. Shrunken kidneys indicate chronic underlying renal disease.

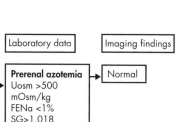

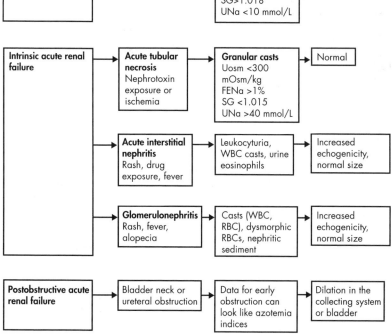

**FIGURE 38–1.**   Diagnostic algorithm for azotemia.

*Note.*   FENa=fractional excretion of sodium; RBC=red blood cell; SG=specific gravity; UNa=urine sodium; Uosm=urine osmolarity; WBC=white blood cell.

If the clinical, urine, and serum studies are consistent with prerenal azotemia from volume loss, it is reasonable to give fluid boluses and monitor urine output, blood pressure, and daily weight. If prerenal azotemia occurs in the setting of congestive heart failure, a trial of diuretics can be attempted.

Renal replacement therapy with dialysis is indicated for the patient with acidosis, volume overload, and hyperkalemia that is unresponsive to medical therapy. For lithium toxicity, dialysis is indicated in 1) any symptomatic patient, 2) when the serum lithium level is >4 mEq/L in the setting of normal renal function, and 3) when the serum lithium level is >2.5 mEq/L in a patient with renal insufficiency.

With respect to preventing acute renal failure, maintaining euvolemia will preclude hemodynamic causes of prerenal azotemia. NSAIDs and metformin should be avoided completely in patients with underlying renal insufficiency, but they can be used sparingly in patients with otherwise normal renal function. Patients with underlying renal disease may benefit from taking acetylcysteine or sodium bicarbonate before any imaging study that uses intravenous contrast agents. The dose of medications that are renally cleared should be adjusted for use in patients with renal insufficiency. For any patient who develops kidney disease, evaluation by a nephrologist is advisable.

## References

Barceloux DG, Krenzelok EP, Olson K, et al: American Academy of Clinical Toxicology Practice Guidelines on the Treatment of Ethylene Glycol Poisoning. J Toxicol Clin Toxicol 37:537–560, 1999

Bjorck S, Svalander CT, Aurell M: Acute renal failure after analgesic drugs including paracetamol (acetaminophen). Nephron 49:45–53, 1988

Blakely P, McDonald BR: Acute renal failure due to acetaminophen ingestion: a case report and review of the literature. J Am Soc Nephrol 6:48–53, 1995

Cobden I, Record CO, Ward MK, et al: Paracetamol-induced acute renal failure in the absence of fulminant liver damage. Br Med J 284:21–22, 1982

Elias TJ, Bannister KM, Clarkson AR, et al: Clozapine-induced acute interstitial nephritis. Lancet 354:1180–1181, 1999

Parks JM, Reed G, Knochel JP: Cocaine-associated rhabdomyolysis. Am J Med Sci 297:334–336, 1989

Spital A, Panner B, Sterns R: Acute interstitial nephritis: report of two cases and review of the literature. Am Kidney Dis 9:71–78, 1987

Zamora-Quezada JC, Kinerman H, Stadecker MJ, et al: Muscle and skin infarction after free-basing cocaine (crack). Ann Intern Med 108:564–566, 1988

Zarich S, Fong LS, Diamond JR: Fractional excretion of sodium: exceptions to its diagnostic value. Arch Intern Med 145:108–112, 1985

# CHAPTER 39

# Hematuria

## Hitesh Shah, M.D.

## Clinical Presentation

Hematuria (or blood in the urine) is defined as the excretion of an abnormal amount of either intact or damaged red blood cells (RBCs) (or erythrocytes) in the urine. Hematuria may be grossly visible or microscopic and can occur in transient, persistent, or recurrent patterns (Glassock 2001). Gross hematuria is suspected because of the presence of red or brown urine. Microscopic hematuria is defined by the presence of two or more RBCs per high-power field on microscopic examination (Cohen and Brown 2003). Urine dipstick testing is highly sensitive for detecting hemoglobin from one to two RBCs per high-power field. However, it lacks specificity, because the presence of myoglobin or hemoglobin may result in a positive test. After dipstick testing, the presence of erythrocytes must be confirmed by microscopic examination of the urine. Hematuria may be associated with symptoms referable to the urinary tract (such as dysuria or pelvic or flank pain) or may be asymptomatic.

## Differential Diagnosis

Abnormal quantities of RBCs in the urine may originate from the glomerular capillaries to the tip of the distal urethra. Causes of hematuria are usually classified as glomerular or nonglomerular, depending on the site of origin of erythrocytes. Causes of nonglomerular hematuria can be further classified as systemic, upper tract, and lower tract disorders. The glomerular bleeding usually arises from small breaks or discontinuities in the integrity of the glomerular capillary wall (Glassock 2001). The presence of dysmorphic RBCs tends to be strongly associated with glomerular hematuria. Abnormal quantities of protein in the urine should also increase the suspicion of underlying glomerular disease. Glomerular diseases presenting with hematuria could be either associated with systemic disorders (e.g., systemic lupus erythematosus, vasculitis, malignancy, and infections such as viral hepatitis) or be exclusively localized to the kidney (e.g., IgA nephropathy, basement membrane disease, and glomerulonephritis).

Abnormalities in the urinary tract (from the renal pelvis to the distal urethra) can lead to microscopic or macroscopic hematuria; however, the RBCs are normomorphic. The differential diagnosis of nonglomerular hematuria involving the upper urinary tract and the kidney includes nephrolithiasis, tumors, cystic diseases, pyelonephritis, papillary necrosis, and metabolic defects such as hypercalciuria or hyperuricosuria (Cohen and Brown 2003). The causes of hematuria involving the lower urinary tract include diseases of the bladder, urethra, and prostate. Urological malignancies, mainly of the bladder and the prostate, can present with gross or microscopic hematuria (Cohen and Brown 2003; Heney and Young 2003). Several drugs that are associated with interstitial nephritis can cause hematuria. Clozapine has been reported to cause hematuria and proteinuria, in addition to other clinical manifestations (Thompson et al. 1998). In these cases, the clinical and urinary findings were resolved after the drug was discontinued. The common causes of hematuria are listed in Table 39–1.

## Risk Stratification

Transient microscopic hematuria is a common problem in young adults (Froom et al. 1984). No obvious cause can usually be identified in most cases of transient hematuria. Fever, infection, trauma to the urinary tract, sexual activity, and vigorous exercise just before urine collections are potential causes of transient hematuria. The urinalysis should be repeated after a few days in cases of asymptomatic isolated microscopic hematuria before any evaluation is initiated, especially if there is a clinical suspicion of transient microscopic hematuria (Cohen and Brown 2003; Grossfeld et al. 2001). An important exception occurs in older patients in whom even transient hematuria carries an appreciable risk of urological malignancy (assuming no evidence of glomerular bleeding). Underlying urological malignancy is an even greater concern in patients with persistent hematuria for which no obvious cause can be identified from the history and in whom no evidence supporting underlying glomerular disease is present (Messing et al. 1992).

**TABLE 39–1.**   Common causes of hematuria

| Glomerular causes | Nonglomerular causes |
|---|---|
| Primary glomerular disease | Upper urinary tract |
|   IgA nephropathy |   Nephrolithiasis |
|   Thin basement membrane disease |   Tumors (renal-cell cancer, renal-pelvis cancer, ureteral transitional-cell cancer) |
|   Hereditary diseases (Alport's syndrome, Fabry`s disease) |   Pyelonephritis |
|   Membranoproliferative glomerulonephritis |   Acute (drug-induced) interstitial nephritis |
| Secondary glomerular disease |   Polycystic kidney disease |
|   Lupus nephritis |   Medullary sponge kidney |
|   ANCA-mediated vasculitis |   Trauma |
|   Goodpasture's syndrome |   Papillary necrosis |
|   Postinfectious glomerulonephritis |   Sickle cell trait or disease |
|   Hepatitis-associated glomerulonephritis |   Renal infarction or arteriovenous malformation |
|   Thrombotic microangiopathies (hemolytic-uremic syndrome) |   Ureteral stricture and hydronephrosis |
| |   Hypercalciuria, hyperuricosuria, or both, without nephrolithiasis |
| |   Renal tuberculosis |
| | Lower urinary tract |
| |   Infection and inflammation (bladder, prostate, and urethra) |
| |   Benign and malignant tumors (bladder, ureter, and prostate) |
| |   Polyps (bladder and ureter) |
| |   Urethral strictures |
| | Systemic |
| |   Febrile illness |
| |   Strenuous exercise |
| |   Coagulopathies |

*Note.*   ANCA=antineutrophil cytoplasmic antibody.

## Assessment and Management in Psychiatric Settings

The initial evaluation of hematuria usually does not require the consultation of a specialist (nephrologist or urologist). The initial steps in evaluating hematuria are to obtain a thorough history and perform a physical examination. Initial laboratory testing should include evaluation of the urine for proteinuria, bacteriuria, and pyuria. Blood urea nitrogen and serum creatinine should be measured in order to determine if underlying renal dysfunction is present (Glassock 2001; Grossfeld et al. 2001).

Several clues from the history or physical examination may suggest a particular diagnosis. Concurrent dysuria and pyuria are usually indicative of a urinary tract infection. A urine culture should be obtained if either dysuria or pyuria is present. Patients with urinary tract infections should be treated with appropriate antibiotics, and urinalysis should be repeated approximately 6 weeks after treatment. A recent history of vigorous exercise, fever, or trauma can cause transient hematuria. Contamination with menstrual blood is always a possibility and should be ruled out by repeating the urinalysis when menstruation has ceased. A recent upper respiratory infection, may suggest either postinfectious glomerulonephritis or IgA nephropathy. A history of nephrolithiasis or the presence of flank pain, which may radiate to the groin, may suggest ureteral obstruction due to a calculus. Older men should be evaluated for a history or symptoms of prostatic enlargement, such as urinary hesitancy and dribbling. The clinician should not be discouraged from pursuing further evaluation of hematuria in older men with benign prostatic hypertrophy, as they are more likely to have fatal diseases such as cancer of the bladder or prostate. Hematuria in a patient taking anticoagulant therapy should generally be evaluated in the same way as in other patients unless there is evidence of markedly abnormal coagulation studies with bleeding from multiple sites (Van Savage and Fried 1995). The patient's history of medication use is also important, because several drugs that might cause acute interstitial nephritis (nonsteroidal anti-inflammatory drugs, antibiotics) can also cause hematuria. Papillary necrosis with hematuria is a relatively common manifestation of sickle cell anemia.

The other question to be asked during evaluation of hematuria is whether the bleeding is glomerular or extraglomerular. The identification of the glomeruli as the source of bleeding is important both for determining the prognosis and for optimizing the subsequent investigation (Cohen and Brown 2003). Microscopic examination of urine is the single most important test in the evaluation of hematuria, as it often helps to distinguish glomerular from nonglomerular bleeding. An additional important abnormality that may help to differentiate glomerular from nonglomerular hematuria is the presence of blood clots (see Table 39–2). Clots usually are not seen in glomerular disease, perhaps because of the presence of urokinase and tissue-type plasminogen activators in the glomeruli and in the renal tubules.

Signs of glomerular bleeding include a predominance of dysmorphic RBCs, red cell casts (essentially pathognomonic for glomerular disease), and significant protein excretion that exceeds 1,000 mg in a 24-hour

**TABLE 39–2.** Features distinguishing nonglomerular and glomerular hematuria

| Feature | Glomerular hematuria | Nonglomerular hematuria |
|---|---|---|
| Erythrocyte morphology | Dysmorphic | Normomorphic |
| Red blood cell casts | May be present | Absent |
| Proteinuria | Usually >500 mg/day | Usually ≤500 mg/day |
| Clots | Absent | May be present |

urine collection (or a spot urinary protein-to-creatinine ratio exceeding 1.0) at a time when there is no gross bleeding. However, the absence of these findings does not exclude underlying glomerular disease.

Patients with glomerular hematuria should be referred to a nephrologist for a decision regarding the need for renal biopsy. A biopsy is not usually performed for isolated glomerular hematuria, because the management of these patients is rarely affected by the biopsy results (Cohen and Brown 2003). However, a biopsy should be considered if there is evidence of progressive renal disease, such as findings of an increasing plasma creatinine concentration or worsening protein excretion.

Radiological evaluation of the upper and lower urinary tracts should be pursued in cases in which a glomerular source of hematuria has been excluded (Grossfeld et al. 2001). The purpose of the evaluation is to look for lesions in the kidney, renal pelvis, ureters, and bladder. Although an intravenous pyelogram (IVP) or renal ultrasound has been routinely used to evaluate the upper urinary tract in cases of nonglomerular hematuria, computed tomography (CT) is highly sensitive in detecting diseases in the upper urinary tract and the bladder. An ultrasound or a helical (spiral) CT scan, first without and then with contrast medium, would be an appropriate initial test for the detection of upper urinary tract or bladder mass and occult stone disease. The patient should be referred to a urologist if nephrolithiasis or a suspicious lesion is identified. A nephrological evaluation is recommended for patients with polycystic kidney disease.

Cystoscopy should be done if the urine cytology examination has revealed cancer cells or if the patient has risk factors for bladder cancer. Risk factors for transitional-cell cancer of the urinary tract and bladder include heavy cigarette smoking, heavy phenacetin use, occupational exposure to certain chemicals used in certain industries (rubber, tire, leather, or dye manufacturing), analgesic abuse, long-term administra-

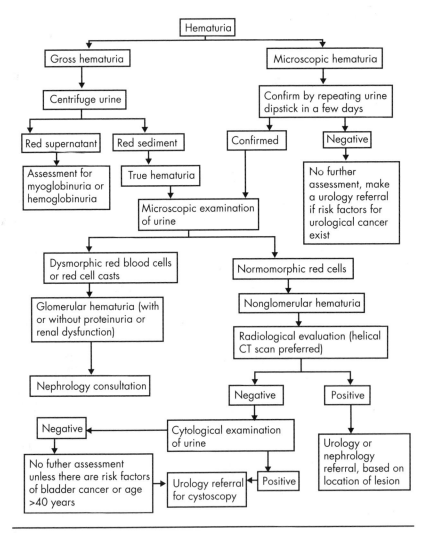

**FIGURE 39–1.**    Algorithm for evaluation of hematuria.

*Note.*    CT=computed tomography.

tion of cyclophosphamide, and ingestion of aristolochic acid, which is found in some herbal weight loss preparations (Cohen and Brown 2003; Glassock 2001). The risk for bladder cancer also increases significantly with age. Hence, cystoscopy is recommended for patients older than age 40 years who have persistent isolated hematuria and negative findings from radiological imaging (Grossfeld et al. 2001). Cystoscopy is also recommended for patients with gross hematuria, as this finding is associated with a higher risk of urological cancer, compared to microscopic hematuria (Grossfeld et al. 2001). Figure 39–1 outlines a suggested approach to hematuria.

Although only a few patients with negative findings in the initial evaluation of asymptomatic microscopic hematuria eventually develop serious urological disease, the American Urological Association recommends repeating urinalysis, voided urine cytology examination, and blood pressure measurement at 6, 12, 24, and 36 months after the initial evaluation. A complete urological reevaluation is recommended for patients with unexplained dysuria or urinary frequency, gross hematuria, or abnormal urinary cytology findings. Patients with persistent hematuria who develop hypertension, proteinuria, or renal insufficiency should be referred to a nephrologist for further evaluation (Grossfeld et al. 2001).

## References

Cohen RA, Brown RS: Microscopic hematuria. N Engl J Med 348:2330–2338, 2003

Froom P, Ribak J, Benbassat J: Significance of microhaematuria in young adults. Br Med J 288:20–22, 1984

Glassock RJ: Hematuria and proteinuria, in Primer on Kidney Diseases, 3rd Edition. Edited by Greenberg A. San Diego, CA, Academic Press, 2001, pp 38–46

Grossfeld GD, Wolf JS Jr, Litwin MS, et al: Asymptomatic microscopic hematuria in adults: summary of the AUA best practice policy recommendations. Am Fam Physician 63:1145–1154, 2001

Heney NM, Young RH: Case 39–2003: a 33-year-old woman with gross hematuria. N Engl J Med 349:2442–2447, 2003

Messing EM, Young TB, Hunt VB, et al: Home screening for hematuria: results of a multiclinic study. J Urol 148:788–790, 1992

Thompson J, Chengappa KN, Good CB, et al: Hepatitis, hyperglycemia, pleural effusion, eosinophilia, hematuria and proteinuria occurring early in clozapine treatment. Int Clin Psychpharmacol 13: 95–98, 1998

Van Savage JG, Fried FA: Anticoagulant associated hematuria: a prospective study. J Urol 153:1594–1596, 1995

# CHAPTER 40

# Hyponatremia

Ananea Adamidis, M.D.

Hitesh Shah, M.D.

## Clinical Presentation

Hyponatremia is usually defined as a serum sodium concentration of less than the lower limit of normal as specified by the laboratory (usually <135 mEq/L). It occurs in 10%–15% of hospitalized patients (Schrier and Berl 2000). Despite its name, hyponatremia actually represents a state of excess free water and has little to do with total body sodium content. As will be discussed in more depth later, total body sodium concentration may be increased, decreased, or normal in patients with hyponatremia. Hyponatremia in psychiatric patients may result from the psychiatric disorder itself, from its treatment, or from concomitant medical conditions. Symptoms may include lethargy, disorientation, generalized weakness, muscle cramps, anorexia, hiccups, nausea and vomiting, agitation or delirium, stupor, coma, depressed deep tendon reflexes, hypothermia, positive Babinksi responses, Cheyne-Stokes respirations, pseudobulbar palsy, seizures, orthstatic hypotension, or cranial nerve palsies.

## Differential Diagnosis

Despite its simple definition, hyponatremia has a broad differential diagnosis (Table 40–1). The first step in narrowing the differential is to stratify hyponatremia according to serum osmolarity. Serum osmolarity may be measured directly or calculated by the following formula:

$$\text{serum osmolarity} = 2 \times [Na^+] + [glucose]/18 + BUN/2.8,$$

where $[Na^+]$ is the serum sodium concentration, [glucose] is the serum glucose concentration, and BUN is the blood urea nitrogen concentration.

**TABLE 40−1.**  Differential diagnosis of hyponatremia

| Hyperosmolar | Iso-osmolar | Hypo-osmolar | | |
| --- | --- | --- | --- | --- |
| | | Hypervolemic | Hypovolemic | Isovolemic |
| Hyperglycemia | Pseudohyponatremia | Cirrhosis | Renal losses | Hypothyroidism |
| Hypertonic mannitol infusion | Isotonic mannitol infusion | Congestive heart failure | Extrarenal losses | Adrenal insufficiency |
| | | Nephrotic syndrome | | Primary polydipsia |
| | | | | Syndrome of inappropriate antidiuretic hormone |

## Hyperosmolar Hyponatremia

When the serum osmolarity is elevated, the diagnosis is hyperosmolar hyponatremia. In this situation, there are osmotically effective solutes besides sodium in the serum. Osmotically effective solutes are solutes that are impermeable to cell membranes, such as mannitol, and therefore draw water. The water entering the serum then dilutes the serum sodium concentration. The most common examples of this process are found in diabetic patients with severe hyperglycemia (Kumar and Berl 1998). To calculate serum osmolarity in patients with hyperglycemia, a correction is needed for the serum sodium concentration, as follows:

$$[Na^+]_{corrected} = 1.6 \times ([glucose] - 100)/100 + [Na^+]_{measured}$$

## Iso-Osmolar Hyponatremia

When the serum osmolarity is within normal limits (270–290 mOsm/L), hyponatremia is classified as iso-osmolar hyponatremia. The most common cause of iso-osmolar hyponatremia is pseudohyponatremia. Pseudohyponatremia arises when there are severe increases in triglycerides or proteins in the serum or after an isotonic mannitol infusion. Sodium does not dissolve into the portion of serum containing the triglycerides or proteins. Any increase in the volume of serum in which sodium cannot dissolve results in a falsely low measure of sodium concentration.

## Hypo-Osmolar Hyponatremia

Hypo-osmolar hyponatremia occurs when the serum osmolarity is less than normal. Hypo-osmolar hyponatremia is the most common form of hyponatremia. Unfortunately, it is sometimes very difficult to discern its etiology. To further aid in this endeavor, hypo-osmolar hyponatremia is subclassified according to volume status. Volume status is a marker for total body sodium concentration, because sodium is the principal solute in the serum.

When there are clinical signs of volume overload such as jugular venous distention, S3 gallop, peripheral edema, or pulmonary edema, the patient most likely has hypervolemic hypo-osmolar hyponatremia. Common causes of this form of hyponatremia are congestive heart failure, cirrhosis, and nephrotic syndrome. In these cases, the effective circulating volume is usually low, and therefore blood flow to the kidneys is decreased. The decreased blood flow to the kidneys stimulates secretion of antidiuretic hormone and results in the retention of sodium and water in the body, with water retention in excess of sodium retention (Kumar and Berl 1998). On the other hand, patients with volume depletion usually exhibit dry mucous membranes, poor skin turgor, loss of axillary sweat, or orthostatic hypotension. These patients have salt and water losses, with salt losses exceeding water losses. These losses may be either renal or extrarenal. With extrarenal losses, blood flow to the kidneys is again decreased; as a result, sodium and water is retained in the body and the urine sodium concentration is <10 mEq/L. Examples of patients with volume depletion include those with gastrointestinal losses from vomiting or diarrhea or losses into a "third space" in pancreatitis or severe burns. Renal losses may also occur, as in salt-losing nephropathy or with thiazide diuretic ingestion. In these cases, the urine sodium concentration will exceed 20 mEq/L. Salt-losing nephropathy generally occurs in patients with various chronic kidney diseases and creatinine levels >3 mg/dL (Kumar and Berl 1998; Schrier and Berl 2000). Thiazide diuretics act to disturb the kidney's urine-diluting capacity in the distal convoluted tubule. Volume depletion itself worsens the hyponatremia by stimulating secretion of antidiuretic hormone (Kumar and Berl 1998).

A patient who lacks the clinical signs of either volume overload or volume depletion is characterized as having isovolemic hypo-osmolar hyponatremia. One must first exclude hypothyroidism or adrenal insufficiency as etiologies by measuring the patient's thyroid-stimulating hormone and cortisol levels, respectively. These disorders result in enhanced antidiuretic hormone secretion and alter renal handling of sodium and water by mechanisms not fully understood (Kumar and Berl 1998). After these two states have been excluded, the differential becomes either the syndrome of inappropriate antidiuretic hormone (SIADH) or primary polydipsia. SIADH is the most common cause of hyponatremia in hospitalized patients (Kumar and Berl 1998).

The easiest way to differentiate SIADH from primary polydipsia is to measure urine osmolarity. In primary polydipsia, urine osmolarity is low (<100 mOsm/L), as the kidneys appropriately try to excrete a maximally dilute urine. However, hyponatremia arises because the patient ingests such a large volume of water (10–15 L/day) that the kidney's capacity to excrete it is overwhelmed (Rose 2000). However, it has been found that antidiuretic hormone may not be fully suppressed and therefore the urine will not be maximally diluted in certain psychiatric patients with this disorder (Goldman et al. 1988; Kramer and Drake 1983). This effect compounds the effects of excessive water intake on the development of hyponatremia. In addition, many antipsychotic agents cause dry mouth, which leads to increased thirst and even more water intake (Rao et al. 1975). Primary polydipsia is such an important diagnostic consideration in psychiatric patients, especially those with schizophrenia, that it has also been called psychogenic polydipsia.

In SIADH, an inappropriately high level of antidiuretic hormone is secreted. Antidiuretic hormone acts to make the collecting duct permeable to water, thereby increasing water reabsorption. Therefore, the urine osmolarity in patients with SIADH will be inappropriately elevated (>100 mOsm/L), compared to the serum osmolarity. SIADH itself has various causes, including nausea, pain, acute psychosis, tumors (especially small-cell lung cancer), various central nervous system or pulmonary disorders, and numerous drugs (see Table 40–2) (Adrogue and Madias 2000; Kumar and Berl 1998; Schrier and Berl 2000). Many of the drugs listed are commonly used in treating psychiatric patients.

## Hyponatremia in Psychiatric Patients

Many commonly used medications in psychiatry can cause hyponatremia. In a retrospective study of 199 elderly psychiatric inpatients in Australia, patients taking selective serotonin reuptake inhibitors (SSRIs) or venlafaxine were noted to be 5.6 times as likely as patients who were not taking these drugs to develop hyponatremia (Kirby et al. 2002). Furthermore, this elevated risk of hyponatremia persisted although the researchers controlled for age, sex, severity of depression, concomitant use of medications likely to cause hyponatremia, and severity of medical illness. This study provided evidence that SSRIs and venlafaxine independently predispose elderly psychiatric inpatients to hyponatremia. Elderly psychiatric patients treated with these medications should be monitored for the development of hyponatremia.

Some data show that SSRIs cause hyponatremia in outpatients. In a case-control study of 811 patients in the Netherlands, patients who started taking SSRIs as outpatients were four times as likely to be admitted to the hospital for hyponatremia as were matched control subjects (Movig et al. 2002). The authors noted that the increased risk for hyponatremia was greatest during the first 2 weeks after initiation of SSRI therapy. Therefore, SSRI-associated hyponatremia is also very important in the outpatient setting, and patients' serum sodium concentrations should be closely monitored, especially in the first 2 weeks after initiating these drugs.

**TABLE 40-2.**    Drugs that cause hyponatremia, by mechanism

| ADH release | ADH potentiation | ADH analogues | Other |
|---|---|---|---|
| Nicotine | Chlorpropamide | Desmopressin | MDMA (Ecstasy) |
| SRIs | Prostaglandin- | Vasopressin | Bromocriptine |
| Tricyclics | synthesis | Oxytocin | Barbiturates |
| Antipsychotics | inhibitors | | Thiazides |
| Carbamazepine | Methylxanthines | | |
| Chemotherapy | | | |
| Opiate derivatives | | | |

*Note.*    ADH=antidiuretic hormone; MDMA=3, 4-methylenedioxymethamphetamine; SRI=serotonin reuptake inhibitor.

More recently, a 12-week prospective longitudinal study of paroxetine and its contribution to the development of hyponatremia in elderly patients was conducted (Fabian et al. 2004). Hyponatremia developed in 12% of 75 outpatients who received paroxetine for the treatment of major depressive episode. In these patients, hyponatremia was associated with a lower body mass index and a lower baseline serum sodium concentration.

Numerous reports have associated carbamazepine with hyponatremia. In one small study of six psychiatric inpatients who developed hyponatremia after exposure to carbamazepine, hyponatremia resolved after discontinuation of carbamazepine (Brewerton and Jackson 1994). These patients were then given demeclocycline, a treatment for certain forms of hyponatremia (discussed later in this chapter, under "Assessment and Management in Psychiatric Settings"). Afterward, the patients were reexposed to carbamazepine. Five of the six patients were protected from the development of recurrent hyponatremia. Thus, carbamazepine is also an important contributor to hyponatremia.

## Risk Stratification

The severity of the clinical signs and symptoms of hyponatremia is dependent not only on the absolute degree of hyponatremia but perhaps more importantly on the rate of fall in the serum sodium concentration. In the setting of acute hypernatremia (<48 hours), rapid correction of the hyponatremia will lead to normalization of serum osmolarity, causing fluid to leave the swollen cells and reenter the serum. The cells will return to normal size, and symptoms will be alleviated.

However, in chronic hyponatremia, rapid correction is dangerous and can result in the serum osmolarity's exceeding the intracellular osmolarity because of the presence of a normalized serum sodium concentration as well as the additional solutes secreted by the brain cells. Water will therefore exit the cells and enter the serum. The normal-sized brain cells then shrink, producing the osmotic demyelination syndrome (also known as central pontine myelinolysis), which may lead to quadriplegia, pseudobulbar palsy, seizures, coma, and death (Adrogue and Madias 2000).

## Assessment and Management in Psychiatric Settings

The treatment of hyponatremia varies depending on severity, cause, and acuity of the disorder. For severe symptomatic hyponatremia the treatment consists of administration of 3% saline solution to bring the serum sodium concentration to approximately 120 mEq/L (Adrogue and Madias 2000). Recommended rates of correction are 1–2 mEq/L/hour for several hours and up to 8 mEq/L/day (Adrogue and Madias 2000). To calculate the rate of infusion and the volume of sodium chloride required to correct hyponatremia in this and other situations, the following approach can be used:

1. Calculate total body water (TBW):
   a. TBW=0.6×weight (in kg) for males
   b. TBW=0.5×weight (in kg) for females
2. Measure milliequivalents of sodium required (Na required):
   a. Na required=TBW×(Na$^+$ $_{desired}$−Na$^+$ $_{measured}$)
3. Measure volume of replacement fluid needed (V):
   a. V=Na required/osmolarity (in mEq/L) of replacement fluid
      i. 3% saline solution=513 mEq/L
      ii. 0.9% (normal) saline solution=154 mEq/L
      iii. 0.45% (half-normal) saline solution=77 mEq/L
4. Determine rate of fluid replacement (rate):
   a. rate=V/desired time of correction

It is very important to frequently monitor the concentration of serum sodium and other electrolytes during correction of hyponatremia because the formulas do not take into account ongoing salt and water losses or shifts. In addition, a loop diuretic may be added to prevent volume overload; the medication also aids in correction of hyponatremia by interfering with the urine concentrating mechanism in the ascending limb of the loop of Henle (Kumar and Berl 1998).

For chronic hyponatremia, the treatment depends on the type of hyponatremia. In general, the rate of correction should be more gradual than in acute hyponatremia. For hyperosmolar and iso-osmolar hyponatremia, treatment of the underlying disorder will generally correct the serum sodium concentration.

For hypovolemic hypo-osmolar hyponatremia, the treatment consists of volume replacement with infusion of normal saline solution. Alternatively, salt tablets may be used. Discontinuation of thiazide diuretics and treatment of hypokalemia will also aid in correction of the hyponatremia.

For hypervolemic hypo-osmolar hyponatremia, the treatment consists of fluid restriction of usually 1 L/day as well as loop diuretics. In addition, sodium intake must also be restricted.

For euvolemic hypo-osmolar hyponatremia, treatment also consists of fluid restriction. Alternatively, salt tablets combined with loop diuretics may be used. It is also important to correct any underlying hypothyroidism or adrenal insufficiency. SIADH that is resistant to the treatment described earlier may be treated with 600–1,200 mg/day of demeclocycline, a drug that interferes with the action of antidiuretic hormone in the collecting tubule (Verbalis 1998). It is also important to discontinue any medications that may cause SIADH unless they are absolutely necessary. Fluid restriction in patients with primary polydipsia is possible only if access to water is restricted, and such restriction is rarely possible. Treatment of the underlying psychiatric disorder is therefore valuable in addressing polydipsia. There is also some evidence to suggest that clozapine may be useful in patients with primary polydipsia. Clozapine is thought to correct the intracerebral biochemical disturbance responsible for both the psychiatric disorder and the abnormal stimulation of thirst (Lee et al. 1991).

# References

Adrogue H, Madias N: Hyponatremia. N Engl J Med 342:1581–1589, 2000

Brewerton TD, Jackson CW: Prophylaxis of carbamazepine-induced hyponatremia by demeclocycline in six patients. J Clin Psychiatry 55:249–251, 1994

Fabian TJ, Amico JA, Kroboth PD, et al: Paroxetine-induced hyponatremia in older adults: a 12-week prospective study. Arch Intern Med 164:327–332, 2004

Goldman MB, Luchins, DJ, Robertson GL: Mechanisms of altered water metabolism in psychotic patients with polydipsia and hyponatremia. N Engl J Med 318:397–403, 1988

Kirby D, Harrigan S, Ames D: Hyponatraemia in elderly psychiatric patients treated with selective serotonin reuptake inhibitors and venlafaxine: a retrospective controlled study in an inpatient unit. Int J Geriatr Psychiatry 17:231–237, 2002

Kramer DS, Drake ME Jr: Acute psychosis, polydipsia, and inappropriate secretion of antidiurec hormone. Am J Med 75:712–714, 1983

Kumar S, Berl T: Sodium. Lancet 352:220–228, 1998

Lee HS, Kwon KY, Alphs LD, et al: Effect of clozapine on psychogenic polydipsia in chronic schizophrenia (letter). J Clin Psychopharmacol 11:222, 1991

Movig KL, Leufkens HG, Lenderink AW, et al: Serotonergic antidepressants associated with an increased risk for hyponatraemia in the elderly. Eur J Clin Pharmacol 58:143–148, 2002

Rao KJ, Miller M, Moses A: Water intoxication and thioridazine (Mellaril) (letter). Ann Intern Med 82:61, 1975

Rose BD: Polydipsia and hyponatremia in patients with mental illness. [UpToDate Web site]. August 28, 2000. Available at: http://www.utdol.com/application/topic.asp?file=fldlytes/21479. Accessed December 29, 2003.

Schrier RW, Berl T: The patient with hyponatremia or hypernatremia, in Manual of Nephrology, 5th Edition. Edited by Schrier RW. Philadelphia, PA, Lippincott Williams & Wilkins, 2000, pp 21–30

Verbalis JG: Hyponatremia and hypoosmolar disorders, in Primer on Kidney Diseases, 2nd Edition. Edited by Greenberg A. San Diego, CA, Academic Press, 1998, pp 57–63

# CHAPTER 41

# Hypernatremia and Polyuric States

## Joseph Mattana, M.D.

## Clinical Presentation

Hypernatremia and polyuric states are commonly encountered in hospitalized patients (Palevsky et al. 1996) and psychiatric practice. The frequent mechanistic overlap of these disorders makes it reasonable to consider them together, as will be done in this chapter. The work of the clinician in approaching these disorders and choosing effective and safe therapies can be facilitated by remembering the following general principles: 1) hypernatremia is a deficiency of total body water relative to sodium—an elevated serum sodium level has no relationship whatsoever with the total body sodium level, which could be normal, increased, or decreased; 2) hypernatremia and polyuric states are predominantly disorders of water metabolism and much less commonly of sodium metabolism; and 3) the cellular response to acute and chronic hypernatremia is an important consideration in choosing a therapeutic regimen.

The development of hypernatremia is the result of 1) a lack of water intake, 2) increased water losses (renal or extrarenal), 3) a shift of water into cells, or 4) an excess (usually iatrogenic or hormonally mediated) of total body sodium concentration in relation to water. It is important to remember that individuals who have an intact thirst mechanism and have adequate access to water will not develop a significant rise in the serum sodium level. Thus, for a patient to develop sustained hypernatremia, a lack of water intake is necessary. Individuals with nephrogenic diabetes insipidus, for example, who have resistance to the action of antidiuretic hormone (ADH) on the collecting duct, will essentially manage their disorder through their thirst mechanism, which will stimulate a large intake of water to compensate for urinary water losses.

Signs and symptoms of hypernatremia generally correlate with the extent of electrolyte balance and can include thirst, restlessness, irritability, disorientation, delirium, coma, convulsions, flushed skin, fever, oliguria or anuria, hyperventilation, hyperreflexia, or brain hemorrhage.

## Differential Diagnosis

### Hypernatremia Due to Inadequate Water Intake

Hypernatremia may be encountered in the presence of normal urinary concentrating mechanisms when there is inadequate water intake. Inadequate water intake may occur when access to water is prevented or when the normal thirst mechanisms are impaired. Primary hypodipsia may be encountered with aging (Phillips et al. 1991) and may result from malignant disease, vascular disease, or infiltrative disorders involving hypothalamic osmoreceptors. In addition, hypernatremia of nonrenal etiology may result when there is loss of water in excess of solute, such as in the fluid losses encountered in patients with diarrhea. Whether hypernatremia due to inadequate water intake occurs with or without nonrenal loss of hypotonic fluids, the urine will be concentrated.

### Hypernatremia Associated With Abnormal Urinary Concentration

Concentrated urine is typically encountered in states of hyperosmolality and in states characterized by low effective arterial volume. Concentrating defects can be caused by one or more of several mechanisms. Osmolalities in excess of 1,000 mOsm/L found in the normal renal medulla allow for a large volume of water reabsorption, a process impaired by renal diseases such as papillary necrosis and chronic tubulointerstitial diseases. In such patients, maximum urinary concentrating ability may be impaired and water conservation may be limited, predisposing some of these patients to the development of hypernatremia. Impaired water conservation may result from a lack of secretion of ADH in the context of a partial or complete disorder. Hereditary disorders as well as several acquired conditions, including granulomatous disease, malignancy, pituitary surgery, infections, autoimmune disease, and vascular events, may impair ADH secretion and give rise to the syndrome termed central diabetes insipidus. In central diabetes insipidus, the collecting duct is functionally intact, but water reabsorption is impaired because of a lack of ADH. ADH replacement therapy with desmopressin acetate allows such patients to reabsorb water effectively, and, as long as adequate water intake is achieved, normonatremia can be maintained in these patients. In other patients with hypernatremia, the primary problem is unresponsiveness of the collecting duct to ADH, a condition termed nephrogenic diabetes insipidus, which is caused by lithium carbonate and other drugs, urinary tract obstruction, hypercalcemia, and hypokalemia. This effect of lithium may persist long after the drug is discontinued (Guirguis and Taylor 2000). Despite an intact medulla and abundant ADH, the collecting duct does not respond normally to ADH or to administration of desmopressin acetate in patients with nephrogenic diabetes insipidus. The patient with nephrogenic diabetes insipidus will maintain normonatremia as long as there is an intact thirst mechanism and access to water, although the patient will experience polyuria (defined as a urine volume of more than 2.5 L/day). The polyuria in patients with nephrogenic diabetes insipidus can be difficult to treat.

Excessive renal water loss may also take place in patients with normal kidney function when there is excretion of an osmotically active substance, such as glucose in uncontrolled diabetes, or when drugs such as mannitol are taken. Renal water loss by this process is termed osmotic diuresis.

## Hypernatremia Associated With Sodium Excess

Rarely, hypernatremia may be seen in settings where the primary driving force is an excess of total body concentration of sodium (Kahn 1999). This process may occur in disease states such as primary hyperaldosteronism or may be an iatrogenic consequence of administration of hypertonic intravenous fluids (e.g., hypertonic saline solution or hypertonic sodium bicarbonate solution).

## Risk Stratification

Aggressive treatment and urgent nephrology consultation are required for all hypernatremic patients with symptoms or physical findings suggestive of hemodynamic instability (dizziness, weakness, syncope, hypotension, or orthostatic hypotension), acute deterioration of renal function, change in mental status, and neurological deficits.

## Assessment and Management in Psychiatric Settings

A careful history, thorough physical examination, and some simple laboratory testing can reveal the cause of hypernatremia in the vast major-

**TABLE 41–1.** Approach to hypernatremia

| | Volume status | | | |
|---|---|---|---|---|
| | Volume depleted | | Euvolemic | Hypervolemic |
| Total body water | Decreased | | Decreased | Increased |
| Total body sodium | Decreased | | Normal | Increased |
| Etiologies | Renal losses caused by osmotic diuresis (e.g., hyperglycemia), loop diuretics (e.g., furosemide), postobstructive diuresis | Extrarenal losses through skin (sweating, burns), diarrhea, enterocutaneous fistulas | Renal losses caused by central and nephrogenic diabetes insipidus | Extrarenal losses through skin and respiratory tract; inadequate water intake | Administration of hypertonic intravenous fluids (sodium bicarbonate, hypertonic saline, parenteral nutrition), primary hyperaldosteronism, Cushing's syndrome |
| Urine sodium concentration | Usually >20 mEq/L | Usually <20 mEq/L | Variable | Decreased | Usually >20 mEq/L |
| Urine osmolality | Less than or equal to plasma osmolality (hypotonic or isotonic) | Greater than plasma osmolality (hypertonic) | Usually hypotonic | Usually hypertonic | Hypertonic or isotonic |

**TABLE 41–1.**  Approach to hypernatremia *(continued)*

|  | Volume status | | |
|---|---|---|---|
|  | **Volume depleted** | **Euvolemic** | **Hypervolemic** |
| **Initial treatment** | 0.9% or 0.45% saline solution | Water replacement (intravenous or orally) | Loop diuretics (to achieve loss of water and sodium) and water replacement |
| **Long-term treatment** | Treat underlying cause | Treat central diabetes insipidus with desmopressin acetate; treat nephrogenic diabetes insipidus with thiazide diuretics | Treat underlying cause; ensure adequate water intake |  Treat underlying cause |

ity of cases. An important as well as challenging part of the evaluation is to determine whether the extracellular fluid volume is normal or abnormally high or low. Useful laboratory data include findings from serum chemistry measures (at minimum, electrolytes, glucose, urea nitrogen, creatinine, and calcium levels), serum osmolality, urinalysis findings, urine electrolytes measures (sodium, potassium, and chloride levels), and urine osmolality. In hospitalized patients, strict measurement of intake and output should be obtained as well. Table 41–1 outlines a suggested approach to the hypernatremic patient.

The hypernatremic patient presents a number of management questions that the clinician must consider: 1) Is this patient's volume depleted, and if so what initial therapy should be given? 2) Is the hypernatremia acute or chronic? 3) What is the patient's water deficit? 4) How rapidly should the hypernatremia be corrected? and 5) Is this problem chronic, and, if so, will it require ongoing medical therapy with or without consultation?

The most important principle in the initial treatment of hypernatremia, as for the treatment of hyponatremia, is to treat hypovolemia if it is present. It is easy to become distracted by alarming electrolyte findings and to overlook a state of volume depletion that may be a far greater immediate threat to the patient's outcome. A safe initial approach is to administer normal saline solution (0.9% sodium chloride) or half-normal saline solution (0.45% sodium chloride) until the patient is thought to be hemodynamically stable.

Calculation of the water deficit is appropriate in treating a patient in whom the main disorder is loss of water, as opposed to a derangement in the sodium level. For example, calculation of the water deficit would be appropriate in the case of a patient with impaired thirst and central or nephrogenic diabetes insipidus.

The water deficit can be determined as follows:

1. Calculate total body water (TBW): TBW $= 0.5 \times$ weight (in kg)
2. Calculate the water deficit: Water deficit in liters $= TBW \times (Na^+_{current} - Na^+_{target})/Na^+_{target}$ [where $Na^+$ is the serum sodium concentration].

For example, a 60-kg woman with serum sodium concentration of 160 mmol/L and a target serum sodium concentration of 140 mmol/L would have a water deficit of 4.3 liters—$60(0.5) \times (160-140)/140$. To lower her serum sodium concentration by 0.5 mmol/L/hour, one would give water (e.g., a solution of 5% dextrose in water) at a rate of $60(0.5) \times (0.5)/140 = 0.107$ L/hour, or 107 mL/hour.

Calculations may not always predict actual changes in serum sodium level. Serum sodium levels must be measured frequently during
therapy. For the severely hypernatremic patient, the consultation of a
nephrologist should be obtained to aid in these determinations.

A common and complex question is how rapidly to correct hypernatremia. Administration of water, if excessive, entails the danger of cell
swelling and neurological complications. Acute, symptomatic hypernatremia that develops over several hours presents a danger because of
cell shrinkage resulting from water being drawn into the hypertonic extracellular space. Intracranial hemorrhage can result. Under these circumstances, it makes sense that initial therapy is directed toward a
rapid decrease in serum sodium concentration through water administration. Hence, in the patient with acute symptomatic hypernatremia, a
decrease in serum sodium concentration of 1 mmol/L/hour can be targeted (Adrogue and Madias 2000). If neurological changes occur during
treatment, it is likely that cell swelling is occurring; in this situation, water administration should be stopped while additional tests are done to
determine the cause of the neurological change (Palevsky 2001). Clinicians are frequently faced with hypernatremia of longer duration or
unknown duration, and the cells may have adjusted to their hypertonic environment by increasing their solute content to match that of
the plasma (McManus et al. 1995). Although the patient with acute hypernatremia is in danger from cell shrinkage that has taken place (and
therapy is directed toward restoring cell volume through water administration), the patient with chronic hypernatremia may develop cell
swelling if water is rapidly administered, leading to complications because of increased intracranial pressure. Here, a conservative approach
is recommended, with water administration limited to achieve a reduction in serum sodium concentration of 0.5 mmol/L/hour (Adrogue and
Madias 2000).

In hypernatremia caused by impaired water intake, the treatment
depends on the etiology. Hypernatremia caused by impaired thirst can
be challenging to address. After acute management, the patient can be
given prescribed amounts of water to ingest, although if the patient is
debilitated, he or she may require assistance in drinking the prescribed
amounts. One should also consider whether the patient's overall dietary intake is adequate, as inadequate water intake could be part of a
more global problem with feeding.

Patients who are hypernatremic as a result of nonrenal losses of water and electrolytes are likely to be volume depleted. Initial fluid therapy should be directed at expanding the extracellular volume. Greater

care should be exercised in use of fluid therapy for patients with cardiac disease. Isotonic saline solution (a normal 0.9% solution) is generally preferred as an initial intravenous fluid. The underlying condition resulting in water and sodium depletion must be addressed, or the problem will recur.

For central diabetes insipidus, once any overt water deficits are corrected, intranasal desmopressin acetate (10–20 µg intranasally every 12–24 hours) is an effective treatment. Underdosing is not dangerous as long as the patient has an intact thirst mechanism. Overdosing can lead to hyponatremia. Development of hyponatremia can be avoided by careful attention to serum sodium levels and by adjusting dosages to allow for the sensation of thirst at least once a day. Central diabetes insipidus may exist as a partial defect, and in such patients, potential therapies include chlorpropamide, clofibrate, and carbamazepine, as well as desmopressin acetate. Therapy for complete or partial central diabetes insipidus should be done with subspecialty consultation.

Patients with nephrogenic diabetes insipidus will not develop hypernatremia as long as they have an intact thirst mechanism and access to water. The aim of treatment is not so much to affect serum sodium levels (which the patient's thirst essentially regulates) as it is to control polyuria, which can be extremely disruptive to these patients because it impairs their ability to work and travel. Thiazide diuretics, including hydrochlorothiazide (which is not potassium sparing) and amiloride (which is potassium sparing), have been found to decrease urinary volume in patients with nephrogenic diabetes insipidus. The rationale for this treatment should be carefully explained to the patient, who may find the idea of taking a diuretic as a treatment for polyuria illogical and might not adhere to the treatment. If a patient's potassium level tends to be high, hydrochlorothiazide (non-potassium-sparing diuretic) might be preferable, whereas for patients who have lower potassium levels amiloride (potassium sparing) might be better. Reductions in solute intake may also help reduce urinary volumes.

## References

Adrogue HJ, Madias NE: Hypernatremia. N Engl J Med 342:1493–1499, 2000
Guirguis AF, Taylor HC: Nephrogenic diabetes insipidus persisting 57 months after cessation of lithium carbonate therapy: report of a case and review of the literature. Endocr Prac 6:324–328, 2000
Kahn T: Hypernatremia with edema. Arch Int Med 159:93–98, 1999

McManus ML, Churchwell KB, Strange K: Regulation of cell volume in health and disease. N Engl J Med 333:1260–1266, 1995

Palevsky PM: Hypernatremia, in Primer on Kidney Diseases, 3rd Edition. Edited by Greenberg A. San Diego, CA, Academic Press, 2001, pp 64–71

Palevsky PM, Bhagrath R, Greenberg A: Hypernatremia in hospitalized patients. Ann Int Med 124:197–203, 1996

Phillips PA, Bretherton M, Johnston CI, et al: Reduced osmotic thirst in healthy elderly men. Am J Physiol 261:R166–R171, 1991

# CHAPTER 42

# Hypokalemia

### Michael Gitman, M.D.

## Clinical Presentation

Potassium is the main intracellular cation and is an integral determinant of the resting membrane potential, which is vital to many cellular functions, including cardiac conduction and muscle contraction. Hypokalemia is defined as a potassium level of <3.5 mEq/L. Because of the innate ability of the kidney to retain potassium and the abundance of potassium in the United States diet, hypokalemia is rare in the general U.S. population, occurring in less than 1% of healthy individuals (Wingo and Weiner 2000). Hypokalemia was found in 33% of acutely schizophrenic patients (Hatta et al. 1999) and 50% of patients who take thiazide diuretics (Bloomfield et al. 1986).

Most patients with mild hypokalemia (serum potassium level of 3–3.5 mEq/L) are asymptomatic. When the serum potassium level drops below 3 mEq/L, the symptoms are varied. Because potassium is the main determinant of the resting membrane potential, many of the symptoms of hypokalemia are manifest in electrically excitable tissues such as the heart, nerves, and muscle.

The cardiac manifestations include hypertension, precipitation of digoxin toxicity, ventricular arrhythmia, and U waves in an electrocardiogram. The skeletal muscle manifestations include weakness, myalgias, and cramping. Severe cases can cause rhabdomyolysis and/or paralysis. The renal manifestations of hypokalemia are numerous and include nephrogenic diabetes insipidus, metabolic alkalosis (Soleimani et al. 1990; Tizianello et al. 1991), hyperphosphaturia, and hypercalciuria. If hypokalemia is chronically present, it can precipitate chronic interstitial nephritis and result in renal failure (Cremer and Bock 1977). The endocrine manifestations include impaired insulin release and decreased end-organ sensitivity to insulin, resulting in hyperglycemia in diabetic patients (Andersson et al. 1991). The gastrointestinal manifestations can range from constipation to paralytic ileus to worsening hepatic encephalopathy in patients with cirrhosis (Artz et al. 1966).

Hypokalemia has been reported to cause neuropsychiatric symptoms, including fatigue, dystrophic mood, irritability, and nervousness, although this association appears to be uncommon (Hafez et al. 1984). Hatta et al. (1999) showed that in acutely psychotic patients, hypokalemia was associated with elevated agitation scores. In one report, potassium repletion alone reversed an episode of acute decompensated schizophrenia in a chronically schizophrenic patient (Hafez et al. 1984).

# Differential Diagnosis

## Spurious Hypokalemia

Both laboratory error and severe leukocytosis can result in factitious hypokalemia. When severe leukocytosis is present, the white blood cells continue to absorb potassium even as the blood sample is transported to the laboratory, resulting in a low potassium value. To avoid this effect, the blood sample should be centrifuged immediately after phlebotomy and refrigerated until it is analyzed.

## Intracellular Shift

Because renal excretion of a potassium load takes hours to occur, the shift of potassium from the extracellular compartment to the intracellular compartment is an important survival mechanism. Shift of potassium from the blood into the cells occurs in minutes and is mainly controlled by insulin release, catecholamine release, and metabolic or respiratory alkalosis.

Hypokalemic periodic paralysis is another cause of intracellular potassium shift. It is a disease characterized by acute attacks of muscle weakness and hypokalemia preceded by periods of normokalemia. It is precipitated by exercise, stress, and high-carbohydrate meals, which are all events associated with increased release of epinephrine or insulin. The condition can be inherited or acquired. The acquired form is seen most commonly in Asian males with thyrotoxicosis. This disease is treated with potassium supplementation during the attack, but one must use caution in this supplementation because rebound hyperkalemia has been reported. The long-term treatment of acquired hypokalemic periodic paralysis includes treatment of any thyroid disease that is present and avoidance of high-carbohydrate meals; some patients benefit from β-blockers or acetazolamide (Palmer 2003).

## Potassium Deficit

A deficit in the total body concentration of potassium can be caused by either decreased potassium intake or excessive potassium losses. Decreased potassium intake is rare in patients who eat a typical American diet, which contains approximately 60–80 mEq/day of potassium (Hajjar et al. 2001).

Most commonly hypokalemia is the result of excessive potassium losses through the gastrointestinal tract or the kidneys. Gastrointestinal losses occur with diarrhea, because of the high concentration of potassium in stool. Vomiting and nasogastric suction can cause hypokalemia by promoting renal potassium loss. Both vomiting and nasogastric suction result in the loss of hydrochloric acid from the stomach, leading to alkalemia, which overwhelms the ability of the proximal tubule to reabsorb sodium bicarbonate. When this unabsorbed sodium bicarbonate reaches the principal cell under the action of aldosterone, sodium is reabsorbed, and potassium is lost into the urine, resulting in hypokalemia.

Renal loss of potassium can occur as a result of an impaired ability of the renal tubules to absorb potassium or as a consequence of mineralocorticoid excess. Postobstructive diuresis, magnesium depletion, recovery from acute tubular necrosis, and use of diuretics lead to a decreased ability to absorb potassium. Renal potassium losses can also occur if potassium forms a complex with nonabsorbable anions in the tubular lumen, such as occurs in β-hydroxybutyrate production in diabetic ketoacidosis.

Mineralocorticoid excess is usually associated with hypertension and can occur from primary hyperaldosteronism as seen in Conn's syndrome, bilateral adrenal hyperplasia, or glucocorticoid-remediable hyperaldosteronism. Secondary hyperaldosteronism can be seen with renal artery stenosis, renin-secreting tumors, and malignant hypertension. Cushing's disease and congenital adrenal hyperplasia also lead to a high mineralocorticoid state and hypokalemia. Lastly, ingestion of black licorice and certain types of chewing tobacco cause apparent mineralocorticoid excess, leading to hypertension and hypokalemia.

It is common for dialysis patients to have potassium values of less than 3 mEq/L immediately after dialysis. The majority of these patients have an overload of total body potassium; over several hours, the potassium level normalizes as potassium leaves the cells and enters the circulation. Unless the patient has symptomatic hypokalemia, the potassium should not be repleted, and the potassium level can be checked the following day.

## Risk Stratification

Most patients with mild hypokalemia are asymptomatic; symptoms usually do not occur until the serum potassium concentration falls below 3 mEq/L. The psychiatric team can manage the vast majority of cases of hypokalemia in the outpatient setting.

Patients should be sent to the emergency department or transferred to the medical ward if they are having an arrhythmia, if they are having significant ongoing losses of potassium that cannot be repleted adequately, or if they cannot take potassium orally. A medical consultation should be obtained if the patient's potassium level is less than 3 mEq/L, if the patient is taking digoxin, if the patient has hypokalemia along with hypertension and is not taking diuretics, or if the hypokalemia is not correcting rapidly.

## Assessment and Management in Psychiatric Settings

The evaluation of hypokalemia should address both the clinical stability of the patient and the cause of the abnormality. The patient should be asked about muscle weakness, myalgias, polyuria, and constipation. Gastrointestinal losses secondary to diarrhea, vomiting, or both should be ruled out. A review of the patient's past medical history for diseases that are associated with hypokalemia, including hypertension, bulimia, laxative abuse, and hyperthyroidism, should be performed. A review of both historical and current medication use for diuretics, laxatives, cisplatin, or amphotericin is essential. The blood pressure should be measured. Laboratory evaluation should include measurement of serum bicarbonate, potassium, and magnesium. Analysis of urine for potassium and chloride levels can be performed by using a spot urine sample. A urinary potassium level <20 mEq/L suggests that the kidney is conserving potassium adequately and that the cause of the hypokalemia is secondary to either low potassium intake or nonrenal potassium losses. A urinary potassium level >20 mEq/L suggests renal loss of potassium.

The initial goal in treatment of hypokalemia is to replete the current potassium deficit. The long-term goal is to prevent the recurrence of hypokalemia by either increasing the patient's potassium intake or de-

**TABLE 42-1.** Potassium repletion protocol

| Initial potassium level (mEq/L) | Intravenous replacement | Oral replacement | Repeat measurement of potassium level |
|---|---|---|---|
| 3.3–3.5 | | 20 mEq of potassium chloride (KCl) every 2 hours for three doses | Following morning |
| 3.0–3.2 | | 20 mEq of KCl every 2 hours for four doses | Following morning |
| <3.0 | 10 mEq of KCl in 100 mL of normal saline solution administered by intravenous Soluset over 1 hour for three infusions | | 1 hour after the last infusion |

creasing the patient's potassium losses. The potassium deficit in patients with hypokalemia can only be approximated. Experimentally, a decrease from a potassium level of 4 mEq/L to 3 mEq/L requires the loss of 200–400 mEq of potassium (Rose 2003; Sterns et al. 1981).

Oral potassium repletion can be used when the potassium level is ≥3 mEq/L, as long as there are no significant ongoing losses (Table 42–1). The potassium level should be rechecked a day or two after supplementation is started. If the patient's renal function is abnormal, potassium repletion should be continued carefully, with smaller amounts of potassium given and blood levels of potassium checked frequently.

Intravenous replacement should be used if the patient is symptomatic, cannot tolerate oral replacement, or has excessive ongoing losses. Intravenous potassium should not be given at a more rapid rate than 10 mEq/hour (Kruse et al. 1994). The patient should be rapidly transferred to a medical unit, because the intravenous replacement requires electrocardiographic monitoring and frequent blood draws to recheck the potassium level.

Because 7%–50% of patients who are taking potassium-losing diuretics develop hypokalemia (Bloomfield et al. 1986), it is reasonable to initiate potassium supplementation at the time of diuretic initiation in patients with normal renal function. Patients who are taking loop or thiazide diuretics and who become hypokalemic often require at least 40 mEq of potassium chloride per day (Schnaper et al. 1989). An alternative is to give a potassium-sparing diuretic (amiloride, triamterene, or spironolactone) in conjugation with the loop or thiazide diuretic. This strategy has the advantage of maintaining magnesium balance and may be more effective than administration of potassium chloride in maintaining the potassium balance (Maronde et al. 1983). The accepted risk, with the addition of a potassium-sparing diuretic, is that the patient will no longer respond to potassium loading with an appropriate kaluresis and will become predisposed to developing hyperkalemia.

# References

Andersson OK, Gudbrandsson T, Jamerson K: Metabolic adverse effects of thiazide diuretics: the importance of normokalaemia. J Intern Med Suppl 735:89–96, 1991

Artz SA, Paes IC, Faloon WW: Hypokalemia-induced hepatic coma in cirrhosis: occurrence despite neomycin therapy. Gastroenterology 51:1046–1053, 1966

Bloomfield RL, Wilson DJ, Buckalew VM Jr: The incidence of diuretic-induced hypokalemia in two distinct clinic settings. J Clin Hypertens 2:331–338, 1986

Cremer W, Bock KD: Symptoms and course of chronic hypokalemic nephropathy in man. Clin Nephrol 7: 112–119, 1977

Hafez H, Strauss J, Aronson M, et al: Hypokalemia-induced psychosis in a chronic schizophrenic patient. J Clin Psychiatry 45:277–279, 1984

Hajjar I, Grim C, George V, et al: Impact of diet on blood pressure and age-related changes in blood pressure in the US population. Arch Intern Med 161:589–593, 2001

Hatta K, Takahashi T, Nakamura H, et al: Hypokalemia and agitation in acute psychotic patients. Psychiatry Res 96:85–88, 1999

Kruse JA, Clark VL, Carlson RW, et al: Concentrated potassium chloride infusions in critically ill patients with hypokalemia. J Clin Pharmacol 34:1077–1082, 1994

Maronde RF, Milgrom M, Vlachakis ND, et al: Response of thiazide-induced hypokalemia to amiloride. JAMA 249:237–241, 1983

Palmer B: Potassium: key physiologic principles: hypokalemic and hyperkalemic disorders [Hypertension, Dialysis, and Clinical Nephrology Web site]. August 2003. Available at: http://www.hdcn.com/symp/03asnb/ 03asnb.htm

Rose B: Treatment of hypokalemia. [UpToDate Web site]. 2003. Available at: http://www.utdol.com. Accessed December 2003.

Schnaper HW, Freis ED, Friedman RG, et al: Potassium restoration in hypertensive patients made hypokalemic by hydrochlorothiazide. Arch Intern Med 149:2677–2681, 1989

Soleimani M, Bergman JA, Hosford MA, et al: Potassium depletion increases luminal Na+/H+ exchange and basolateral NA+:CO3- cotransport in rat renal cortex. J Clin Invest 86:1076–1083, 1990

Sterns RH, Cox M, Feig PU, et al: Internal potassium balance and the control of the plasma potassium concentration. Medicine 60:339–354, 1981

Tizianello A, Garibotto G, Robaudo C, et al: Renal ammoniagenesis in humans with chronic potassium depletion. Kidney Int 40:772–778, 1991

Wingo C, Weiner D: Disorders of potassium inbalance, in Brenner and Rector's The Kidney, 6th Edition. Edited by Brenner BM. Philadelphia, PA, WB Saunders, 2000, pp 1015–1020

# CHAPTER 43

# Hyperkalemia

## Madhu C. Bhaskaran, M.D.

## Clinical Presentation

In an average-sized adult with a normal serum potassium concentration, a total body potassium excess of 100–200 mEq is required to produce a 1 mEq/L rise in serum potassium concentration. The factors that affect potassium secretion in the distal nephron are plasma potassium concentration, tubular blood flow rate, transepithelial potential difference, acid-base status, mineralocorticoids, and sodium chloride concentration in the tubular lumen.

The clinical presentation is as important as the absolute value of serum potassium in defining the severity of hyperkalemia. However, for descriptive purposes, an absolute value of 5.5–6 mEq/L may be considered mild, 6–6.5 mEq/L moderate, and >6.5 mEq/L severe hyperkalemia.

Clinical manifestations of hyperkalemia are highly variable among individuals. Patients can be asymptomatic, have vague and nonspecific complaints involving the gastrointestinal system, or complain of paresthesia or muscle weakness. Electrocardiogram (ECG) changes include peaked T waves, prolonged P–R interval, widened QRS complex, atrial and ventricular arrhythmia, and evidence of pacemaker malfunction. Factors that can potentially contribute to the clinical syndrome include the rate at which hyperkalemia ensues, the presence of other electrolyte abnormalities, coexisting acid-base disorders, and the presence of cardiovascular, neuromuscular, pulmonary, and renal diseases. ECG changes and neuromuscular abnormalities warrant immediate therapy. On the other hand, gradually ensuing or chronic asymptomatic hyperkalemia may be better tolerated and may not require dramatic interventions (Mount and Zandi-Nejad 2004; Evans and Greenberg 2005) (see Figure 43–1).

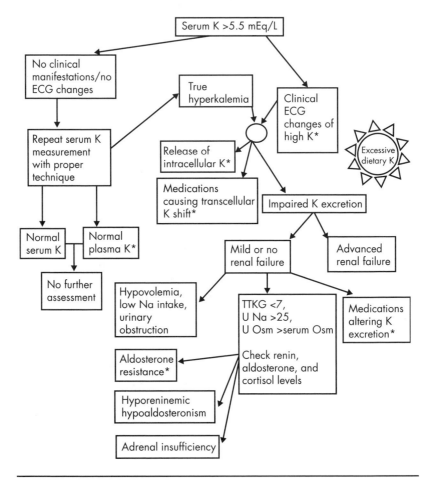

**FIGURE 43–1.** Algorithm for the evaluation of hyperkalemia.

*Note.* ECG=electrocardiogram; K=potassium; Na=sodium;
Osm=osmolarity; TTKG=transtubular potassium gradient; U=urine.
*See text for details.

## Differential Diagnosis

### Spurious Hyperkalemia

Pseudohyperkalemia can occur as a result of release of intracellular potassium from white blood cells (WBCs), platelets, or red blood cells (RBCs) during blood sample collection. Intracellular potassium can also be released after prolonged storage of a blood sample, as well as after breach of RBC membranes because of enzymatic defects. The likelihood of spurious hyperkalemia is greater when blood is collected with the use of a tourniquet, when the platelet count is higher than $500,000/\mu L$, or when the WBC count is more than $100,000/\mu L$. Measurement of plasma potassium concentration rather than serum potassium concentration can help to differentiate spurious hyperkalemia from the true hyperkalemia (Howard et al. 2000).

## Hyperkalemia From Changes in Transcellular Potassium Distribution

### Release of Intracellular Potassium

Hypercatabolic states, such as trauma, tumor lysis, rhabdomyolysis, and large hematomas, cause the release of cellular potassium and lead to marked elevations in plasma potassium concentration, especially when renal excretion is impaired. A similar exit of intracellular potassium can be induced by succinylcholine, a muscle relaxant, especially in patients with severe burns and spinal cord injuries (Mount and Zandi-Nejad 2004; Evans and Greenberg 2005).

Inherited defective potassium channels can lead to a marked elevation in plasma potassium concentration that is associated with periodic skeletal muscle paralysis (Mount and Zandi-Nejad 2004; Evans and Greenberg 2005).

Hyperkalemia in the setting of metabolic acidosis is caused by a transcellular shift of the cation. Exercise, fasting, hyperosmolality, and use of $\alpha$-adrenergic agonists, $\beta$-adrenergic blockers, and digitalis are also known to enhance efflux of cellular potassium (Mount and Zandi-Nejad 2004; Evans and Greenberg 2005).

### Decreased Cellular Uptake of Potassium

Potassium-depleted patients are relatively intolerant to high potassium loads, possibly because the muscular $Na^+$-$K^+$-ATPase pump is diminished in these patients. Digitalis directly inhibits the $Na^+$-$K^+$-ATPase pump, and use of this drug may lead to hyperkalemia. $\beta_2$-Adrenergic blockers are also known to impair cellular potassium uptake.

### Decreased Potassium Excretion

If the excretion of potassium by the kidneys occurs at a normal rate, large potassium loads can be managed without hyperkalemia. However, any factors that affect potassium excretion—including glomerular filtration rate (GFR), rate of distal delivery of sodium, distal tubular flow, availability and response to aldosterone, and renal tubular function—can manifest as impairment of renal potassium excretion (Allon 1995).

**Defect in renal tubular secretion.** Broadly, defective renal excretion of potassium can result from intrinsic causes (local or systemic diseases) or extrinsic causes (medications). Defective potassium excretion can result from either a primary defect in tubular potassium secretion or a mineralocorticoid deficiency that leads to a secondary defect in potassium secretion by the tubules.

**Hypoaldosteronism.** The most common clinical syndrome associated with aldosterone deficiency is hyporeninemic hypoaldosteronism. This condition is characterized by hyperkalemia disproportionate to the GFR, low renin levels as well as low aldosterone levels, and normal cortisol levels. Hyperchloremic metabolic acidosis with a preserved ability to reduce urine pH below 5.5 is seen in these patients. A heterogeneous group of conditions, including diabetic nephropathy, use of nonsteroidal anti-inflammatory drugs (NSAIDs), urinary tract obstruction, HIV-associated nephropathy, lupus nephritis, and paraproteinemias, can lead to this clinical syndrome. Pseudohypoaldosteronism type I is characterized by unresponsiveness to mineralocorticoids. This unresponsiveness in turn leads to salt wasting and high renin and aldosterone levels. Studies have linked this disorder to defective sodium channels. These patients respond to sodium chloride therapy and may grow out of the defect as they age. Pseudohypoaldosteronism type II is characterized by low or normal aldosterone levels secondary to enhanced sodium absorption, hypertension, hyperkalemia, and hyperchloremic metabolic acidosis (Sterns et al. 1981).

**Other factors affecting potassium excretion.** Angiotensin-converting enzyme (ACE) inhibitors, angiotensin-receptor blockers, spironolactone, heparin, and β-blockers act predictably to reduce potassium excretion.

In renal failure, hyperkalemia is known to ensue once the GFR drops below 25 mL/minute, depending on potassium intake, tubular function defects, and urinary volume. Volume depletion promotes hyperkalemia by reducing distal tubular flow, thereby limiting potassium excretion. Reduced sodium intake limits the amount of potassium excreted at the distal tubule by diminishing the amount of sodium reaching the distal tubule. Potassium-sparing diuretics such as triamterene and amiloride interrupt the sodium channel at the distal tubule, leading to a less favorable electrical gradient for potassium secretion.

Hyperkalemia as a part of the syndrome of rhabdomyolysis can occur in alcohol users as well as cocaine users. In addition, compartment syndrome produced by intravenous substance use can cause hyperkalemia. Succinylcholine, a depolarizing muscle relaxant used by anesthesiologists during electroconvulsive therapy, can induce malignant hyperthermia associated with severe hyperkalemia in some individuals (Halliday 2003; Hanlon et al. 1993).

## Risk Stratification

Although any serum potassium value above 5.5 mEq/L is considered evidence of hyperkalemia, the physiological consequences of hyperkalemia and therefore the urgency and even necessity of intervention depend on the significance of the ECG changes. An individual who is taking an ACE inhibitor and who has controlled hypertension and good kidney function may need dietary adjustment or even addition of a non-potassium-sparing diuretic. On the other hand, mild hyperkalemia in an elderly individual with compromised cardiac status and acute renal failure should prompt aggressive management measures. Other reasons for aggressive intervention irrespective of the absolute level of hyperkalemia include obvious physiological consequences of hyperkalemia such as bradycardia or abnormal ECG findings, particularly changes involving the QRS complex.

## Assessment and Management in Psychiatric Settings

The diagnostic approach to the psychiatric patient with significant hyperkalemia should include assessment for the presence of renal failure, urinary obstruction, and volume depletion; a review of patient's medications and diet; a metabolic profile, including measurement of serum osmolality, calcium level, and acid-base status; measurement of the creatine phosphokinase level; urinalysis; and measurement of urinary electrolytes and osmolality (see Figure 43–2). If the transtubular potassium gradient (urine/plasma potassium ratio divided by the urine/plasma osmolality ratio) is less than 7, the patient's renin, aldosterone, and cortisol levels should be measured. Low renin and aldosterone levels indicate hyporeninemic hypoaldosteronism. A high renin level coupled with low aldosterone and cortisol levels suggests adrenal insufficiency.

All patients with symptomatic hyperkalemia or with ECG changes should be transferred immediately to the nearest emergency department for continuous cardiac monitoring and definitive treatment. The

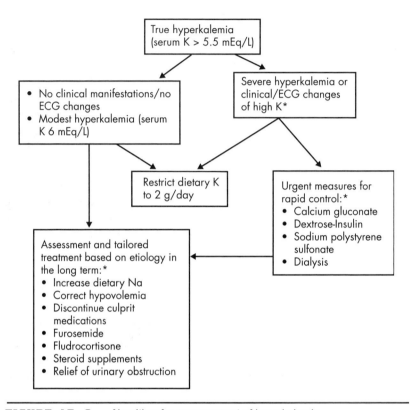

**FIGURE 43-2.** Algorithm for management of hyperkalemia.

*Note.* ECG=electrocardiogram; K=potassium; Na=sodium.
*See text for details.

protocols for emergency treatment of hyperkalemia include the intravenous administration of calcium gluconate (10 mL of a 10% solution over 2–3 minutes), dextrose-insulin (25 g of dextrose in a 50% solution and 10 units of regular insulin), and sodium bicarbonate (45 mEq or one standard vial of 7.5% solution). Albuterol nebulizer (20 mg in 4 mL of normal saline solution) is also effective.

Asymptomatic patients with normal ECG findings should be treated either with 20–30 g po of sodium polystyrene sulfonate every 4–6 hours in 100 mL po of 20% sorbitol solution or with 50 g of sodium polystyrene sulfonate in 50 mL of 70% sorbitol solution and 150 mL of water as an enema. This therapy enhances elimination of potassium from the body. Onset of action occurs about 2 hours after treatment. Each gram of resin binds with up to 1 mEq of potassium. Dietary modifications in-

**TABLE 43-1.**    Common high- and low-potassium foods

**High potassium**

Fruits: Orange, banana, plantain, mango, papaya, guava, apricots, dried fruits, nectarine, kiwi, pomegranate, prunes, tamarind, honeydew, raisins, cantaloupe

Fish and seafood: Flounder, scallop, sole, halibut

Vegetables: Tomato, mushroom, fresh cauliflower, fresh broccoli, fresh spinach, collard, artichokes, pumpkin, squash, bamboo shoots, carrots, potato, corn, dried beans, nuts

Miscellaneous: Salt substitute

**Low potassium**

Fruits: Apple, cranberries, blueberries, blackberries, cherries, figs, grapes, grapefruit, passion fruit, peach, plums, raspberries, strawberries, watermelon, pears

Vegetables: Asparagus, bean sprouts, cabbage, cucumber, rhubarb, celery, string beans, turnips, lettuce, okra, radishes, frozen or canned carrots, frozen spinach, summer squash, frozen broccoli, frozen cauliflower

clude reducing potassium in the diet to 2 g/day (see Table 43–1 for a list of high-and low-potassium foods), increasing daily sodium intake (if not contraindicated), and avoiding dehydration. The patient's medications should be evaluated and replaced with non-hyperkalemia-causing agents if appropriate. Special attention must be paid to NSAIDs, potassium-sparing diuretics, and ACE inhibitors, which may cause hyperkalemia (Kamel and Wei 2003; Weiner and Wingo 1998).

# References

Allon M: Hyperkalemia in end-stage renal disease: mechanisms and management. J Am Soc Nephrol 6:1134–1142, 1995

Evans KJ, Greenberg A: Hyperkalemia: a review. J Intensive Care Med 20:272–290, 2005

Halliday NJ: Malignant hyperthermia. J Craniofac Surg 14:800–802, 2003

Hanlon MJ, Espeland K, Knudson PB: Chemical dependency and hyperkalemia in adolescents and adults: supportive findings. Alcohol 10:541–543, 1993

Howard MR, Ashwell S, Bond LR, et al: Artefactual serum hyperkalaemia and hypercalcaemia in essential thrombocythaemia. J Clin Pathol 53:105–109, 2000

Kamel KS, Wei C: Controversial issues in the treatment of hyperkalaemia. Nephrol Dial Transplant 18:2215–2218, 2003

Mount DB, Zandi-Nejad K: Disorders of potassium imbalance, in Brenner and Rector's The Kidney, 7th Edition. Edited by Brenner BM. Philadelphia, PA, WB Saunders, 2004, pp 997–1008

Sterns RH, Cox M, Feig PU, et al: Internal potassium balance and the control of the plasma potassium balance. Medicine (Baltimore) 60:339–351, 1981

Weiner ID, Wingo CS: Hyperkalemia: a potential silent killer. J Am Soc Nephrol 9:1535–1543, 1998

# CHAPTER 44

# Urinary Tract Obstruction

### Mary C. Mallappallil, M.D.

## Clinical Presentation

Urinary tract obstructions are common and may occur anywhere in the urinary tract, from the kidney to the tip of the urethra. The term "obstructive nephropathy" refers to the renal disease caused by the blockage of urine flow. The obstruction may be a structural or functional interference anywhere along the urinary tract. The upper urinary tract is the area above the vesicoureteric junction, and obstruction in this area is usually unilateral. The lower urinary tract is below the vesicoureteric junction, and obstruction in this area can be bilateral. Up to 5% of end-stage kidney disease is caused by obstruction (Sacks et al. 1989).

The symptoms of urinary tract obstruction vary depending on how rapidly they develop (acute vs. chronic) and on the extent of obstruction (i.e., partial vs. complete, unilateral or bilateral). Symptoms may include colic referred to testicles or vulva (acute obstruction), change in urine output (hesitancy, dribbling), urinary tract infections, decreased force of urine stream, nocturia, abdominal mass, frequency and urgency of urination, thirst, hypertension, edema, epididymitis, acute or chronic urinary retention. Chronic hydronephrosis may be asymptomatic.

## Differential Diagnosis

### Anatomical Obstruction

Causes of obstruction are age related. In patients younger than age 10 years, causes of obstruction include congenital malformations (more commonly in boys), which consist mostly of abnormalities in the posterior urethral valves and pelvic-ureteric junction. If the obstruction occurs early enough in development and is bilateral, severe renal failure can occur. In the adult population, the most common causes of urinary tract obstruction are acquired conditions, including renal calculi, blood clots, tumors (especially related to the reproductive tract), urethritis secondary to infection (e.g., gonococcal infection), vascular system defects such as aneurysms, retrocaval ureter, fibrosis (including fibrosis secondary to radiation therapy) and gastrointestinal diseases such as Crohn's disease and pancreatitis.

Neurogenic bladder can be seen with spinal cord defects, diabetes, Parkinson's disease, and cerebrovascular disease.

One of the most common sites of obstruction in elderly men is at the level of the prostate. In the aging population, the incidence of lower urinary tract disorders, including benign prostatic hypertrophy, prostate cancer, and incontinence, increases significantly (Sutaria and Staskin 2000).

## Functional and Drug-Related Obstruction

Medications can cause functional or structural urinary tract obstruction. The key to identifying the cause is the temporal relationship of the obstruction after the addition of medications, especially anticholinergic agents, levodopa, and certain antiarrhythmic drugs such as disopyramide. A case of urinary tract obstruction in a patient with cerebrovascular disease treated with baclofen has been reported (White 1985). Cessation of baclofen resulted in relief of the urinary tract obstruction; however, a withdrawal syndrome consisting of agitation, hallucinations, and convulsions persisted for about 1 week. Antipsychotic medications have been known to cause urinary tract obstruction. A case report from Germany discusses a patient with newly diagnosed schizophrenia who developed an acute functional bladder obstruction while receiving initial therapy with haloperidol (Ulmar et al. 1988). Urological examination showed no pathological finding except for a urinary tract infection. After haloperidol was discontinued, the patient's bladder function returned to normal. The mechanism appears to be related to the anticholinergic side effects of haloperidol. Rare cases of contraceptive-mediated acute urinary tract obstructions have also been reported (Saborio et al. 1997).

## Pseudo-Obstruction

In some situations, hydronephrosis can be seen without obstruction. One example is pregnancy, in which hormonally mediated dilation of the urinary tract takes place. An ultrasound scan may show hydronephrosis, although the finding is not pathological. Other patients in whom hydronephrosis may be present without an obstruction include patients with a dilated "megaureter" secondary to urinary reflux that has developed over time and patients with a extrarenal urinary pelvis (a urinary renal pelvis located outside the kidney; this occurs when there is an obstruction of the uteropelvic junction of the ureter) that is not obstructed.

In patients with certain disorders, a dilated urinary tract may be seen without an obstruction. These conditions include high urine flow states such as diabetes insipidus and psychogenic polydipsia. Anatomical and physiological defects secondary to polydipisia may be seen in up to 50% of patients who consume large amounts of fluid (Blum and Friedland 1983). The defects noted in these patients include urine with low specific gravity, a large bladder, large postvoid residual of urine, hydronephrosis, and increased back flow pressures, leading to atrophy in the kidney.

## Psychogenic Obstruction

Psychogenic urinary retention was first clearly described in adults (Williams and Johnson 1956) and in subsequent reports in which urinary retention was noted to be a symptom of an underlying emotional disease (Norden and Friedman 1961). Psychogenic urinary retention has been described as a hysterical or conversion disorder that develops in response to stress and that occurs in a greater number of women than men. Most cases of psychogenic urinary retention are diagnosed after negative findings in medical, neurological, and urological evaluations and are confirmed by psychiatric consultation. The disorder is managed by biofeedback-monitored relaxation and visualization combined with self-catheterization on a fixed schedule (Montague and Jones 1979). The use of a β-adrenergic blocker is not effective in this disorder (Zgourides and Warren 1990).

## Risk Stratification

The greatest risk for obstructive uropathy exists among elderly men with prostate problems, hospitalized patients, patients with recent cerebrovascular accidents, and patients who have dementia or who are otherwise unable to communicate their needs.

Compulsive water drinkers with psychogenic polydipsia may develop hydronephrosis. Although psychogenic polydipsia is recognized by the presence of hyponatremia, a sudden self-correction of the hyponatremia should alert the physician to the possibility of urinary tract obstruction.

## Assessment and Management in Psychiatric Settings

The first and most important step is to measure the postvoid residual volume. After the patient spontaneously voids, a bladder catheter is placed to see if any urine is left over. An amount >100 mL is suggestive of obstruction. The obtained urine should be sent for urinalysis, cytology examination, and culture. An alternative to placing a bladder catheter is to check the postvoid residual with a bladder ultrasound. The physician should also look for evidence of renal failure and electrolyte abnormalities. Routine serum chemistry analysis can be used to detect acute renal failure, hyperkalemia, and a low bicarbonate level. In patients with hyperkalemia (serum potassium level >5.5 mEq/L), an electrocardiogram is required to test for the presence of life-threatening cardiac arrhythmias. If the hyperkalemia is not amenable to medical management, acute hemodialysis may be needed. The presence of electrolyte abnormalities and acute or chronic renal failure with elevated blood urea nitrogen and creatinine levels are indications for a nephrology consultation.

The next priority is to define the level (the location in the upper or lower urinary tract) and cause of the obstruction. The most frequently used test is the renal ultrasound. If bilateral hydronephrosis is seen, a bladder ultrasound and, in men, a prostate ultrasound should be conducted. Retrograde urography can be done if a high-grade obstruction is suspected. Upper tract obstruction is more likely to be unilateral. If hydronephrosis is observed in the imaging studies, placement of a nephrostomy tube may be necessary. Although an ultrasound gives quick information about the presence of an obstruction, it does not determine the cause or often the level of obstruction. Once a nephrostomy is in place, a retrograde urogram can be performed to determine the cause and level of obstruction more definitely. A computed tomography scan without contrast can yield clues, including the presence of retroperitoneal fibrosis. The gold standard is the intravenous urogram, which is used in evaluation of patients with suspected upper tract obstruction who do not have acute renal failure. If the results of the urogram are normal, a diuretic renal scan may be performed.

After the cause of the obstruction is determined, a more definitive therapeutic plan can be designed. Stones can be removed, and the patient can begin medical therapy to help slow further stone formation. Strictures may be dilated with a balloon, and, if needed, stents can be placed. Benign prostatic hypertrophy is usually managed with medications in the early phases. Two categories of medications are often used.

The first category includes the α-adrenergic blockers, which relax the smooth muscle of the bladder neck and prostate and decrease ureteral pressure. The second group consists of the 5α-reductase inhibitors, which inhibit the conversion of testosterone to its most active metabolite, dihydrotestosterone. Because these medications may have a slow onset of action, the bladder catheter should be kept in place. These medications either reduce prostate size or relax the prostate (Anderson 1995).

In the case of neurogenic bladder, both functional and urodynamic studies are needed to define the problem. For an atonic bladder with lower motor neuron injuries, the treatment is intermittent self-catheterization to keep the bladder from overfilling with the maximal amount of about 400–500 mL of urine, which is retrieved with each catheterization. For a hypertonic/unstable bladder from an upper motor neuron injury, anticholinergic agents and possibly self-catheterization may be needed.

There is no definitive rate at which urine output should be allowed to continue once the obstruction is resolved. The conservative approach places an emphasis on prevention of volume depletion when the obstruction is initially relieved. After placement of a catheter, a "postobstructive diuresis" can be observed in patients who were anuric. Excessive volume and electrolytes are rapidly excreted. Even if the obstruction is rapidly removed, the tubular defects may take weeks to months to improve, and continued nephrogenic diabetes insipidus may cause significant volume depletion, dehydration, and worsening of renal function. These effects can be avoided by monitoring the urine output on an hourly basis and by using volume repletion. Electrolytes should be replaced as necessary. Although decompression of an enlarged bladder should be done gradually, an ideal rate of decompression has not been established in the literature. The practice of attempting to control the patient's urine output by clamping a bladder catheter after the removal of a specific amount of urine each hour remains controversial.

# References

Anderson JT: Alpha-1-blockers vs. 5-alpha-reductase inhibitors in benign prostatic hyperplasia: a comparative review. Drugs Aging 6:388–396, 1995

Blum A, Friedland GW: Urinary tract abnormalities due to chronic psychogenic polydipisia. Am J Psychiatry 140:915–916, 1983

Montague DK, Jones LR: Psychogenic urinary retention. Urology 13:30–35, 1979

Norden CW, Friedman EA: Psychogenic urinary retention: report of two cases. N Engl J Med 264:1096–1097, 1961

Saborio DV, Kennedy WA 2nd, Hoke GP: Acute urinary retention secondary to urethral inflammation from a vaginal contraceptive suppository in a 17-year-old boy. Urol Int 58:128–130, 1997

Sacks SH, Aparicio SA, Bevan A, et al: Late renal failure due to prostatic outflow obstruction: a preventable disease. BMJ 298:156–159, 1989

Sutaria PM, Staskin DR: Hydronephrosis and renal deterioration in the elderly due to abnormalities of the lower urinary tract and ureterovesical junction. Int Urol Nephrol 32:119–126, 2000

Ulmar G, Schunck H, Kober C: Urinary retention in the course of neuroleptic therapy with haloperidol. Pharmacopsychiatry 21:208–209, 1988

White WB: Aggravated CNS depression with urinary retention secondary to baclofen administration. Arch Intern Med 145:1717–1718, 1985

Williams GE, Johnson AM: Recurrent urinary retention due to emotional factors: report of a case. Psychosom Med 18:77–80, 1956

Zgourides GD, Warren R: Propranolol treatment of paruresis (psychogenic urinary retention): a brief case report. Percept Mot Skills 71(3 Pt 1):885–886, 1990

# PART XI

# Endocrine and Metabolic Abnormalities

Section Editor:

Harvey L. Katzeff, M.D.

# CHAPTER 45

# Diabetes Mellitus

Terry Gray, Ph.D.

Harvey L. Katzeff, M.D.

## Clinical Presentation

According to the American Diabetes Association (2004), diabetes is defined as a "group of metabolic diseases" that occurs because of defects in either or both insulin secretion and insulin action. Defects in carbohydrate, fat, and protein metabolism characterize the essence of the disease process. Diabetes is a chronic disorder accompanied by complications that affect the cardiac, cerebral, vascular, and neurological systems. End-organ damage is manifested in the microvasculature as diabetic retinopathy and diabetic nephropathy and neuropathy and in the macrovascular tree as an aggressive and accelerated form of atherosclerosis.

## Differential Diagnosis

### Type 1 and Type 2 Diabetes Mellitus

The pathological process of diabetes, and the subsequent hyperglycemia with its symptoms and deleterious effects, is centered around either an absolute or a relative insulin deficiency. An absolute insulin deficiency defines the person with type 1 diabetes, and the person with type 2 diabetes exhibits a relative insulin deficiency. Type 1 diabetes is characterized by an autoimmune destruction of the pancreatic β-cells and is often diagnosed after a dramatic presentation of clinical symptoms, frequently in the form of diabetic ketoacidosis. The initial presentation usually occurs in children age <20 years, but approximately 10% of adults presenting with diabetes have type 1 diabetes. In adults, there is a prolonged period of ongoing β-cell destruction preceding the diagnosis during which euglycemia or mild hyperglycemia is maintained despite a progressively decreasing β-cell mass and function. The presence of autoantibodies can be detected during this period of β-cell destruction, and that time period can be as long as 9–13 years.

As opposed to the sudden clinical onset of type 1 diabetes, type 2 diabetes may remain undiagnosed for many years. The relative insulin deficiency found in the person with type 2 diabetes results in a state in which the normal amount of insulin is no longer able to produce an appropriate biological response. Insulin resistance plays a major role in type 2 diabetes. Almost every person with type 2 diabetes progresses from euglycemia, through a period of impaired glucose homeostasis known as the stage of "prediabetes," to finally reach the stage in which the diagnostic criteria of type 2 diabetes are met.

## Schizophrenia and Diabetes Mellitus

Individuals with schizophrenia are at an increased risk of developing diabetes, as has been reported in the literature even as early as the 1960s (Cohen 2004; Dynes 1969; Felker et al. 1996; McKee et al. 1986; Mukherjee et al. 1996). This susceptibility may be caused by a direct genetic link between diabetes and schizophrenia, but weight gain, poor dietary habits, and decreased physical activity attributable to schizophrenia are probably the major risk factors for diabetes in this population. However, the risk of diabetes initially increased with the introduction of conventional antipsychotics and has increased even further with the introduction of atypical antipsychotics. In 1996, for example, the prevalence of diabetes was estimated to be 24.5% among schizophrenic outpatients in the United States (Mukherjee et al. 1996).

Use of the atypical antipsychotics has been associated with the appearance of diabetes, cardiovascular disease, dyslipidemia, hyperprolactinemia, and weight gain (Abidi and Bhaskara 2003). Cases of diabetes were reported soon after patients began taking medication (Lindenmayer et al. 2003), and some cases presented in the form of diabetic ketoacidosis (Liebzeit et al. 2001). The literature includes reports of these effects within as little as 3–6 months of drug initiation (Henderson et al. 2000; Jin et al. 2002). Early onset was reported after only 6 months of therapy with olanzapine in a majority (73%) of the cases evaluated by Koller and Doraiswamy (2002). These authors have evaluated 237 cases of olanzapine-associated diabetes. Eighty patients had metabolic acidosis or ketosis, 41 had glucose levels of 1,000 mg/dL or greater, and 15 patients died. Glucose levels stabilized after discontinuation of the medication.

**TABLE 45–1.** Risk factors for type 2 diabetes

Age ≥45 years

Overweight (body mass index ≥25 kg/m²)

Family history of diabetes (i.e., parents or siblings with diabetes)

Habitual physical inactivity

Race/ethnicity (e.g., African American, Hispanic American, and Native American)

Previously identified impaired fasting glucose or impaired glucose tolerance

History of gestational diabetes or delivery of a baby weighing >9 lb at birth

Hypertension (≥140/90 mm Hg in adults)

High-density lipoprotein (HDL) cholesterol ≤35 mg/dL (0.90 mmol/L) and/or triglyceride level ≥250 mg/dL (2.82 mmol/L)

Polycystic ovary syndrome

*Source.* Adapted from American Diabetes Association 2004.

## Risk Stratification

Patients for whom atypical antipsychotic therapy is being considered must be evaluated for any characteristics that would influence the decision to prescribe a medication regimen (i.e., for traits that would increase the patient's risk of developing diabetes in the future). Table 45–1 lists characteristics that put a person at greater risk for the development of type 2 diabetes mellitus (American Diabetes Association 2004). The likelihood of developing diabetes is greater in patients with a greater number of risk factors. Identification of multiple risks in the same patient may influence the practitioner's therapeutic decisions.

The challenge of prescribing appropriate medication for the person with schizophrenia is a fundamental undertaking in and of itself. The added burden of identifying those persons at risk for developing the aforementioned maladies, and thus hopefully avoiding potentially grave problems, increases the responsibilities shouldered by the practitioner. As a reminder of the impact of this problem, the United States Food and Drug Administration requires drug manufacturers to include a warning on the labels of atypical antipsychotics about the risk of associated hyperglycemia and diabetes (Rosack 2003).

Once the decision is made to treat the patient with atypical antipsychotics and the therapy is instituted, the patient must be monitored at timely intervals for the appearance of any diabetogenic side effect attributed to this class of agents (Bonanno et al. 2001; Goldstein et al. 1999).

**TABLE 45–2.**    Glycemic control

| Parameter | Target range |
|---|---|
| Hemoglobin $A_{1c}$ | <7.0% (normal: 4.0%–6.0%) |
| Preprandial plasma glucose | 90–130 mg/dL (5.0–7.2 mmol/L) |
| Postprandial plasma glucose (1–2 hours after meal) | <180 mg/dL (<10.0 mmol/L) |

*Source.*   Adapted from American Diabetes Association 2004.

Suggested parameters for follow-up monitoring include measurement of weight, waist circumference, body mass index (BMI), and glucose and lipid levels; in addition, the patients' baseline prolactin level may be measured, and testing may be repeated if the patient exhibits symptoms of prolactin disturbance (Chue and Dovacs 2003). Risk ranges for lipid parameters and target ranges for glucose parameters are presented in Table 45–1 and Table 45–2, respectively.

The American Diabetes Association's guidelines for target ranges for blood glucose level recommend that patients be evaluated on an individual basis and that specific goals be established for each patient. Special attention is needed by patients who experience frequent or severe hypoglycemia, elderly patients, and children. For safety reasons, glycemic targets may be more stringent in these groups. Striving for the lowest glucose levels possible, without significant hypoglycemic events, provides the best avenue for prevention of the chronic complications associated with diabetes.

Obesity and overweight contribute significantly to the development of type 2 diabetes. Persons with schizophrenia manifest more of a propensity toward weight gain than those not afflicted, and that characteristic in itself may subsequently place them at greater risk for a diabetes diagnosis. A study evaluating the presence of obesity and overweight in schizophrenia patients demonstrated an increased incidence of a significantly elevated mean BMI in the schizophrenia versus the nonschizophrenia cohort (Allison et al. 1999). Improper dietary habits, sedentary lifestyle, and the weight gain associated with atypical antipsychotics have been identified as modifiable factors potentially responsible for increased weight in patients with schizophrenia (Dixon and Wohlheiter 2003).

In addition to increased weight and lack of physical activity, many other characteristics prevalent in the schizophrenic population put patients at greater risk for the development of diabetes. Included among these characteristics are social withdrawal, communication and cognitive difficulties, and poor health habits such as smoking. Antipsychotics may cause weight gain, elevated serum glucose levels, movement abnormalities, and an apathetic state, all of which could intensify a sense of social isolation and self-neglect.

The proposed physiological mechanism underlying the onset of diabetes in schizophrenia is as yet unidentified. However, several possibilities have been proposed, including hypothalamic dysregulation involving the dopamine antagonistic effect of the atypical antipsychotics. Dopamine agonists (such as bromocriptine) decrease elevated blood glucose levels, and it follows that the antipsychotics may counter that effect (Liebzeit et al. 2001). Other proposals include the effects of weight gain (Hagg et al. 1998; Wirshing et al. 1998) and direct damage to pancreatic β-cells (Goldstein et al. 1999).

## Assessment and Management in Psychiatric Settings

### Assessment

It is usually unnecessary to screen for the presence of type 1 diabetes, because patients typically present in a compromised metabolic state that can be diagnosed fairly easily by the astute practitioner. However, because type 2 diabetes may be undiagnosed for years, during which the person remains vulnerable to the debilitating effects of the undetected hyperglycemia, screening for the presence of this disease process is in many cases a prudent decision. Screening is especially appropriate for persons with characteristics that make them more likely to develop the disease. The clinical practice recommendation of the American Diabetes Association (2004) for screening for type 2 diabetes is a fasting plasma glucose test every 3 years for anyone age 45 years or older. However, the person whose characteristics suggest a higher level of suspicion for the development of type 2 diabetes should be screened earlier (see Table 45–3).

The screening process would also identify those in the prediabetic phase and offer the clinician an opportunity to intervene in the hopes of preventing or delaying the progression to a diagnosis of type 2 diabetes.

A diagnosis of diabetes is made when one of three diagnostic criteria are met on two separate occasions: fasting plasma glucose level ≥ 126 mg/dL or symptoms (polyuria, polydypsia, unexplained weight loss) plus random plasma glucose level ≥200 mg/dL or 2-hour plasma glucose level ≥200 mg/dL during 75 g oral glucose tolerance test (Ex-

**TABLE 45–3.**    Screening for adult onset (type 2) diabetes using fasting plasma glucose level[a]

Screening is recommended for all persons age ≥45 years at 3-year intervals. Earlier testing is recommended if the person has any of the following risk factors:
- Overweight (body mass index ≥25 kg/m²)
- History of impaired glucose tolerance or impaired fasting glucose
- Member of at-risk racial/ethnic group
- History of gestational diabetes
- First-degree relative with diabetes
- History of delivery of baby weighing >9 lb at birth
- Hypertension
- Manifestations of insulin resistance
- High density lipoprotein (HDL) cholesterol ≤35 mg/dL
- Triglyceride level ≥250 mg/dL

[a]Normal level is <100 mg/dL.
*Source.*   Adapted from American Diabetes Association 2004.

pert Committee on the Diagnosis and Classification of Diabetes Mellitus 1997) . A person meets the criteria for inclusion in the prediabetic category when the blood glucose levels are elevated but are not high enough to satisfy the diagnostic criteria for diabetes. The prediabetic parameters are as follows: a fasting glucose level greater than 99 mg/dL but no greater than 125 mg/dL or a 2-hour oral glucose tolerance test result ranging from 140 mg/dL to 199 mg/dL.

## Management

Persons with type 1 diabetes require insulin for survival, whereas the person with type 2 diabetes can be treated with a variety of oral agents, combined with insulin if necessary, that address the physiological defects of type 2 diabetes, namely insulin resistance, insulin deficit, and increased hepatic glucose production.

In patients with type 2 diabetes, a combination of agents aimed at the aforementioned multiple defects of the disorder can be used for effective management. The combination of oral medications taken during the daytime hours with insulin administered at the hour of sleep has proved a most effective approach to therapy. Multiple forms of insulin and oral agents are available.

## Insulin Therapy

The form of insulin currently prescribed is human insulin, as opposed to the beef and pork preparations used previously. Insulin preparations with various timing properties can be combined in a single mode of administration. Combination preparations are premixed and are easier for some patients to use. A drawback is that these preparations limit the ability of the practitioner to manipulate the dose of one component of the mixture without changing the dose of the other components. Examples of insulin mixtures include 70% neutral protamine Hagedorn (NPH)/30% regular, 50% NPH/50% regular, and 75% NPH/25% lispro, among others.

## Oral Agents

The oldest oral agents, the sulfonylureas, have been in use since the early 1940s and act to increase insulin secretion through direct stimulation of the β-cell. A major side effect associated with sulfonylurea preparations is hypoglycemia. Weight gain can also accompany the use of these agents. Despite the side effects, the sulfonylureas are very effective agents and are usually inexpensive. Various preparations are available, including the second-generation formulations of glimepiride, glipizide, and glyburide. The first-generation preparations are now rarely prescribed as a first line of treatment.

The meglitinides, nonsulfonylurea insulin secretagogues, also stimulate β-cell secretion but act at a different receptor site, compared to the sulfonylureas. The advantages of this class of agents include a quicker onset and shorter duration of action, compared to the sulfonylureas. They are responsive to glucose levels and cause fewer problems with hypoglycemia than the older agents. They are taken 0–30 minutes before a meal and are withheld if the person decides not to eat. Persons with renal disease, inconsistent dietary habits, early postprandial hyperglycemia, or late postprandial hypoglycemia can benefit from using these agents. Examples of this class include repaglinide and nateglinide.

The thiazolidinediones, relatively new agents for the treatment of diabetes, primarily decrease insulin resistance in the peripheral sites and have a minor role in diminishing hepatic glucose production. A desirable consideration is the fact that hypoglycemia is not a major side effect of the thiazolidinediones, unless hypoglycemic medications are used concomitantly. The thiazolidinediones should be used selectively, and their use should be avoided in patients with liver conditions. These agents may cause significant fluid retention and weight gain, especially when used in combination with insulin or insulin secretagogues, and these conditions are especially contraindicated in persons with heart disease. The therapeutic response to thiazolidinediones may be delayed, and the benefits of treatment may not appear for 6–12 weeks.

Ongoing evaluation of liver function is required with the thiazolidinediones. The liver function tests should be obtained bimonthly for 1 year after initiation of therapy and four times a year thereafter. Usage should be discontinued if the alanine transaminase value increases to greater than three times the upper limit of normal (ULN) values. These agents should not be prescribed for patients with hepatic dysfunction or in the presence of elevated findings on liver function tests (>2.5×ULN). Thiazolidinedione preparations now available in the United States include rosiglitazone and pioglitazone.

The biguanides have their primary effect on hepatic glucose output and are most effective in persons who are obese or overweight. They should not be used in cases where there is a history of alcohol abuse, renal disease (with a creatinine level ≥1.5 in males and ≥1.4 in females), hepatic disease, or congestive heart failure. The biguanide metformin is approved for use in the United States; different preparations can be prescribed in other countries.

One effect that may be seen with the biguanides in some cases is weight loss, a welcome effect in obese patients. The gastrointestinal side effects of the biguanides may preclude their use in a number of patients. A major, but rare, side effect is lactic acidosis, which usually occurs in patients for whom the drug was prescribed inappropriately. Lactic acidosis, should it occur, can be recognized by the symptoms of malaise, somnolence, myalgias, respiratory distress, abdominal discomfort, hypothermia, hypotension, and bradycardia. Like the thiazolidinediones, metformin does not usually cause hypoglycemia. Additional benefits of this agent include decrease in insulin resistance, improvement in lipid profiles, and weight loss or weight neutrality, all of which are desirable effects in persons who are candidates for the metabolic syndrome.

α-Glucosidase inhibitors, including acarbose and miglitol, inhibit the action of the gastrointestinal enzymes responsible for carbohydrate metabolism and interfere with absorption of carbohydrates. The primary effect is to lower postprandial glucose elevation after a meal containing carbohydrates. If the agent is administered with hypoglycemic agents, any episodes of hypoglycemia must be treated with a glucose-containing preparation (i.e., glucose tablets), as α-glucosidase inhibitors interfere with the absorption of sucrose and other starches. Unfortunately, the gastrointestinal side effects of flatulence, bloating, and diarrhea associated with these medications often cause patients to discontinue their use despite their potential efficacy. The side effects can be lessened if the agent is titrated slowly to the effective dose, usually requiring a period of 6–12 weeks.

# References

Abidi S, Bhaskara SM: From chlorpromazine to clozapine—antipsychotic adverse effects and the clinician's dilemma. Can J Psychiatry 48:749–755, 2003

Allison DB, Fontaine KR, Heo M, et al: The distribution of body mass index among individuals with and without schizophrenia. J Clin Psychiatry 60:215–220, 1999

American Diabetes Association: 2004 Clinical practice recommendations: diagnosis and classification of diabetes mellitus. Diabetes Care 27 (supp 1):S5–S10, 2004

Bonanno DG, Davydov L, Botts SR: Olanzapine-induced diabetes mellitus. Ann Pharmacother 35:563–565, 2001

Chue P, Dovacs CS: Safety and tolerability of atypical antipsychotics in patients with bipolar disorder: prevalence, monitoring and management. Bipolar Disord 5 (suppl 2):62–97, 2003

Cohen D: Atypical antipsychotics and new onset diabetes mellitus: an overview of the literature. Pharmacopsychiatry 37:1–11, 2004

Dixon LB, Wohlheiter K: Diabetes and mental illness: factors to keep in mind. Consultant 12:337–344, 2003

Dynes JB: Diabetes in schizophrenia and diabetes in nonpsychotic medical patients. Dis Nerv Syst 30:341–344, 1969

Expert Committee on the Diagnosis and Classification of Diabetes Mellitus: Report of the Expert Committee on the Diagnosis and Classification of Diabetes Mellitus. Diabetes Care 20:1183–1197, 1997

Felker B, Yazel JJ, Short D: Mortality and medical comorbidity among psychiatric patients: a review. Psychiatr Serv 47:1356–1363, 1996

Goldstein LE, Sporn J, Brown S, et al: New-onset diabetes mellitus and diabetic ketoacidosis associated with olanzapine treatment. Psychosomatics 40:438–443, 1999

Hagg S, Joelsson L, Mjorndal T, et al Prevalence of diabetes and impaired glucose intolerance in patients treated with clozapine compared with patients treated with conventional depot neuroleptic medications. J Clin Psychiatry 59:294–299, 1998

Henderson DC, Cagliero E, Gray C, et al: Clozapine, diabetes mellitus, weight gain, and lipid abnormalities: a five-year naturalistic study. Am J Psychiatry 157:975–981, 2000

Jin H, Meyer JM, Jeste DV: Phenomenology of and risk factors for new-onset diabetes mellitus and diabetic ketoacidosis associated with atypical antipsychotic medications: an analysis of 45 published cases. Ann Clin Psychiatry 14:59–64, 2002

Koller EA, Doraiswamy PM: Olanzapine-associated diabetes mellitus. Pharmacotherapy 22:841–852, 2002

Liebzeit KA, Markowitz JS, Caley CF: New onset diabetes and atypical antipsychotics. Euro Neuropsychopharmacol 11:25–32, 2001

Lindenmayer JP, Czobor P, Volavka J, et al: Changes in glucose and cholesterol in patients with schizophrenia treated with typical and atypical antipsychotics. Am J Psychiatry 160:290–296, 2003

McKee HA, D'Arcy PF, Wilson PJ: Diabetes and schizophrenia: a preliminary study. J Clin Hosp Pharm 11:297–299, 1986

Mukherjee S, Decina P, Bocola V, et al: Diabetes mellitus in schizophrenic patients. Compr Psychiatry 37:68–73, 1996

Rosack J: FDA to require diabetes warning on antipsychotics. Psychiatr News 38(20):1, 2003

Wirshing DA, Spellberg BJ, Erhart SM, et al. Novel antipsychotics and new onset diabetes. Biol Psychiatry 44:778–783, 1998

# CHAPTER 46

# Hyperlipidemia

Harvey L. Katzeff, M.D.

## Clinical Presentation

Hyperlipidemia is a general term that defines an increase in the serum concentration of various lipoproteins. Lipoproteins are usually classified into three major categories. Low-density lipoproteins (LDLs) are cholesterol-rich particles whose serum concentration is directly correlated with the risk of myocardial infarction and death. The serum concentration of very-low-density lipoproteins (VLDLs), which are triglyceride-rich particles, is strongly correlated with the level of insulin resistance and inversely proportional to the serum concentration of high-density lipoproteins (HDLs). HDL particles are antiatherogenic lipid particles, and high serum levels of HDL are protective against coronary artery disease.

Conventional antipsychotics are associated with hypercholesterolemia. The majority of atypical antipsychotics produce an increase in body weight and hyperlipidemias. Recent studies have demonstrated the role of clozapine and olanzapine in producing hypertriglyceridemia and the insulin resistance syndrome.

## Differential Diagnosis

To evaluate the patient for hyperlipidemia, a blood sample for a lipid profile should be drawn after a 10–12-hour fast. A lipid profile consists of total serum cholesterol, serum triglyceride, and serum HDL cholesterol measurements. The LDL cholesterol value is calculated as follows: LDL cholesterol = total cholesterol − (HDL cholesterol + triglyceride/5).

**TABLE 46–1.**  Suggested cholesterol guidelines

| Lipoprotein and serum concentration | Status |
|---|---|
| Low-density lipoprotein (LDL) cholesterol (primary target of therapy) | |
| <100 mg/dL | Optimal |
| 100–129 mg/dL | Near optimal |
| 130–159 mg/dL | Borderline high |
| ≥160 mg/dL | High |
| Total cholesterol | |
| <200 mg/dL | Desired |
| 200–239 mg/dL | Borderline high |
| ≥240 mg/dL | High |
| High-density lipoprotein (HDL) cholesterol[a] | |
| <40 mg/dL | Low |
| ≥40 mg/dL | Desired |
| ≥60 mg/dL | High |
| Triglyceride | |
| ≤150 mg/dL | Desired |
| >200 mg/dL | Treatment advised |

[a]For women, it has been suggested that the HDL goal be increased by 10 mg/dL.
*Source.*  Modified from Expert Panel on the Detection, Evaluation, and Treatment of High Blood Cholesterol in Adults 2001.

This formula is not accurate for triglyceride values >400 mg/dL. In those situations, LDL levels may be measured directly. Patients can be broadly classified into two groups on the basis of their lipid profiles: those with an elevation of LDL cholesterol alone and those with both an elevated triglyceride level and a low HDL cholesterol level. However, a significant proportion of individuals have abnormal values of all three parameters.

A variety of medical conditions and drugs can exacerbate hyperlipidemias. Elevations of the serum LDL cholesterol level can occur in response to hypothyroidism and nephrotic syndrome. Hypertriglyceridemia and decreased HDL levels are commonly seen in patients with insulin resistance, diabetes, and the metabolic syndrome. Individuals are characterized by their coronary risk profile according to the National Cholesterol Education Program Adult Treatment Panel III guidelines, as shown in Table 46–1.

# Risk Stratification

The risk assessment of dyslipidemia has been defined by a group of experts in the third report of the National Cholesterol Education Program (Expert Panel on Detection, Evaluation, and Treatment of High Blood Cholesterol in Adults 2001). All patients older than 20 should have a fasting lipoprotein profile (i.e., total cholesterol, LDL cholesterol, HDL cholesterol, and triglyceride). The LDL cholesterol is the primary target for therapeutic intervention and the risk level is calculated by taking into account the following factors: age (men older than 44 years, women older than 54 years) cigarette smoking, blood pressure greater than 139/89, HDL cholesterol level lower than 40 mg/dL, family history of premature coronary heart disease (i.e., coronary heart diseas in a male first-degree relative younger than 55 years or in a female first-degree relative younger than 65 years). Patient with zero or one risk factors should be treated if their LDL cholesterol level is greater 160 mg/dl. Patients with two or more risk factors require intervention if their LDL cholesterol level is greater than 130 mg/dL. Finally, patients with history of coronary heart disease or coronary heart disease equivalents (e.g., diabetes, peripheral artery disease, abdominal aortic disease, and symptomatic coronary artery disease) benefit from lowering the LDL cholesterol level to less than 100 mg/dL.

# Assessment and Management in Psychiatric Settings

The discovery and employment of a variety of classes of therapeutic agents and the dramatic effects these agents have on serum lipid fractions have dramatically altered clinical practice. The discovery of these agents was followed by an explosion of epidemiological and prospective, randomized, interventional clinical studies that have demonstrated the significant effects of these agents in reducing both the morbidity and mortality of coronary heart disease and cerebrovascular stroke.

The pathophysiogical basis of each form of dyslipidemia also dictates the type of therapy to be used. Diet therapy usually involves decreasing cholesterol and saturated fat intake. With this intervention, the serum LDL cholesterol level decreases by an average of 15%, but there is significant variability in that response (0%–30%). Diet therapy alone usually does not allow individuals to reach their goal. The 3-hydroxy-3-methylglutaryl coenzyme A (HMG-CoA) reductase inhibitors, the so-called "statins," are potent, well-tolerated agents that primarily lower LDL cholesterol levels. For individuals who already show signs of dia-

**TABLE 46–2.** Medications to treat hyperlipidemia

| Drug class | Lipid/lipoprotein effects | Selected side effects | Selected contraindications/ warnings | Outcomes trial results |
|---|---|---|---|---|
| HMG-CoA reductase inhibitors (statins) | LDL ↓ 18%–55%<br>HDL ↑ 5%–15%<br>TG ↓ 7%–30% | Myopathy, elevated liver enzyme values | Active or chronic liver disease, concomitant use of certain drugs | Reduction in major coronary events, deaths due to coronary heart disease, need for coronary procedures, stroke, and total mortality |
| Bile acid sequestrants | LDL ↓ 15%–30%<br>HDL ↑ 3%–5%<br>TG no change or ↑ | Gastrointestinal distress, constipation, decreased absorption of other drugs | Dysbetalipoproteinemia, TG>200 mg/dL | Reduction in major coronary events and deaths due to coronary heart disease |
| Nicotinic acid | LDL ↓ 5%–25%<br>HDL ↑ 15%–35%<br>TG ↓ 20%–50% | Flushing; hyperglycemia, hyperuricemia (or gout), upper gastrointestinal distress, hepatotoxicity | Chronic liver disease, severe gout, diabetes, hyperuricemia, peptic ulcer disease | Reduction in major coronary events and possibly in total mortality |

**TABLE 46–2.** Medications to treat hyperlipidemia *(continued)*

| Drug class | Lipid/lipoprotein effects | Selected side effects | Selected contraindications/ warnings | Outcomes trial results |
|---|---|---|---|---|
| Fibric acids | LDL ↓ 5%–20% (may be ↑ in patients with high TG) HDL ↑ 10%–20% TG ↓ 20%–50% | Dyspepsia; gallstones, myopathy | Severe renal disease, severe hepatic disease | Reduction in major coronary events |
| Ezetimibe | LDL ↓ 15%–20% | Elevated liver enzyme values in combination with statins | Liver disease | No outcomes data |

*Note.* HMG-CoA=3-hydroxy-3-methylglutaryl coenzyme A; LDL=low-density lipoprotein; HDL=high-density lipoprotein; TG=triglyceride betes or macrovascular disease of the heart or brain, there is evidence supporting the need to lower the LDL cholesterol level to 70 mg/dL. If a single agent is unable to reduce the LDL cholesterol to such a level, combination therapy using agents that inhibit cholesterol reabsorption from the gut is efficacious. Other agents such as niacin also may lower the LDL cholesterol level but are less well tolerated.

The treatment of hypertriglyceridemia is usually more responsive to diet therapy and exercise. Even a modest weight loss of 10–20 lb can result in a significant decline in the serum triglyceride level. Diet modification also includes reduction in simple carbohydrates and alcohol. Even one or two drinks of alcohol in an individual with hypertriglyceridemia can raise the level of triglyceride significantly. In a patient with diabetes, improved blood sugar control is also effective in lowering the serum triglyceride level. Drug therapy usually starts with a fibric acid derivative such as gemfibrozil or fenofibrate. These agents usually produce a drop in the serum triglyceride level of 50%. Niacin is also effective but may raise the blood glucose level in diabetic patients. Fish oil supplements that include omega-3 fatty acids are also effective in lowering serum triglyceride levels.

Raising the HDL cholesterol level to 40 mg/dL or greater is also an important component of hyperlipidemia therapy but is the most difficult goal to achieve. In studies in which the HDL cholesterol level was raised to 45 mg/dL, rates of myocardial infarction and death were decreased up to 40% (Israeli Society for Prevention of Heart Attacks 2000). Statin therapy can raise the HDL cholesterol level by 10%–12%, but it is usually not able to raise the level to 45 mg/dL. Niacin is the most potent agent, and it should be employed in this clinical condition more frequently. Fibrates, which are also partially effective in increasing the HDL cholesterol level, can be used in combination with other agents. Table 46–2 presents a list of agents used in the treatment of hyperlipidemia.

# References

Expert Panel on the Detection, Evaluation and Treatment of High Blood Cholesterol in Adults: Executive Summary of the Third Report of the National Cholesterol Education Program Expert Panel on Detection, Evaluation, and Treatment of High Blood Cholesterol in Adults (Adult Treatment Panel III). JAMA 285:2486–2497, 2001

Israeli Society for Prevention of Heart Attacks: Secondary prevention by raising HDL cholesterol and reducing triglycerides in patients with coronary artery disease: bezafibrate infartion prevention study. Circulation 102:21–27, 2000

# CHAPTER 47

# Thyroid Abnormalities

Harvey L. Katzeff, M.D.

Optimal concentrations of thyroid hormones are necessary for the regulation of normal function of most organ systems, especially the brain and central nervous system (CNS). The tightly coordinated regulation of thyroid hormone metabolism is executed at various levels of control. The release of thyrotropin-releasing hormone (TRH) from the hypothalamus stimulates the release of thyroid-stimulating hormone (TSH) from the anterior pituitary gland, which then regulates the synthesis and release of thyroxine ($T_4$) from the thyroid gland. $T_4$ is then deiodinated to triiodothyronine ($T_3$) in peripheral tissues, including the brain, through the action of the enzyme 5'-deiodinase, of which there are three isoforms. $T_4$ is considered to be a prohormone and $T_3$ the active thyroid hormone, because $T_3$ is the more specific ligand for thyroid hormone receptors in all tissues (Surks and Oppenheimer 1977).

Alterations in thyroid hormone metabolism can occur in a variety of illnesses. Conditions that are associated with increased serum cortisol levels frequently suppress TRH and decrease the conversion of $T_4$ to $T_3$. Thus, nonthyroidal illness can have profound effects on tissue concentrations of $T_3$, despite relatively normal serum levels of $T_4$. This effect can lead to a decrease in concentration of $T_3$ in the brain in a variety of medical conditions, including undernutrition, which may alter brain function and lead to altered mental states.

Abnormalities in thyroid hormone action can lead to serious and permanent alterations in brain growth and development in children, as well as altered brain function as adults. Thyroid hormones stimulate and inhibit the action of specific genes that are responsive to these hormones. The presence of adequate thyroid hormone levels within the developing brain is necessary to stimulate normal myelin synthesis and neuronal development. In adults, regulation of protein synthesis and nutrient metabolism within brain cells by thyroid hormones is an important modulator of CNS activity.

In adults, approximately one-half of the $T_3$ in the brain is synthesized from deiodination of $T_4$ within the brain through the action of type II 5'-deiodinase. The activity of this enzyme decreases in hyperthyroid states and increases in hypothyroidism; thus the enzyme serves as an autoregulator that attempts to maintain stable levels of intracellular $T_3$ within the brain.

## Hyperthyroidism

### Clinical Presentation

Hyperthyroidism is the state in which an increase in the serum thyroid hormone level results in a suppression of the serum TSH concentration. An almost complete absence of a response in TSH after TRH administration is normally observed in hyperthyroidism. In younger individuals, diffuse goiter or Graves' disease is the most common cause of hyperthyroidism. In older individuals, autonomous nodules and diffuse goiter both commonly lead to hyperthyroidism. This disorder affects women much more frequently than men and usually presents in the third and fourth decade. The signs and symptoms of hyperthyroidism are frequently the result of a combination of the direct effects of the increased thyroid hormone concentrations and secondarily of an increase in adrenergic activity (Table 47–1).

**TABLE 47–1.**    Signs and symptoms of hyperthyroidism

| Signs | Symptoms |
| --- | --- |
| Eye stare | Heat intolerance |
| Lid lag | Palpitations |
| Warm, smooth skin | Weight loss |
| Onycholysis | Muscle weakness |
| Goiter | Diarrhea |
| Tachycardia | Anxiety |
| Atrial fibrillation | Restlessness |
| Fine tremor | Labile mood |
| Brisk reflexes | Diaphoresis |

*Subclinical hyperthyroidism* is the association of a suppressed TSH level (<0.03 mIU/mL) in the blood with normal $T_4$ and $T_3$ levels and no clinical symptoms. These patients do not have overtly hyperthyroid characteristics and frequently are not treated, although they have an increased risk of atrial fibrillation. This condition needs to be differentiated from *apathetic hyperthyroidism,* in which patients have suppressed TSH and elevated $T_4$ and $T_3$ levels but do not have any evidence of adrenergic hyperactivity. Apathetic hyperthyroidism is more commonly observed in older patients, and these patients may present with weight loss and resting tachycardia. The predominant psychiatric abnormality in this condition appears to be overt psychomotor depression without the agitation frequently seen in hyperthyroidism.

Symptoms of increased adrenergic activity in hyperthyroid patients can include heat intolerance, fine tremor, and sweats, which are unlike panic reactions in that the skin is usually warm and moist rather than cool and clammy. In patients with hyperthyroidism, the resting heart rate is elevated, whereas in patients with panic attacks, the heart rate is usually elevated only during the panic episodes. Hyperthyroidism has direct effects on appetite and resting metabolic rate and frequently leads to weight loss, although an increase in appetite can produce weight neutrality and even weight gain in 15% of individuals. Hyperthyroidism also has direct effects on affect and behavior that may mimic the symptoms of primary psychological disorders. Anxiety, irritability, and a tense dysphoria are frequently observed in patients with symptomatic hyperthyroidism. In addition, motor acceleration, pressured speech, and disorganized thought content are found in patients with hyperthyroidism. Additional cognitive symptoms include decreased attention span, impaired recent memory, and exaggerated startle response in proportion to the degree of increase in the serum $T_4$ concentration. Patients with hyperthyroidism may also have sleep difficulties, and the overall clinical picture may be confused with mania.

Thyrotoxicosis secondary to the surreptitious administration of excessive doses of oral $T_4$ or $T_3$ preparations is called *thyrotoxicosis factitia.* This condition is usually observed in young men and women who are trying to lose weight and who may present with atrial tachyarrhythmias. These individuals have been reported to ingest up to 20–30 times the daily maintenance dose of $T_4$ or $T_3$ preparations. However, because of the binding properties of $T_3$ to its receptor, the maximal effect of $T_3$ is usually observed at a plasma concentration five times the normal level, and higher concentrations do not have any greater metabolic action.

## Assessment and Treatment

The treatment of hyperthyroidism must be planned by an endocrinologist. The options include pharmacological approaches (with propylthiouracil or methimazole), radioiodine ablation, or surgery.

# Hypothyroidism

## Clinical Presentation

Overt primary hypothyroidism is the condition of decreased levels of $T_4$ and $T_3$ in the blood in association with an elevation of the serum TSH. This condition is commonly observed in young women (ages 20–40 years), but has also been observed in 5%–19% of individuals older than age 65 years in several studies. *Chronic lymphocytic thyroiditis* (Hashimoto's thyroiditis) resulting in lymphocytic infiltration and fibrosis of the thyroid gland is the most common cause of permanent hypothyroidism in industrialized countries, and iodine deficiency is the major cause of hypothyroidism in nonindustrialized countries. In adults, the diagnosis of chronic lymphocytic thyroiditis is established by the presence of antithyroid antibodies in the blood. Approximately 40% of adult women in the United States have positive antithyroid antibodies, and 1%–3% of these individuals go on to develop overt hypothyroidism each year. Chronic lymphocytic thyroiditis exists as either hypothyroidism, painless goiter, or both.

*Secondary hypothyroidism* exists when there is a decrease in TSH secretion that results in a decrease in serum $T_4$ and $T_3$ levels. This condition is usually caused by destruction of the pituitary gland and/or hypothalamus as a result of tumor, trauma, or surgery. Secondary hypothyroidism should be differentiated from the *sick euthyroid syndrome* (or low $T_3$ syndrome), which is the result of impaired TSH secretion brought on by acute and chronic stress. This syndrome results in low serum $T_4$ levels and especially low serum $T_3$ levels in association with a low or normal TSH level. Patients with secondary hypothyroidism need $T_4$ replacement therapy, but it is controversial whether thyroid hormone replacement with either $T_4$ or $T_3$ is indicated in sick euthyroid syndrome.

The signs and symptoms of hypothyroidism are listed in Table 47–2. Of all the signs and symptoms presented, the presence of cold intolerance is the most specific symptom, occurring in approximately 40% of individuals with hypothyroidism and in only 5% of healthy subjects (Cooper et al. 1984).

**TABLE 47–2.**   Signs and symptoms of hypothyroidism

| Signs | Symptoms |
|-------|----------|
| Dry skin | Fatigue |
| Depression | Lethargy |
| Bradycardia | Sleepiness |
| Hoarseness | Cold intolerance |
| Mild weight gain | Constipation |
| Delayed relaxation of reflexes | Muscle cramps |
| Metromenorrhagia | Arthralgias |
| | Anorexia |
| | Paresthesia |

*Subclinical hypothyroidism* is diagnosed when the $T_4$ and $T_3$ levels are completely normal, but the serum TSH level is elevated to 4–10 mIU/mL. These individuals do not have increased somatic symptoms, compared with the general population, but whether they have an increased risk of depressive symptoms is highly controversial. It is important to follow patients with subclinical hypothyroidism, because they have a high risk of developing overt hypothyroidism over time.

A relatively transient form of hypothyroidism is frequently observed (in 5%–10% of new mothers), starting approximately 3 months postpartum and lasting for up to 9 months. *Postpartum thyroiditis* may present initially as a short-lived episode of hyperthyroidism, lasting up to 2 months, followed by 7–9 months of hypothyroidism. This form of thyroiditis is usually asymptomatic and is not normally accompanied by the presence of antithyroid antibodies. If antithyroid antibodies are present in the postpartum state, the patient is considered to have chronic lymphocytic thyroiditis, which is likely to be a permanent condition.

*Myxedema* is a severe, life-threatening form of hypothyroidism that is more likely to occur in elderly patients. These patients usually have long-standing hypothyroidism in addition to a precipitating event such as an infection, congestive heart failure, medication effect, or metabolic event. The combination can lead to myxedema coma, which usually includes altered mental status, respiratory failure, and hypothermia. Cardiac contractility is impaired, and pericardial effusions may be present and can lead to cardiovascular collapse. A considerable proportion of patients who develop myxedema coma may have seizures (~25%) because of the direct effects of CNS dysfunction or in response to a metabolic encephalopathy secondary to hyponatremia or hypoxia. The treatment of myxedema is replacement of thyroid hormone. However, because of the high mortality rate associated with myedema coma and because $T_4$ replacement therapy alone may take several days to achieve its desired effects, there is controversy about the role of $T_3$ therapy in this disorder. The onset of action of $T_3$ occurs in hours, versus days for $T_4$, and intravenous treatment with a combination of $T_3$ and $T_4$ appears to be reasonable, although there are no clinical study findings that recommend this approach.

The neuropsychiatric features of hypothyroidism are frequently nonspecific and include both somatic and cognitive deficits (see Table 47–1). The cognitive abnormalities include impaired short-term memory, the inability to concentrate, slowing of mental calculations, slower speech patterns, and in some cases visual and hallucinatory disturbances. The hypothyroid state may be confused with primary depression and difficult to diagnose in the absence of specific somatic features of hypothyroidism. A proportion of hypothyroid individuals present with psychosis and suicidal ideation, and the differentiation of primary versus secondary depressive states should therefore be part of the standard evaluation of depressed individuals.

Postpartum depression and *postpartum thyroiditis* are common disorders that can occur separately or in combination. The prevalence of depression among patients with postpartum thyroid dysfunction is no greater than among postpartum women with normal thyroid function (Lucas et al. 2001).

A rare clinical condition called *Hashimoto's encephalopathy* is found in patients who present with chronic autoimmune thyroiditis and a variety of neurological symptoms and signs, including recurrent severe migraine headache, psychoses, seizures, ataxia, dementia, stupor, and coma (Chaudhuri and Behan 2004). These patients have high titers of antithyroid antibodies, and their cerebral blood flow is decreased. This condition usually responds to glucocorticoid therapy. The pathogenesis of this disorder is uncertain, but its response to glucocorticoid therapy suggests that it probably originates in an autoimmune process.

## Assessment and Treatment

In the large majority of individuals with hypothyroidism, treatment with $T_4$ results in complete resolution of the behavioral and somatic disturbances. In patients who have an underlying depressive disorder, cognition may be improved by $T_4$ replacement therapy, but the depressive affect may still persist. The goal of $T_4$ replacement therapy is to normalize the serum TSH level. With the sensitive third-generation assay for serum TSH level, the range of normal values is 0.3–4.0 mIU/mL, including two standard deviations around the mean. However, when the mean is determined on the basis of measures from young adults without positive serum antibodies, the range of normal values is 0.5–2.0 mIU/mL. Lowering the TSH value to this range should be the goal of thyroid hormone replacement therapy. Care should be taken in instituting thyroid hormone replacement therapy in patients with ischemic heart disease or in elderly patients. Hypothyroidism can mask ischemic heart disease and rapid replacement may provoke symptoms of cardiac ischemia.

Some patients complain of persistent symptoms despite having normal TSH values while receiving $T_4$ replacement therapy. Some of these individuals may have previously been given excessive doses of $T_4$, but the continuation of this therapy may lead to excessive bone loss or cardiac arrhythmias and should be discouraged. There is little evidence that excessive doses of $T_4$ lead to healthy weight loss. Data indicate that hyperthyroid individuals lose proportionately more protein than fat, compared to individuals without hyperthyroidism who are on weight loss diets; thus excessive doses of $T_4$ may lead to osteoporosis (Faber and Galloe 1994).

There has been interest in combining $T_3$ and $T_4$ replacement therapy for individuals who have persistent symptoms of hypothyroidism while receiving $T_4$ replacement therapy alone. The results of randomized trials, however, are contradictory. In one study, 50 μg of patients' usual dose of $T_4$ was replaced with 12.5 μg of $T_3$ (Bunevicius et al. 1999). Serum TSH values were similar during both the $T_4$ phase and the combination therapy phase, but the combination therapy was associated with improvement on some scores in assessment of cognitive performance and mood. Similarly, for 10 of the 15 visual analogue scales used to measure mood and physical status, the results were significantly better after treatment with $T_4$ plus $T_3$. However, resting heart rates were increased with the combination therapy, suggesting that elevated thyroid hormone levels may be intermittently present for a portion of each day. In a second study that used a lower $T_3$-to-$T_4$ ratio of hormone replacement (14:1), there were no differences between treatment arms (Siegmund et al. 2004).

Both hyper- and hypothyroidism are associated with alterations in affect and thought processes that are similar to the primary disorders of mood and thought. Depression is a common disorder, as is hypothyroidism, so it is not surprising that the two diseases may coexist. It is self-evident that if hypothyroidism is present, thyroid hormone replacement should be initiated and continued until the TSH level is completely normal. The main question for both clinicians and researchers is whether primary major depressive disorder without evidence of a primary thyroid disorder is associated with changes in the hypothalamic-pituitary-thyroidal axis.

Some studies have suggested that the response to antidepressant therapy (both tricyclic and selective serotonin reuptake inhibitor agents) is augmented with $T_3$ (Altshuler et al. 2001). The reason may be that the $T_3$ content of the brain may be somewhat decreased because of high cortisol levels, which can inhibit the type II 5'-deiodinase in the brain. This hypothesis, although attractive, has not been proved.

A substantial proportion of patients with bipolar disorder resistant to pharmacologic interventions have been reported to have decreased serum-free $T_4$ levels, as well as higher serum TSH values (Cole et al. 2002). What appears to be consistent is the mania-promoting effect of thyroid hormone supplementation in patients with rapid cycling. Lithium, which has been a mainstay of bipolar disorder treatment, can produce mild hypothyroidism, which may worsen the mood. Patients who are taking lithium should have their thyroid hormone levels checked routinely.

## References

Altshuler LL, Bauer M, Frye MA, et al: Does thyroid supplementation accelerate tricyclic antidepressant response? a review and meta-analysis of the literature. Am J Psychiatry 158:1617–1622, 2001

Bunevicius R, Kazanavicius G, Zalinkevicius R, et al: Effects of thyroxine as compared with thyroxine plus triiodothyronine in patients with hypothyroidism. N Engl J Med 340:424–429, 1999

Cooper DS, Halpern R, Wood LC, et al: L-Thyroxine therapy in subclinical hypothyroidism: a double-blind, placebo-controlled trial. Ann Intern Med 101:18–24, 1984

Cole DP, Thase ME, Mallinger AG, et al: Slower treatment response in bipolar depression predicted by lower pretreatment thyroid function. Am J Psychiatry 159:116–121, 2002

Chaudhuri A, Behan PO: The clinical spectrum, diagnosis, pathogenesis and treatment of Hashimoto's encephalopathy (recurrent acute disseminated encephalomyelitis). Eur J Neurol 11:711–713, 2004

Faber J, Galloe AM: Changes in bone mass during prolonged subclinical hyper-thyroidism due to L-thyroxine treatment: a meta-analysis. Eur J Endocrinol 130:350–356, 1994

Lucas A, Pizarro E, Granada ML, et al: Postpartum thyroid dysfunction and postpartum depression: are they two linked disorders? Clin Endocrinol (Oxf) 55:809–814, 2001

Siegmund W, Spieker K, Weike AI, et al: Replacement therapy with levothyrox-ine plus triiodothyronine (bioavailable molar ratio 14:1) is not superior to thyroxine alone to improve well-being and cognitive performance in hy-pothyroidism. Clin Endocrinol (Oxf) 60:750–757, 2004

Surks MI, Oppenheimer JH: Concentration of L-thyroxine and L-triiodothyro-nine specifically bound to nuclear receptors in rat liver and kidney: quanti-tative evidence favoring a major role of $T_3$ in thyroid hormone action. J Clin Invest 160:555–562, 1977

# CHAPTER 48

# Hypercalcemia

## Stuart Morduchowitz, M.D.

## Clinical Presentation

In the human body calcium plays an important role in neuromuscular function, blood coagulation, and intracellular signaling. The circulating calcium concentration is closely regulated and maintained in a narrow physiological range. Disturbances of the calcium level can affect all aspects of organ systems. The calcium concentration in the blood is closely regulated by two main hormones: parathyroid hormone (PTH) and calcitriol. Parathyroid cells sense extracellular calcium by means of a calcium sensing receptor on the cell membrane and secrete PTH through a negative feedback loop. PTH increases the calcium concentration in the blood by several mechanisms, including decreases in urinary calcium excretion, increases in the production of calcitriol, and release of calcium from the bone by osteoclast activation and increased bone resorption. The major effect of calcitriol is to augment intestinal calcium and phosphate absorption, but it may also have direct effects on bone turnover. Vitamin D is obtained mainly through dietary sources or is generated in the skin by ultraviolet light. Vitamin D is hydroxylated in the liver and then again in the kidney to produce the active form, calcitriol (Bringhurst et al. 2003).

Hypercalcemia is a relatively common finding in both inpatients and outpatients. Because screening of the serum calcium level has been a routine part of patient evaluations, many asymptomatic hypercalcemic patients have been identified. The most common cause of asymptomatic hypercalcemia is primary hyperparathyroidism; only approximately 20% of patients with primary hyperparathyroidism are symptomatic (Wermers et al. 1998). The nature of the signs and symptoms of hypercalcemia is related to the serum calcium level, as well as the acuteness of

445

the rise in the serum level. Mental status changes, cardiac abnormalities, neuromuscular weakness, lethargy, abdominal pain, and severe dehydration are usually seen with very high levels (>14 mg/dL). With more moderately elevated levels, polyuria and polydipsia may occur because the elevated calcium level causes a decrease in the concentrating capacity of the kidney, leading to a mild nephrogenic diabetes insipidus. Other symptoms can include constipation, apathy, fatigue, anorexia, nausea, and muscle weakness. Vague symptoms of dyspepsia, depression, or mild cognitive impairment may also occur (Bringhurst et al. 2003).

Patients with depression and hypercalcemia have significant improvement after the cause of the elevated calcium level has been corrected by medication or surgery. It is still unclear whether a direct link exists between hypercalcemia and depression or whether the correction of the metabolic derangement improves the person's mood and feeling of well-being. All of the symptoms mentioned earlier may be seen in hypercalcemia regardless of the cause of the elevated calcium level, but osteoporosis and kidney stones are usually seen in chronic PTH-mediated hypercalcemia.

## Differential Diagnosis

The differential diagnosis for hypercalcemia is relatively straightforward. An elevated calcium level with an elevated or nonsuppressed PTH level is consistent with PTH-mediated hypercalcemia. If the PTH level is suppressed, the hypercalcemia is considered to be non-PTH mediated. Malignancy is the most common cause of non-PTH-mediated hypercalcemia and is also the most frequent cause of an elevated calcium level in hospitalized patients. Some neoplasms produce circulating factors that bind to the PTH receptors and significantly increase the serum calcium level. The most common hormone responsible for this syndrome is PTH-related protein (PTH-RP). Tumors known to produce PTH-RP include squamous cell carcinomas of the lung, esophagus, head, and neck. Renal cell carcinomas, T-cell lymphomas, and carcinomas of the breast, ovary, cervix, and bladder can also produce PTH-RP (Inzucchi 2004).

Multiple myeloma has been found to produce osteoclast-activating factors, which can cause hypercalcemia. Lymphomas, as well as granulomatous diseases such as tuberculosis, sarcoidosis, and certain fungal infections elevate calcium levels through the unregulated production of calcitriol. These causes of hypercalcemia are frequently associated with high normal levels of serum phosphate, because they enhance the actions of vitamin D. Other endocrine causes of hypercalcemia include hyperthyroidism, hypothyroidism, adrenal insufficiency, pheochromocytoma, and Paget's disease of the bone with prolonged immobilization (Cox and Haddad 1994).

Certain medications can cause hypercalcemia, but many times this effect actually represents an unmasking of undiagnosed mild hyperparathyroidism. Elevated serum levels of vitamin D and vitamin A along with the presence of milk-alkali syndrome are usually secondary to an overdose of these supplements in combination with renal insufficiency. This combination is being seen more often, as more people address their nutritional needs with megavitamins. Thiazide diuretics and lithium can cause dehydration, but this effect may uncover a subclinical case of hypercalcemia. Besides causing nephrogenic diabetes insipidus, lithium has been found to produce hypercalcemia in approximately 10% of patients who are receiving chronic lithium therapy. Lithium may shift the parathyroid set-point, causing increased PTH secretion. Patients taking chronic lithium therapy have been found to have mild increases in the serum calcium level and PTH secretions, and persistent parathyroid gland hypertrophy (Taniegra 2004). Although lithium can cause four-gland hyperplasia, the majority of patients with lithium-induced hypercalcemia have a single adenoma. If calcium levels rise, discontinuation of the lithium dose may not reverse the hypercalcemia, and surgery may be indicated to correct the abnormality (Bringhurst et al. 2003).

In general, approximately 85% of cases of primary hyperparathyroidism are caused by a single parathyroid adenoma. Four-gland hyperplasia or multiple adenomas make up the rest of the cases, with parathyroid carcinomas accounting for less than 1% of cases. The decision to address this problem with surgery needs to be made by the patient and the physician, but there are indications that can be used for guidance. Patients with hypercalcemia who are symptomatic, including those with kidney stones, bone fractures, and hospitalization for dehydration, should be strongly encouraged to have surgery. Asymptomatic patients may be at risk for complications from hyperparathyroidism, and surgery may provide a cure (Mahadevia et al. 2003). The 2002 National Institutes of Health Consensus Panel identified the following characteristics of patients with asymptomatic primary hyperparathyroidism: age less than 50 years, bone density with a T-score below –2.5 at any site, an unexplained reduction in creatinine clearance by 30%, 24-hour urinary calcium excretion >400 mg, or serum calcium concentration 1.0 mg/dL above the upper limit of normal values (Mahadevia et al. 2003).

## Risk Stratification

Acute symptomatic hypercalcemia and hypercalcemic crisis are life-threatening complications of primary hyperparathyroidism and malignancy-associated hypercalcemia. The conditions must be suspected in hypercalcemic, acutely ill patients who present with change in mental status, muscle weakness, and gastrointestinal symptoms (Marienhagen et al. 2005). In patients with chronic hypercalcemic states, the risk of major complications is predicted by marked hypercalcemia (>1 mg/dL above the upper limit of normal), significant hypercalciuria (>400 mg/day), renal insufficiency and decreased bone density (Boonen et al. 2004).

## Assessment and Management in Psychiatric Settings

Acute symptomatic hypercalcemia (<15 mg/dL), for which hospitalization is required, can be fatal. The four basic goals of therapy for these patients are to correct dehydration, increase renal excretion of calcium, inhibit bone resorption, and treat the underlying disorder. Hydration with normal saline solution is the first step of management, because these patients can have severe intravascular depletion. Loop diuretics such as furosemide, which increase calcium excretion, should not be used until the patient is fully rehydrated. Bisphosphonates, such as pamidronate or zoledronic acid, can be infused to stop bone resorption, but the calcium level does not usually respond to the drug for about 24–48 hours. Calcitonin and glucocorticoids can also be used in certain situations as needed (Bilezikian 1992).

In cases of asymptomatic primary hyperparathyroidism, the criteria mentioned earlier are used to evaluate the patient for surgery. The evaluation should include at least measurement of the serum PTH, calcium, and phosphorus levels; bone density measurement, including density in the forearm, spine, and hip; and a 24-hour urine collection for measurement of calcium excretion. A diagnosis of hyperparathyroidism should never be based on a parathyroid scan, because it is nonspecific. Ultrasound, computed tomography, and magnetic resonance imaging scans are usually not needed, and an experienced endocrine surgeon may perform surgery in a medically stable patient without any radiological testing. However, with the new minimally invasive parathyroid surgery, a parathyroid scan (sestamibi scan) is usually obtained preoperatively to localize the adenoma and decrease operative time. If the scan shows a single enlarged gland, the surgeon is able to remove only the abnormal gland with a small local incision. An intraoperative decrease in the serum PTH level of 50% usually indicates successful removal of the abnormal gland. If the blood level of PTH does not fall, the surgeon may need to look for other abnormal parathyroid glands that are causing the hypercalcemia. The procedure may take only 45 minutes, and the patient can be discharged the same day without the need for an overnight hospital stay. Asymptomatic patients who are not surgical candidates or who refuse surgery can be closely watched with recommendations for adequate hydration and normal calcium intake of 500–1,000 mg/day. Management guidelines include measurement of the serum calcium level every 6 months and yearly measurement of the serum creatinine level and three-site bone density. Even asymptomatic patients can develop complications related to hypercalcemia and studies have shown effective treatment with bisphosphonates for bone protection, although serum calcium levels did not decrease significantly (Viera 2002).

## References

Bilezikian JP: Management of acute hyopercalcemia. N Engl J Med 326:1196–1203, 1992

Boonen S, Vandershueren D, Pelemens W, et al: Primary hyperparathyroidism: diagnosis and management in the older individual. Eur J Endocrinol 151:297–302, 2004

Bringhurst FR, Demay MB, Kronenberg HM: Hormones and disorders of mineral metabolism, in Williams Textbook of Endocrinology, 10th Edition. Edited by Larsen PR, Kronenberg HM, Melmed S, et al. Philadelphia, PA, WB Saunders, 2003, pp 1317–1346

Cox M, Haddad JG: Lymphoma, hypercalcemia, and the sunshine vitamin. Ann Intern Med 121:709–712, 1994

Inzucchi SE: Understanding hypercalcemia: its metabolic basis, signs, and symptoms. Postgrad Med 115:69–70, 73–76, 2004

Mahadevia PJ, Sosa JA, Levine MA, et al: Clinical management of primary hyperparathyroidism and thresholds for surgical referral: a national study examining concordance between practice patterns and consensus panel recommendations. Endocr Pract 9:494–503, 2003

Marienhagen K, Due J, Hanssen TA, et al: Surviving extreme hypercalcemia: a case report and review of the literature. J Intern Med 258:86–89, 2005

Taniegra ED: Hyperparathyroidism. Am Fam Physician 69:333–339, 2004

Viera AJ: Hyperparathyroidism. Clinics in Family Practice 4:627, 2002

Wermers RA, Khosla S, Atkinson EJ, et al: Survival after the diagnosis of hyperthyroidism: a population-based study. Am J Med 104:115–122, 1998

# CHAPTER 49

# Obesity

## Stuart Morduchowitz, M.D.

## Clinical Presentation

Obesity has become increasingly prevalent in industrialized countries, and in the United States obesity is now at epidemic proportions. Over the last 40 years the percentage of obese individuals in the United States has continued to rise, and an estimated 65% of the adult population is overweight. In high-risk populations, such as African Americans and Hispanics, the number may even be higher. Even more alarming, there has also been a steady rise in the proportion of children and adolescents who are either overweight or obese. The health risks linked to obesity include hypertension, type 2 diabetes, cardiovascular disease, and several cancers. These risks can be significantly reduced by awareness and treatment of this problem (Mokdad et al. 2001).

The definition of obesity is any increase in body fat, but exact measurements of height, weight, and waist circumference are used for evaluating the individual patient. The standard epidemiological assessment of body weight is measured by body mass index (BMI), which can be determined by using the formula: weight/height$^2$ or kg/m$^2$. The BMI can also be found by looking up the corresponding height and weight on a standardized chart. The precision of the BMI can be extended to all races and both sexes (Klein 2003).

## Differential Diagnosis

Aging, genetics, smoking cessation, sedentary lifestyle, and poor dietary habits are usually the major factors in weight gain, but clinicians should also consider other less common causes of weight gain, especially if there is a rapid change in the patient's BMI. Hypothyroidism has been implicated by patients and physicians alike as a cause of significant weight gain, but in actuality the weight gain in this disorder is modest. Cushing's syndrome produces central obesity with loss of fat and muscle mass from the extremities, producing the characteristic body habitus, usually over a period of several years. Excessive endogenous cortisol synthesis or exogenous cortisol ingestion can also produce depression or psychosis, which can indirectly affect food consumption and weight regulation. Acromegaly can cause a modest weight gain and should be ruled out if there is adequate clinical suspicion. Hypothalamic obesity, which occurs as a genetic syndrome or is secondary to trauma, tumor, or surgery in the hypothalamic region, can produce obesity because of loss of satiety, leading to excessive and inappropriate food intake. Multiple medications can induce weight gain, including glucocorticoids, certain diabetes medications, specific antiseizure medications, and many commonly used antipsychotics and antidepressants.

Several of the newer antipsychotic agents, such as olanzapine and risperidone, have been associated with a significant increase in body weight and a marked increase in the diagnosis of new-onset type 2 diabetes mellitus. Recent data demonstrate that about 15% of patients treated with olanzapine gain about 4% of their body weight (up to 5 lb) during the first 2 weeks of treatment. These patients are younger, have a lower baseline BMI, and are likely to report an increase in apetite (Kinon et al. 2005; Safer 2004).

## Risk Stratification

Obesity causes or worsens a large number of disorders with life-threatening potential, including type II diabetes, coronary heart disease, atherogenic dyslipidemia, hypertension, stroke, obstructive sleep apnea, nonalcoholic steatohepatitis, gastroesophageal reflux, various malignancies, and major affective disorder (O'Brien and Dixon 2002). For example, persons who gain 11–18 lb as adults are 1.9 times more likely to to be diagnosed with type II diabetes and 1.25 times more likely to have angina, myocardial infarction, or sudden death secondary to coronary heart disease than individuals who maintain a stable weight (Kawachi 1999).

## Assessment and Management in Psychiatric Settings

Both clinical and laboratory information are needed to evaluate overweight patients. The patients' view of their weight, their motivation for weight loss, and findings for any concomitant mental and physical diseases all are integral elements in treatment planning. Measurement of blood pressure is essential because of the close relationship of obesity and hypertension. Laboratory measurements should include lipid profile; thyroid-stimulating hormone, glucose (fasting), and uric acid levels; complete blood count; and a comprehensive profile. Data from the history, physical examination, and laboratory tests should be combined to evaluate the patient for various causes of obesity, as well as for possible anemia, sleep apnea, gout, and osteoarthritis.

After the patient has been fully evaluated, two important questions must be addressed: 1) Is the patient willing to try to lose weight? and 2) Does the patient have any risk factors for future medical problems? It is extremely difficult to help a patient lose weight if the person is unmotivated or mentally unable at the present time to make appropriate lifestyle changes to reach a goal. In this case, the best treatment is to strive for weight maintenance and address the other risk factors until the patient is ready to lose weight. If the person is willing to address the weight problem, setting up a weight loss team that consists of the patient, doctor, nutritionist, and possibly others is the best approach.

For successful weight loss, an appropriate change in diet, as well as exercise and behavior therapy, are needed. Behavioral changes can be extremely difficult for psychiatric patients, compared with other populations. A recent study showed that individuals with schizophrenia and other psychiatric disorders were willing to participate in a weight control program focused on nutrition, exercise, and motivation (Menza et al. 2004). The patients benefited from the intervention, and there were clinically significant reductions in weight, BMI, hemoglobin $A_{1c}$ values, and other risk factors for poor health. The group that did not participate in the program continued to gain weight.

Multiple programs and diets have been tried for all types of people, with disappointing long-term benefits. The popularity of low-carbohydrate diets is a recent example. Although faster initial weight loss occurs with a low-carbohydrate diet, long-term results are no better than those with more conservative treatment because of more rapid weight regain. The possible dangers of ketosis from low-fiber/high-fat diets and the decreased emphasis on regular exercise are also worrisome. A 1-year trial comparing low-carbohydrate to low-fat diets reported that weight loss after 1 year was not significantly different between the two groups (Bonow and Eckel 2003). Until further long-term studies are completed, a common sense approach of fewer carbohydrates, less fat, and more fruits and vegetables may be the best alternative.

Even for a motivated patient who is adherent to the diet and exercise regimen, medical pharmacology may at times be indicated. For certain morbidly obese patients who have made many attempts at weight reduction with diet and medications, bariatric surgery may be the most effective option. This treatment modality is reserved for individuals who are more than 100 lb over ideal body weight and who are psychologically able to follow the postoperative regimen of small frequent liquid meals for several weeks to months. There is a plethora of over-the-counter remedies, and there are numerous charlatans who sell "magical" weight-loss pills. The safety and effectiveness of these medications is almost always in question, and they should never be recommended. Although many drugs are currently being researched, only two drugs—orlistat and sibutramine—are approved by the U. S. Food and Drug Administration for long-term treatment of obesity. Clinically, their effect has been somewhat disappointing, and only mild weight loss has occurred in most patients. Both orlistat and sibutramine have been used for up to 2 years, and an average weight loss of 10–20 lb has been seen. Although no direct comparison studies have been reported, the results with sibutramine have been slightly better that those with orlistat. Sibutramine is a mixed neurotransmitter inhibitor, and its primary effect is appetite suppression. Sibutramine is similar to the selective serotonin reuptake inhibitors (SSRIs) and was first studied as an antidepressant. Many SSRIs and other antidepressants cause weight gain, but sibutramine was found to be associated with significant weight loss. The main side effects of sibutramine are dry mouth, insomnia, and increased blood pressure and pulse, but no cardiac problems have been found. Sibutramine has interactions with antimigraine and other medications and should be used only with a physician's supervision.

Orlistat is a lipase inhibitor that exerts its effect by blocking fat absorption in the gut, but it is not systemically absorbed. Its main side effects are fecal urgency, fatty/oily stools, and possible fecal incontinence. Orlistat can block the absorption of fat-soluble vitamins, and patients taking the medication should take a multivitamin 2–4 hours before or after the last orlistat dose of the day. Numerous other drugs have been used for weight loss with inconsistent results. Metformin therapy in patients with diabetes, impaired glucose tolerance, and polycystic ovarian syndrome is associated with an early (3-month) weight loss and maintenance of this weight loss for up to several years. Drugs with less successful outcomes include acarbose (an α-glucosidase inhibitor that delays absorption of complex carbohydrates) and SSRIs, which are usually ineffectiven for weight loss or cause weight gain. The use of topiramate and nizatidine has also been suggested, but clear evidence of their efficacy has not yet been reported.

After the patient has started a treatment plan, close follow-up is essential. Return visits to a nutritionist or physician for discussion of questions about treatment and for reinforcement of proper dietary behavior are integral to continued weight loss. For certain patients with a BMI ≥40 or a BMI of 35 with current medical diseases such as diabetes mellitus, hypertension, or hypercholesterolemia, gastric bypass surgery may be a reasonable option. Details about the different types of gastric bypass surgery are beyond the scope of this review, but the complications are significantly reduced with the newer procedures as well as with a laparoscopic approach. In a morbidly obese individual, the risks of surgery have to be weighed against the benefit of a weight loss of 100 lb or more and the associated health improvements (Balsiger et al. 1997).

## References

Balsiger BM, Luque de Leon E, Sarr MG: Surgical treatment of obesity: who is an appropriate candidate? Mayo Clin Proc 72:551–557, 1997

Bonow RO, Eckel RH: Diet, obesity, and cardiovascular risk. NEJM 348:2057–2058, 2003

Kawachi I: Physical and psychological consequences of weight gain. J Clin Psychiatry 60 (suppl 21):5–9, 1999

Kinon BJ, Kaiser CJ, Ahmed S, et al: Association between early and rapid weight gain and change in weight over one year of olanzapine therapy in patients with schizophrenia and related disorders. J Clin Psychopharmacology 25:255–258, 2005

Klein S, Romijn J: Obesity, in Williams Textbook of Endocrinology, 10th Edition. Edited by Larsen PR, Kronenberg HM, Melmed S, et al. Philadelphia, PA, WB Saunders, 2003, pp 1619–1635

Menza M, Vreeland B, Minsky S, et al: Managing atypical antipsychotic-associated weight gain: 12-month data on a multimodal weight control program. J Clin Psychiatry 65:471–477, 2004

Mokdad AH, Bowman BA, Ford ES, et al: The continuing epidemic of obesity and diabetes in the United States. JAMA 286:1195–1200, 2001

O'Brien PE, Dixon JB: The extent of the problem of obesity. Am J Surg 184:4S–8S, 2002

Safer DJ: A comparison of risperidone-induced weight gain across the age span. J Clin Psychopharmacol 24:429–436, 2004

# PART XII

# Electrocardiographic Abnormalities

Section Editor:

Gino Farina, M.D.

# CHAPTER 50

# ST Segment and T Wave Abnormalities

Thomas Doohan, M.D.

Gino Farina, M.D.

## Clinical Presentation

The ST segment of the electrocardiogram (ECG) represents the period during which the ventricular myocardium remains in an activated or depolarized state. It begins at the termination of the QRS complex and ends as it merges with the T wave. The J point is the position of the junction between the QRS complex and the ST segment. Normally, the ST segment forms a 90° angle with the QRS complex and then runs horizontally until it joins the T wave. This segment may be abnormal when it becomes elevated or depressed in relation to the baseline. The baseline is a line drawn from the start of the P wave to the end of the T wave (American Heart Association 2001). An example of the J point, ST segment, and the baseline are shown in Figure 50–1.

The T wave represents the portion of the ventricular repolarization in the cardiac cycle. It follows the ST segment and ends as it joins the isoelectric line before initiation of the next P wave. The normal T wave shape should be smooth, rounded, and symmetric. Its axis should be the same as that of the P wave, and thus it is positively directed in all leads except aVR, where it is negative, and in V1, where it is biphasic (initially positive and then negative). The duration of the T wave is considered in the measurement of the Q–T interval (discussed in Chapter 52, "Prolonged Q–Tc Interval"). The amplitude of the T wave is variable among age groups and between the sexes. Normally, it does not exceed 0.5 mV in any limb lead or 1.5 mV in any precordial lead. The upper limits of

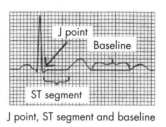
J point, ST segment and baseline

**FIGURE 50–1.**    Normal electrocardiogram.

normal are lower for females. Lastly, the T wave should be inspected to determine if it is upright (positively deflected) or inverted (negatively deflected) (Wagner 2001).

## Differential Diagnosis

An ECG is frequently performed to evaluate a patient who complains of chest pain. Alterations in the ST segment and/or T wave do not provide a definitive diagnosis, but they rapidly influence the physician's suspicion of whether the complaint is of cardiac origin or not. For this reason, an ECG should be performed promptly in the assessment of acute coronary syndrome. Acute coronary syndrome is a spectrum of diseases from myocardial ischemia through myocardial necrosis and including stable angina, unstable angina, and myocardial infarction (Hollander 2000). There are several conditions that may produce similar changes in the morphology of the ST segment and T wave that are not related to either myocardial ischemia or infarction. It is important to be aware of these conditions and their associated changes in these components of the ECG.

### Myocardial Infarction

#### ST Segment Changes

When persistent total coronary occlusion occurs, there is elevation of the ST segment in relation to the baseline. The ST segment is considered to be elevated if the J point of the segment is more than 1 mm above the baseline (Hampton 2003). An elevation in two or more anatomically contiguous leads is suggestive of acute myocardial infarction. The deviated ST segment may be horizontal, up-sloping, or down-sloping. For this reason, the ST segment may have different degrees of deviation with

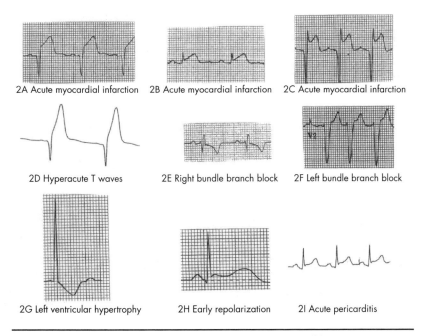

2A Acute myocardial infarction   2B Acute myocardial infarction   2C Acute myocardial infarction

2D Hyperacute T waves   2E Right bundle branch block   2F Left bundle branch block

2G Left ventricular hypertrophy   2H Early repolarization   2I Acute pericarditis

**FIGURE 50–2.**   Examples of electrocardiogram abnormalities.

progression across the segment (Wagner 2001). An example of ST segment elevation in acute myocardial infarction is shown in Figure 50–2, Parts 2A, 2B, and 2C.

The infarct can be localized on the basis of changes in particular leads. To more accurately assess the right ventricular wall, the V4 precordial lead can be moved to its mirror image location on the right chest wall. Elevation of the ST segment in this lead is consistent with a right ventricular infarction. Because the overall vector of depolarization is toward the inferior aspect of the left ventricle, there will be depression of the ST segment in the V1 and V2 leads rather than elevation during a posterior wall myocardial infarction.

Table 50–1 summarizes the locations of myocardial infarction associated with ST segment changes in various leads.

## T Wave Changes

At the onset of acute myocardial infarction, the T waves may become elevated as well. The amplitude of the normal T wave is ≤0.5 mV in any limb lead or ≤1.5 mV in any precordial lead. The T wave elevation may have two forms. In some cases, the height of the T wave is the same as

**TABLE 50–1.** Locations of myocardial infarction associated with electrocardiogram leads and ST segment findings

| Location of myocardial infarction | ECG leads | ST segment finding |
|---|---|---|
| Anterior wall | V1–V4 | Elevation |
| Lateral wall | I, aVL, V5, and V6 | Elevation |
| Inferior wall | II, III, and aVF | Elevation |
| Right ventricle | V4R | Elevation |
| Posterior wall | V1–V3 | Depression |

that of the ST segment. In this case, the T wave elevation is secondary to deviation of the ST segment, as the origin of the T wave is joined to the terminal end of the elevated ST segment. In other patients, the T waves are more markedly elevated and independent of the ST segment. The elevations in the latter case are more characteristic of an acute myocardial infarction and are defined as hyperacute T wave changes. Their presence is usually brief, and they usually occur at the onset of total coronary arterial occlusion and therefore they may be helpful in the timing and progression of an acute myocardial infarction (Wagner 2001). An example of hyperacute T waves is shown in Figure 50–2, Part 2D.

## Reciprocal Changes

Reciprocal changes are horizontal or down-sloping ST segments in leads that are anatomically opposite to leads in which ST segment elevation is seen in patients with acute myocardial infarction. For example, patients with an acute anterior wall infarction may have reciprocal ST depression in the inferior leads (Grauer 1998).

## Infarction Evolution

The ECG changes described in the previous sections are static. They follow a relatively predictable timeline throughout the process of infarction. With that pattern in mind, it is extremely important to be aware that these classic ECG findings may have resolved or may have not yet occured, depending on the progression of the infarction. The earliest change is an increase in the amplitude of the T waves. This change is quickly followed by elevation in the ST segment. The ST elevation falls gradually over 12 hours, followed by a plateau and then slow normalization. Normally, within 9 hours but as early as within 2 hours, there may be loss of the R wave and development of an abnormal Q wave. Over the same time period, there is an inversion of the T wave in the leads containing the ST elevation (Aufderheide and Gibler 1998).

## Abnormalities and Patterns That Resemble Infarction

### Right Bundle Branch Block

Some of the characteristic ECG findings of a right bundle branch block include prolongation of the QRS complex and a T wave that is usually directed opposite to the latter portion of the complex. These findings may be interpreted as ST elevation and T wave inversion. Therefore, they may sometimes resemble the pattern for an anteroseptal, inferior, or posterior wall myocardial infarction. However, if the typical features of the bundle branch block are recognized properly, the right bundle branch block should not obscure the ECG changes of an acute myocardial infarction (Aufderheide and Gibler 1998). An example of the ECG pattern for right bundle branch block is shown in Figure 50–2, Part 2E.

### Left Bundle Branch Block

Several of the ECG features of left bundle branch block may be interpreted as those of an acute myocardial infarction. QS complexes in leads V1–V3 can be mistaken for those of an anterior wall myocardial infarction. Occasionally, these QS complexes may extend to the V5 lead or occur in leads III and aVF and thus resemble extension to the lateral wall and inferior wall myocardial infarction, respectively. The ST segment can be elevated in any lead with a QS or RS pattern. The T wave in these leads can have a convex upward shape or be tall, similar in appearance to hyperacute T waves. Together, these ST segment elevations and tall T waves are easy to misconstrue as changes associated with acute myocardial infarction.

An acute myocardial infarction is difficult to distinguish from a left bundle branch block, but there are criteria that may be applied to aid the diagnosis of an acute myocardial infarction in this situation. The following ECG features, if present, are suggestive of an acute myocardial infarction and should be treated as such: 1) ST segment elevation ≥1 mm and concordant with the QRS complex; 2) ST segment depression ≥1 mm in lead V1, V2 ,or V3; and 3) ST segment elevation ≥5 mm and discordant with the QRS complex (Aufderheide and Gibler 1998). An example of the ECG pattern for left bundle branch block is shown in Figure 50–2, Part 2F.

## Left Ventricular Hypertrophy

A left ventricular strain pattern is a characteristic ECG finding of left ventricular hypertrophy. This strain pattern appears as either biphasic or inverted T waves in leads with a predominant R wave. These inversions may be minimal or may even be greater than 5 mm.

The ECG in left ventricular hypertrophy may also reveal ST segment elevation in the anterior leads. In this case, the T waves may also be prominent, resembling the hyperacute T waves of infarction (Aufderheide and Gibler 1998). An example of an ECG of left ventricular hypertrophy is shown in Figure 50–2, Part 2G.

## Early Repolarization

Early repolarization can give the appearance of an acute myocardial infarction. The ECG shows ST elevation, usually in leads V3–V5. ST elevation may also be present in V6 and the limb leads, although the elevation in these leads will be to a lesser extent. The ST segments of early repolarization appear to be evenly lifted off of the baseline (Aufderheide and Gibler 1998). There may also be tall T waves resembling hyperacute T waves, which further obscure the picture. Clues that may help distinguish early repolarization include the presence of Q waves and reciprocal changes in the inferior leads as well as more marked ST elevation in the V6 lead in the case of acute myocardial infarction. An example of the ECG pattern for early repolarization is shown in Figure 50–2, Part 2H.

## Acute Pericarditis

Acute pericarditis causes a number of ECG changes, but most significantly it can cause ST segment elevation. The ECG in acute pericarditis progresses through a number of stages over a variable time period. The first stage is characterized by ST segment elevation. It may be difficult to distinguish pericarditis from acute myocardial infarction because these ST elevations accompany a clinical picture in which the patient may be complaining of excruciating chest pain. However, acute pericarditis causes diffuse pericardial inflammation, and thus there is diffuse ST segment elevation in leads I, II, aVL, aVF, and V2–V6 (Grauer 1998). In acute myocardial infarction, the ST segment elevation is typically confined to the anatomically contiguous leads (anterior, inferior, or lateral), in contrast to the diffuse pattern in pericarditis. The third stage is characterized by T wave inversion. However, the amplitude of these inversions is usually less than 5 mm, in contrast to those in an acute myocardial infarction, which are normally deeper. Furthermore, the deep T wave inversions of acute myocardial infarction are associated with a prolonged Q–T interval because of a prolonged period of repolarization. Another characteristic ECG finding in acute pericarditis is PR segment depression as a result of inflammation of the atria. In acute pericarditis, the Q–T interval should not be affected (Aufderheide and Gibler 1998). An example of an ECG pattern for acute pericarditis is shown in Figure 50–2, Part 2I.

### Left Ventricular Aneurysm

A left ventricular aneurysm is an area of the myocardium that bulges outward. The aneurysm is normally confined to infarcted myocardium, and thus it normally occurs after an acute myocardial infarction, especially after a large anterior myocardial infarction. Left ventricular aneurysm is most commonly located in the anterior wall, but it can rarely occur in the inferoposterior wall. An ECG typically shows ST segment elevation that persists long after the myocardial infarction. Because left ventricular aneurysm generally occurs in the anterior wall, there will be ST elevations in leads I, aVL, and V1–V6. A left ventricular aneurysm that involves the inferoposterior wall will have persistent ST elevation in leads II, III, and aVF. However, in contrast to the pattern for acute myocardial infarction, there should not be evidence of reciprocal ST depression in the opposite leads (Aufderheide and Gibler 1998).

### Hypertrophic Cardiomyopathy

Hypertrophic cardiomyopathy can cause a number of ST segment and T wave changes that can closely resemble the pattern for an acute myocardial infarction. Furthermore, these changes tend to appear in anatomically contiguous leads. The myocardial hypertrophy will alter the timing of ventricular depolarization, which may result in ST segment elevation, tall T waves, or deeply inverted T waves, as well as patterns associated with bundle branch blocks (Aufderheide and Gibler 1998). It is extremely difficult to determine if these ECG changes are secondary to hypertrophic cardiomyopathy or acute myocardial infarction, and the clinician may need to rely on comparison with the patient's prior ECGs or on further evaluation with an echocardiogram. However, in leads with pathological Q waves, the T waves should be upright in ECGs in patients with hypertrophic cardiomyopathy.

### Hyperkalemia

In the early stages of hyperkalemia, there may be the development of tall symmetric T waves that may be misconstrued as hyperacute T waves. These T waves tend to be narrow, peaked, and symmetric. Furthermore, they are not associated with Q–T prolongation, are most prominent in the V1 and V2 leads, and are generally found in conjunction with the other ECG changes commonly seen with hyperkalemia. The hyperacute T waves of acute myocardial infarction are also symmetric, but they are usually slightly wider, have Q–T prolongation, and are associated with reciprocal T wave inversion in opposite leads (Aufderheide and Gibler 1998).

### Hypothermia

When the core body temperature dips below 32°C, there is an elevation of the J point (Osborne J wave) that is similar to ST segment elevation. The J wave is most prominent in the V3–V6 leads and can be associated with reciprocal J point depression in leads aVR or V1. The amplitude of the J wave is directly proportional to the temperature. Hypothermia is also associated with T wave inversions. The J wave generally causes elevation in the initial portion of the ST segment, in contrast to the elevation of the entire ST segment in acute myocardial infarction. Contrary to the pattern in acute myocardial infarction, the J wave and T wave inversions associated with hypothermia will resolve with rewarming (Aufderheide and Gibler 1998).

### Clozapine Effect

A case report described a 48-year-old male patient who developed ST segment elevations after initiation of treatment with clozapine (Ketch et al. 1996). These elevations were no longer apparent days after discontinuation of the medication. The patient had an extensive cardiac evaluation, which did not reveal any evidence of myocardial injury. Only the history of current clozapine use suggested a noncardiac source of ST segment elevation in this patient.

## Myocardial Ischemia

As in myocardial infarction, a coronary artery occlusion restricts myocardial blood flow. If the occlusion is incomplete, the decreased perfusion is limited to the subendocardial layer, and myocardial ischemia occurs. The process of myocardial ischemia also produces characteristic ST segment and T wave changes on an ECG.

### ST Segment Depression

ST segment depression represents subendocardial noninfarctional ischemia. The segment is depressed when it is more than 1.0 mm beneath

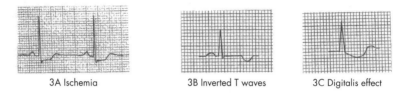

| 3A Ischemia | 3B Inverted T waves | 3C Digitalis effect |

**FIGURE 50-3.** Examples of electrocardiogram abnormalities.

the baseline. The shape of the depressed segment can be down-sloping or horizontal. Smaller depressions of the segment may be secondary to ischemia, but they are not diagnostic until the 1-mm threshold is met in at least one lead. As described earlier, ST segment depression in the V1 and V2 leads is indicative of myocardial infarction rather than ischemia. An example of an ECG pattern for ischemic ST segment depression is shown in Figure 50–3, Part 3A.

### T Wave Inversion

The T wave represents the repolarization process of the myocardium. With myocardial ischemia, there may be delayed myocardial repolarization and thus inversion of the T wave (Wagner 2001). To complicate this picture, T wave inversions may be seen in other conditions. They may be caused by acute myocardial infarction as well as other causes, such as left ventricular hypertrophy, acute myocarditis, pulmonary embolism, cerebrovascular accident, and lithium usage. T wave inversions caused by myocardial ischemia are typically narrow and symmetric. Inversions produced by an acute myocardial infarction normally follow an isoelectric ST segment rather than ST depression. Prominent, deep, and wide T waves are more indicative of noninfarction and nonischemic conditions (Aufderheide and Gibler 1998). An example of an inverted T wave is shown in Figure 50–3, Part 3B.

### Postextrasystolic T Wave Change

Myocardial ischemia can sometimes be identified by a change in T wave morphology and polarity in the beat following a premature ventricular contraction. This phenomenon is very rare and is not specific for ischemia, but when it is seen, further evidence of ischemia should be sought.

## Abnormalities and Patterns That Resemble Myocardial Ischemia

### Digitalis Effect

The digitalis effect refers to the ECG findings that are commonly seen with therapeutic digoxin levels rather than those seen with toxic levels of this medication. Digitalis causes P–R interval prolongation, ST segment depression, T wave depression, and Q–T interval shortening.

The ST segment and T wave changes are most prominent in leads V4–V6. If an individual previously had normal upright T waves, there may be T wave inversion when digitalis levels are therapeutic. In patients who previously had ST depression or T wave inversion, these abnormalities may be emphasized when treatment with digitalis is initiated (Aufderheide and Gibler 1998). The underlying mechanism responsible for these changes is not completely understood. The physician is often unable to differentiate digitalis effect from ischemic ST segment and T wave changes. An example of a digitalis effect is shown in Figure 50–3, Part 3C.

### Pulmonary Embolism/Acute Cor Pulmonale

Acute cor pulmonale secondary to pulmonary embolism may cause the ECG appearance of a pseudoinfarct or ischemic pattern in the inferior or anteroseptal leads. Approximately 12% of patients with acute pulmonary embolism have an S wave in lead I, a Q wave in lead III, and shallow T wave inversions in the inferior leads. There may also be slight ST segment elevations in the inferior and anteroseptal leads, T wave inversions in the inferior leads, and poor R wave progression as a result of acute right ventricular strain. These patterns may resemble those for ischemia.

The S wave in lead I, Q wave in lead III, and poor R wave progression are caused by acute right ventricular dilatation. The ST segment and T wave changes are in fact likely secondary to ischemia. But the ischemia results from hypoxemia, decreased cardiac output, and increased myocardial oxygen demand associated with massive pulmonary embolus (Aufderheide and Gibler 1998).

### Cerebrovascular Accident

Sixty percent of patients with a subarachnoid hemorrhage will have diffuse, deep T wave inversions that may mimic myocardial ischemia. These T wave inversions are one component of the ECG triad of cerebrovascular accidents. The other two are prominent U waves and Q–T interval prolongation. The T wave inversions are different from those associated with ischemia in that they are wide and blunt. These ECG changes may also be seen in patients with cerebral artery occlusion, intracerebral hemorrhage, and cerebral infarction. It is hypothesized that these changes are a result of increased sympathetic and vagal tone from the hemorrhage, which alters myocardial repolarization (Aufderheide and Gibler 1998). To differentiate between cerebrovascular accident and myocardial ischemia, the clinician should examine the ECG closely. The presence of diffuse, deep, wide T wave inversions, the absence of new Q waves, and the presence of the other components of the triad, in addition to an appropriate clinical picture, favor the diagnosis of a cerebrovascular accident.

### Lithium-Induced Changes

Lithium usage is a well-known cause of T wave inversion and flattening (Mitchell and Mackenzie 1982). This effect is a fairly common occurrence, with reported incidences ranging from 13% to 100%. The inversions are entirely benign and have no adverse effects in otherwise healthy patients. In fact, the T wave changes are transient. They often vanish and normalize with either continuation or removal of lithium treatment. However, individuals with a propensity to cardiac arrhythmias should have their ECG reexamined once a lithium steady state is reached.

### Clozapine-Induced Changes

In addition to being associated with ST segment elevation, as described earlier, clozapine use has been linked to ST segment depression as well as T wave inversions (Ketch 1996). Little is known about this linkage, and there is no clear explanation for these ECG changes. Fortunately, these clozapine-induced effects are infrequent.

## Risk Stratification

In 1995, baseline ECGs were obtained in 1,006 patients admitted to a psychiatric hospital and were classified as normal ($N$=765), abnormal ($N$=93), or equivocal ($N$=148) (Hollister 1995). The abnormalities included any definitive deviation from the normal pattern, including any ischemic changes, conduction delays, arrhythmias, and hypertrophy. It is noteworthy that 60 of the abnormal ECGs were obtained in patients who had no preexisting heart disease. The abnormality in 12 of these cases was found to be ischemic ST segment and T wave changes. The other abnormalities included left ventricular hypertrophy, as well as left and right bundle branch blocks. It is important to recognize that a significant portion of psychiatric patients may have an ECG with ischemic ST segment and T wave changes or one of the ECG patterns that may be misinterpreted as indicating an ischemic condition. As in the general population, these finding should be considered real until properly worked up.

The initial risk stratification is achieved by examining the clinical situation in addition to the ECG. Positive cardiac risk factors as well as symptoms that are highly suggestive of an acute myocardial event substantially increase an individual's risk. These symptoms include severe retrosternal chest pain or pressure that radiates to the shoulders, neck, arms, jaw, or back and associated nausea, vomiting, diaphoresis, shortness of breath, or light-headedness. The ECG can be classified into three categories, according to increasing levels of risk (American Heart Association 2001):

1. Nondiagnostic ECG in which there is no change in the ST segment or T wave, corresponding to a low/intermediate risk of unstable angina.
2. ST segment depression or dynamic T wave inversion, which corresponds to high risk of unstable angina or a myocardial infarction without ST segment elevation.
3. ST segment elevation or new (or presumably new) left bundle branch block, which corresponds to a diagnosis or high risk of an acute myocardial infarction with ST segment elevation.

## Assessment and Management in Psychiatric Settings

In patients with chest pain, it is important to carry out a brief history and physical examination with particular attention to the cardiovascular system. Vital signs, including pulse oximetry, should be measured. Lastly, a 12-lead ECG should be performed and evaluated by a physician.

The mainstay of initial treatment for acute coronary syndrome consists of the following elements (American Heart Association 2001): administration of oxygen (4 L/minute), 160–325 mg of aspirin, nitroglycerin in sublingual or spray form, and intravenous morphine (if the pain is not relieved after three doses of nitroglycerin).

While the immediate assessment and treatment are being carried out, arrangements should be made to transport the patient to the nearest emergency department as soon as possible.

# References

American Heart Association: Adult Advanced Cardiac Life Support: ACLS Provider Manual. Dallas, TX, American Heart Association, 2001

Aufderheide TP, Gibler WB: Acute ischemic coronary syndromes, in Emergency Medicine Concepts in Clinical Practice, Vol 2. Edited by Rosen P. St. Louis, MO, Mosby, 1998, pp 1670–1691

Grauer K: A Practical Guide to ECG Interpretation, 2nd Edition. St. Louis, MO, Mosby, 1998, pp 203–208

Hampton JR: The ECG Made Easy, 6th Edition. New York, Churchill Livingstone, 2003, pp 100–105

Hollander JE: ACS: unstable angina, myocardial ischemia, and infarction, in Emergency Medicine: A Comprehensive Study Guide, 5th Edition. Edited by Tintinalli JE, Kelen GD, Stapczynski JS. New York, McGraw-Hill, 2000, pp 356–366

Hollister LE: Electrocardiographic screening in psychiatric patients. J Clin Psychiatry 56:26–29, 1995

Ketch J, Herd A, Ludwig L: ST segment elevations without myocardial infarction in a patient on clozapine. Am J Emerg Med 14:111–112, 1996

Mitchell JE, Mackenzie TB: Cardiac effects of lithium in man: a review. J Clin Psychiatry 43:47–51, 1982

Wagner GS: Marriott's Practical Electrocardiography, 10th Edition. Philadelphia, PA, Lippincott Williams & Wilkins, 2001, pp 140–200

# CHAPTER 51

# Arrhythmias

Sally S. Chao, M.D.

## Clinical Presentation

Cardiac arrhythmia, or dysrhythmia, denotes any abnormality in cardiac rhythm. The dysrhythmias are usually classified on the basis of the heart rate and site of abnormality. Cardiac dysrhythmias can be either too fast, with heart rates in excess of 100 beats per minute (bpm) (tachyarrhythmias), or too slow, with heart rates less than 60 bpm (bradyarrhythmias) (Craig 2003). Heart rates between 40 and 160 bpm are usually well tolerated in healthy adults without cardiac disease, because they are able to maintain an adequate cardiac output and blood pressure. When adults with heart disease have a heart rate less than 50 bpm or above 120 bpm, they may not be able to maintain adequate cardiac output or adequate perfusion pressure (Craig 2003).

In the normal heart, electrical depolarization originates in the sinus node, and depolarization occurs at a regular rate, depending on physiological needs. After a physiological pause at the atrioventricular (AV) node, depolarization proceeds down the AV node, bundle of His, right and left bundle branches, and the Purkinje system. Tachyarrythmias result from mechanisms other than physiological need that drive cardiac depolarization. These conditions include 1) accessory conduction pathways capable of creating sustained circular depolarization, 2) abnormal automaticity, and 3) afterdepolarizations that cause triggered rhythms (Sabatine et al. 1998). Bradyarrhythmias arise from disorders of impulse formation or impaired impulse conduction.

## Differential Diagnosis

Tachyarrhythmias can be divided into broad categories according to the width of the QRS complex on an electrocardiogram (ECG)—in narrow QRS complex rhythms, the QRS complex is less than or equal to 0.12 seconds or less than three small boxes on an ECG; in wide QRS complex rhythms, the QRS complex is greater than 0.12 seconds—and subsequently divided according to the regularity of the rhythm (regular or irregular) (Sabatine et al. 1998).

### Width of the QRS Complex

If the QRS complex is narrow and the rhythm is regular, the differential diagnosis includes sinus tachycardia, supraventricular tachycardia (SVT), and atrial flutter. If there is a wide QRS complex, the differential diagnosis includes monomorphic or polymorphic ventricular tachycardia. Any of the narrow QRS complex rhythms can present with a widened QRS complex if there is a rate-related aberrant conduction (SVT with aberrant conduction), underlying bundle branch block, or the presence of an accessory pathway, as in Wolff-Parkinson-White syndrome (Craig 2003).

Sinus tachycardia is characterized on an ECG by normal sinus P waves and QRS complexes and a heart rate that is usually between 100 and 160 bpm. This rhythm often arises from increased sympathetic stimulation of the sinoatrial (SA) node, usually in response to 1) physiological stimuli (e.g., normal in infants and children, exertion, anxiety/emotion), 2) pharmacological stimuli (e.g., atropine, epinephrine, sympathomimetics), or 3) pathological stimuli (e.g., fever, hypoxia, anemia/hypovolemia, pulmonary embolism) (Green and Hill 2004).

On an ECG, SVT usually has a pattern of regular narrow QRS complexes at a heart rate between 140 and 250 bpm that does not vary over time. P waves may or may not be "hidden" in the QRS complex. When present, P waves are best seen in leads II, III, and aVF, are often negative, and may appear right after the QRS complex. Sinus tachycardia may be distinguished from SVT because the heart rate in sinus tachycardia varies over time and rarely exceeds 150–160 bpm, while in SVT, the heart rate remains constant and often exceeds 150 bpm (Craig 2003).

Atrial flutter is characterized on an ECG by a rapid, coarse, sawtooth pattern that is especially well seen in leads II and V1. The atrial rate is usually 300–320 bpm; however, many of these fast impulses reach the AV node during its refractory period, and the ventricular rate is generally lower (Pollock 2002). For example, if the atrial rate is 300 bpm and a 2:1 block occurs at the AV node, then the ventricular rate would be 150 bpm.

If there are wide QRS complexes on the ECG, the differential diagnosis includes monomorphic ventricular tachycardia, SVT with aberrant conduction, polymorphic ventricular tachycardia, and ventricular fibrillation.

Monomorphic ventricular tachycardia is characterized by wide QRS complexes of uniform morphology at a heart rate >100 bpm. This rhythm usually occurs in the setting of structural heart disease, but it occasionally occurs in healthy individuals. Polymorphic ventricular tachycardia has characteristics similar to those of monomorphic ventricular tachycardia (wide QRS complex and heart rate >100 bpm). However, the QRS complexes in polymorphic ventricular tachycardia are not uniform and have beat-to-beat variations, as if the complexes were "twisting" about the baseline. This pattern usually occurs in patients who have prolonged Q–T intervals. Ventricular fibrillation is characterized on an ECG by a chaotic irregular appearance, with complexes of varying amplitudes and morphology and without discrete QRS waveforms. This rhythm often occurs in patients with severe heart disease, electrolyte imbalances, hypoxemia, or acidosis (Craig 2003). SVT with aberrant conduction can be difficult to differentiate from ventricular tachycardia, even for the experts. Many criteria exist for distinguishing between these two rhythms, but to date no method of ECG analysis consistently differentiates ventricular tachycardia from SVT with aberrant conduction. The odds are usually in favor of ventricular tachycardia rather than SVT with aberrant conduction in patients with previous myocardial infarction, so if there are doubts about the interpretation of the ECG, a wide complex tachycardia can be treated as monomorphic ventricular tachycardia (see Figures 51–1 and 51–2).

## Regularity of the Rhythm

If the rhythm has a narrow QRS complex and is irregular, the two principal diagnoses to consider are atrial fibrillation and multifocal atrial tachycardia. In multifocal atrial tachycardia, the ECG shows an irregular rhythm with at least three distinct P wave morphologies and an average atrial rate of >100 bpm. This arrhythmia often occurs in the setting of severe pulmonary disease and hypoxemia. The usual treatment is to correct the underlying disorder (Pollock 2002).

Atrial fibrillation is characterized by an irregular rhythm without discrete P waves. Because P waves are not visible on the ECG, the base-

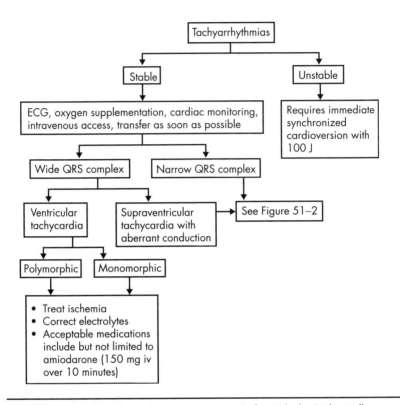

**FIGURE 51–1.**    Diagnosis and management of ventricular tachycardias.

*Note.*    ECG=electrocardiogram.

line shows low-amplitude undulations. The ventricular rate is often 140–150 bpm but may be slower in patients with impaired conduction through the AV node or in patients who are taking cardiac medications. Atrial fibrillation can be chronic or acute. In acute atrial fibrillation, the duration of the rhythm is less than 48 hours. Only in documented atrial fibrillations that occurred less than 48 hours ago can nonemergent chemical or electrical cardioversion be considered (American Heart Association 2000). When the rhythm is more than 48 hours old or the duration is unknown, nonemergent chemical or electrical cardioversion/ shock may cause an atrial thrombus to embolize, unless the patient has been given adequate anticoagulant therapy (Pollock 2002). Chronic atrial fibrillation is usually already rate controlled with medications such as β-blockers, calcium channel blockers, digoxin, or amiodarone. In patients with chronic atrial fibrillation who are hemodynamically sta-

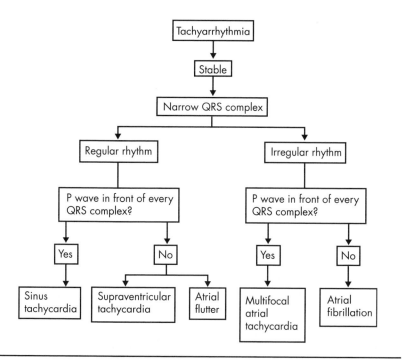

**FIGURE 51–2.** Diagnosis of supraventricular tachycardias.

ble and have a rate between 60 and 100 bpm, no emergent treatment is necessary. These patients may need only routine monitoring of their cardiac medications or any anticoagulation medication they are taking. The common etiologies of atrial fibrillation can be divided into cardiac and noncardiac causes. Cardiac causes include ischemic and valvular heart disease, sick sinus syndrome, congestive heart failure, pericarditis, myocarditis, congenital heart disease, or infiltrative heart disease. Noncardiac causes of atrial fibrillation include pulmonary embolism, medication noncompliance, thyroid disease, acute alcohol intoxication, medication use, metabolic derangements, and chronic pulmonary disease (Green and Hill 2004).

Bradyarrhythmias are abnormal rhythms with a heart rate <60 bpm. These rhythms are caused by one of two mechanisms: 1) decreased intrinsic automaticity of the SA node or 2) a conduction block between the atria and ventricles. For the purpose of this review, only AV blocks will be reviewed, as the need for emergent treatment in bradyarrhythmias is based on two main considerations: 1) the hemodynamic stability of the patient and 2) the potential of the rhythm to degenerate into further bradycardia or asystole.

First-degree AV block is characterized by a prolongation of the P–R interval (>0.2 seconds or more than five small boxes) on the ECG. Reversible causes include heightened vagal tone, transient AV nodal ischemia, and effects of digoxin, β-blockers, or calcium channel blockers. Structural causes include myocardial infarction and chronic degenerative diseases of the conduction system (Green and Hill 2004). Generally, first-degree AV block is a benign, asymptomatic condition that does not require treatment.

Second-degree AV block is characterized by intermittent failure of the AV conduction, such that on an ECG every P wave is not followed by a QRS complex. In Mobitz type I block (also known as Wenckebach block), the ECG shows a progressive increase in the P–R interval from one beat to the next until a single QRS complex is dropped or absent and the cycle repeats itself. Mobitz type I block is usually benign and may be seen in children, trained athletes, and individuals with increased vagal tone; however, this block may also develop during an acute inferior wall myocardial infarction (Green and Hill 2004).

Mobitz type II block is a more serious form of second-degree AV block. The ECG is characterized by P waves that are not followed by QRS complexes. Sometimes there are high-grade blocks that persist for two of more beats with two sequential P waves that are not followed by QRS complexes. Mobitz type II block may be caused by extensive infarction or by chronic degeneration of the conduction pathway. This rhythm may progress to third-degree block without warning.

Third-degree AV block is characterized by P waves and QRS complexes that are independent of each other. The atria and ventricle are activated separately. The most common causes of complete block are acute myocardial infarction, drug toxicity (e.g., digoxin toxicity), and chronic degeneration of the conduction pathway (Green and Hill 2004).

## Risk Stratification

In the prehospital setting the need for emergent treatment of tachyarrhythmias and bradyarrhythmias is guided by the hemodynamic stability of the patient and the potential of bradyarrhythmias to degenerate into further bradycardia or asystole. Signs of hemodynamic instability include hypotension, obtundation, loss of consciousness, pulmonary edema, and ischemic chest pain (American Heart Association 2000, 2001).

## Assessment and Management in Psychiatric Settings

In tachyarrhythmias, if the patient is hemodynamically unstable and the rapid heart rate (usually >150 bpm) is the cause of the signs and symptoms, then the patient should be prepared for immediate cardioversion. The patient may be premedicated with midazolam, diazepam, etomidate, or ketamine, if possible, but cardioversion of the unstable patient should not be delayed (American Heart Association 2000). The prehospital treatment of stable tachycardias includes monitoring of vital signs (i.e., blood pressure, pulse oximetry, heart rate, and respiratory rate), oxygen supplementation, cardiac monitoring, establishment of intravenous access, assessment with a 12-lead ECG, a focused history and physical examination, and transfer of the patient to a hospital setting (i.e., emergency department).

Emergent treatment of bradyarrhythmia is needed only if the patient develops serious signs or symptoms related to the bradycardia. These signs and symptoms include change in mental status, lethargy, and rapidly deteriorating vital signs such as a drop in blood pressure and heart rate. Atropine is the initial agent for treatment of all symptomatic bradycardias. Atropine (0.5–1.0 mg iv) should be given every 5 minutes until the desired response is achieved or a total vagolytic dose (about 0.05 mg/kg) is given. Other agents include dopamine (5–20 μg/kg/minute), epinephrine (2–10 μg/minute), or isoproterenol (2–10 μg/minute) (American Heart Association 2000, 2001). For patients with type II second-degree AV block or third-degree AV block, a transcutaneous pacer should be placed and used if needed. The prehospital treatment of stable bradycardias is similar to that for tachyarrhythmias and includes monitoring the patient's vital signs, oxygen supplementation, cardiac monitoring, establishment of intravenous access, assessment with a 12-lead ECG, a focused history and physical examination, and transfer of the patient to a hospital setting (i.e., emergency department) with a transcutaneous pacer placed on the patient if there is evidence of type II second-degree or third-degree heart block.

Additional tests may include measurement of serum thyroid and electrolyte levels and drug levels, toxicology screens, and measurement of cardiac enzyme levels. A cardiology consultation may be obtained for patients with dysrhythmias. However, all of these tests and the cardiology consultation could be rapidly facilitated in the emergency department. Time should not be wasted conducting these tests, as a patient with dysrhythmia who is currently stable may not continue to be stable and should be transferred to a hospital setting as quickly as possible. Most patients need only be assessed with a 12-lead ECG and rhythm strips. These tracings are more valuable to emergency department personnel than the findings of any laboratory test obtained in the prehospital setting. In addition, the results of a history and physical examination conducted in the prehospital setting and described in a transfer summary would be highly valued by emergency department personnel, especially if the patient is currently unable to give a history.

## References

American Heart Association: International Guidelines 2000 for CPR and ECC. Circulation 102 (suppl I):I1–I370, 2000

American Heart Association: Adult Advanced Cardiac Life Support: ACLS Provider Manual. Dallas, TX, American Heart Association, 2001

Craig SA: Tachyarrhythmias in the ED: best evidence [Emergency Medicine Practice Web site]. February 2003. Available at http://ebmedpractice.net. Accessed June 2004.

Green GB, Hill PM: Approach to chest pain, in Emergency Medicine: A Comprehensive Study Guide, 6th Edition. Edited by Tintinalli JE, Kelen GD, Stapczynski JS. New York, McGraw-Hill, 2004, pp 333–342

Pollock GF: Atrial fibrillation in the ED: cardioversion, rate control, anticoagulation, and more [Emergency Medicine Practice Web site]. August 2002. Available at http://ebmedpractice.net. Accessed June 2004.

Sabatine MS, Antman EM, Ganz LI, et al: Mechanism of cardiac arrythmias, in Pathophysiology of Heart Disease, 2nd Edition. Edited by Lilly LS. Baltimore, MD, Williams & Wilkins, 1998, pp 233–266

# CHAPTER 52

# Prolonged Q–Tc Interval

## Mansoor Khan, M.D.

## Clinical Presentation

The Q–T interval represents the time period from the depolarization to the repolarization of the ventricles. It varies with heart rate to ensure complete repolarization of the ventricle before another cycle begins. Therefore, the Q–T interval shortens when the rate increases to accommodate another cycle. It also varies according to sex and age and is slightly longer in females and in older people.

Because the Q–T interval varies with the heart rate, Bazett's formula is used to obtain a measurement of the Q–T interval with correction for the heart rate. The corrected interval is known as the Q–Tc interval. The Q–Tc interval is obtained by dividing the measured Q–T interval by the square root of the R–R interval, as follows: $Q–Tc = QT / \sqrt{R-R}$. A Q–Tc interval ≥0.45 seconds is considered to be prolonged (Figure 52–1) (Wagner 1994).

The Q–T interval is measured from the beginning of the Q wave to the end of the T wave (Figure 52–1). It should be measured in leads, which have the tallest T waves. The U wave, which is a positive deflection after the T wave but before the P wave, may merge with the T wave. In this situation, the onset of the U wave should be considered the end of the Q–T interval. At faster rates, the T wave may merge with the P wave; in this instance the onset of the P wave should be considered the end of the Q–T interval.

An understanding of normal cell electrophysiology is helpful in fully appreciating the pathophysiology of prolonged Q–T interval. Normal depolarization and repolarization involves five phases (Figure 52–2).

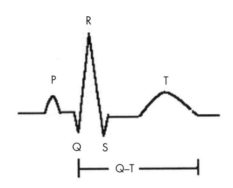

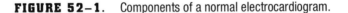

**FIGURE 52-1.**   Components of a normal electrocardiogram.

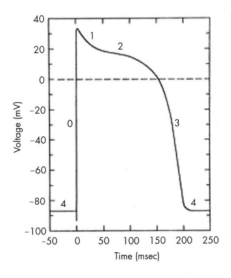

**FIGURE 52-2.**   Cardiac membrane polarization.

Phase 0: Depolarization of the membrane, caused by a rapid influx of sodium
Phase 1: Initial repolarization, which represents the transient outward potassium current
Phase 2: Plateau phase, which represents the influx of calcium
Phase 3: Repolarization, caused by the efflux of potassium current
Phase 4: Resting membrane potential, largely dictated by potassium channels

A prolongation of the Q–T interval results from a net reduction in outward current in phase 2 or 3. Therefore an increase in sodium influx caused by pharmacological agents such as ibutilide can prolong the Q–T interval. A decrease in potassium efflux caused by class IA (e.g., quinidine, procainamide, disopyramide) or class III (sotalol) antiarrhythmic drugs can also prolong the Q–T interval.

There is no consensus on the best way to measure Q–T in a setting of atrial fibrillation. Some authors recommend averaging the measurement over 10 beats. There are also no data on the measurement of the Q–T interval in the setting of a widened QRS interval; some authors recommend that a Q–T interval >500 msec be considered prolonged (Al-Khatib et al. 2003).

## Differential Diagnosis

Many factors can influence the Q–T interval and cause it to become abnormally prolonged. These factors include acquired causes, such as hypokalemia, hypocalcemia, myocardial infarction, and the effects of many pharmacological agents. Prolongation may also be secondary to congenital causes, such as Jervell and Lange-Nielsen syndrome and Romano-Ward syndrome (Table 52–1).

Many pharmacological interventions lead to a prolonged Q–T interval. They include antimicrobials (such as erythromycin, levofloxacin, fluconazole, and quinine) and psychiatric medications (such as thioridazine, sertindole, and ziprasidone). Figure 52–3 shows the average changes some of these medications cause in the Q–Tc interval. Antihistamines, such as fexofenadine, can also prolong the Q–T interval (Viskin 2003).

Prolongation of the Q–T interval can lead to the development of torsades de pointes, which can cause sudden cardiac death. Until the 1960s torsades de pointes was thought to be caused primarily by congenital abnormalities or by cardiac medications. In 1963 two cases of sudden death were reported in patients who were taking thioridazine. In 1991, a study of medicolegal autopsies performed in Finland found 49 cases of sudden death. Of these, 46 involved phenothiazines, mainly thioridazine (28 of the 46). The authors of the study concluded that sudden death in apparently healthy adults was associated with low-potency phenothiazines, especially thioridazine. Thioridazine was involved in 61% of cases of sudden death, versus only 13% for haloperidol, even though haloperidol was used with equal frequency (Glassman et al. 2001).

**TABLE 52–1.**    Major causes of prolonged Q–T interval

| | |
|---|---|
| **Antihistamines** | **Metabolic** |
| Astemizole | Hypocalcemia |
| Terfenadine | Hypokalemia |
| **Congenital** | Hypomagnesemia |
| Jervell and Lange-Nielsen syndrome | **Psychotropic drugs** |
| Romano-Ward syndrome | Butyrophenones |
| **Antiarrhythmic drugs** | Haloperidol |
| Amiodarone | High-dose methadone |
| Disopyramide | Phenothiazines |
| Quinidine | Risperidone |
| Procainamide | Selective serotonin reuptake inhibitors |
| Sotalol | Thioridazine |
| **Antimicrobial drugs** | Tricyclic antidepressants |
| Ampicillin | **Other medications/substances** |
| Erythromycin, azithromycin, | Arsenic |
| clarithromycin | Cisapride |
| Fluconazole | Cocaine |
| Ketoconazole, itraconazole | Droperidol |
| Levofloxacin | Organophosphates |
| Quinine | **Other** |
| Pentamidine | Hypothermia |
| Trimethoprim-sulfamethoxazole | Intracranial hemorrhage |
| | Mitral valve prolapse |
| | Myocardial ischemia or infarction |

Other antipsychotics, such as pimozide and droperidol, also cause prolongation of the Q–T interval. Droperidol was previously used extensively by emergency physicians, psychiatrists, and anesthesiologists. In December 2001, the U. S. Food and Drug Administration required a "black box warning" on droperidol packaging because of its association with prolongation of the Q–T interval, leading to the development of torsades de pointes (Richards and Schneir 2003). In January 2001, distribution of droperidol was discontinued in Europe.

## Risk Stratification

Q–T interval prolongation predisposes the patient to deadly arrhythmias such as torsades de pointes, which is associated with a characteristic electrocardiogram (ECG) pattern in which the tracing appears to be twisting around the isoelectric line (Figure 52–4).

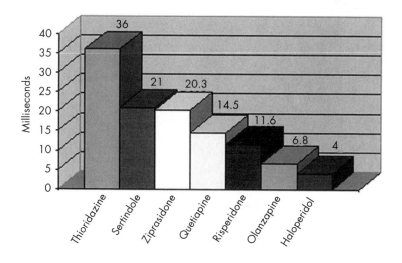

**FIGURE 52–3.**    Mean changes in the Q–Tc interval from baseline associated with antipsychotic medications.

*Source.*    Adapted from Zimbroff et al. 1997 and Pfizer Inc. 2000.

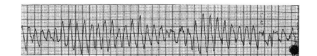

**FIGURE 52–4.**    Torsades de pointes.

Many risk factors have been described for drug-induced torsades de pointes (Roden 2004). They include

- Female sex
- Hypokalemia
- Bradycardia
- Recent conversion from atrial fibrillation, especially with a drug known to prolong the Q–T interval
- Congestive heart failure
- Digitalis therapy

- High drug concentrations
- Rapid rate of intravenous infusion with a drug known to prolong the Q–T interval
- Baseline Q–T interval prolongation
- Subclinical long Q–T interval syndrome
- Severe hypomagnesemia

A prognostic measurement in the setting of Q–T interval prolongation is the Q–T dispersion. Q–T dispersion is the variability in the Q–T interval between different leads on the ECG. In one study, the Q–T dispersion was most prolonged in patients who were symptomatic; in addition, a Q–T dispersion of 0.10 or less had an 80% sensitivity and specificity for identifying patients who responded to β-blocker therapy (Priori et al. 1994).

In another study involving patients with congenital causes of Q–T interval prolongation, the Q–Tc interval was a strong predictor of cardiac event rates (Zareba et al. 1998). The odds ratio was 2.18 for a Q–Tc interval >0.44 to 0.46 seconds, 3.93 for a Q–Tc interval >0.46 to 0.50 seconds, and 9.66 for a Q–Tc interval >0.50 seconds. In a retrospective analysis of pediatric patients with congenital long Q–T interval syndrome, the presence of a Q–Tc interval >0.60 seconds was strongly associated with sudden cardiac death or syncope (Garson et al. 1993). Major risk factors found to be associated with sudden cardiac death in probands were congenital deafness, history of syncope, family history of sudden cardiac death, female gender, and a Q–Tc interval >0.60 seconds (Schwartz and Locati 1985).

## Assessment and Management in Psychiatric Settings

Acquired Q–T interval prolongation differs slightly from congenital Q–T interval prolongation. Bradycardia usually leads to torsades de pointes in the acquired form, whereas catecholamine surges lead to torsades de pointes in the congenital form. However, the emergent treatment of prolonged Q–T interval leading to torsades de pointes is the same in the acquired and congenital forms.

Assessment of an unresponsive patient always starts with the ABCs: (checking if the airway is clear), breathing (listening for breath sounds), and circulation (feeling for a pulse). If no pulse is present, the defibrillator paddles can be used to detect heart rhythm. If a polymorphic wide-complex tachycardia is present, an initial unsynchronized cardioversion with 200 J is delivered. If no pulse is present, the initial cardioversion is followed by a 300-J and subsequently a 360-J cardioversion. Magnesium (2 g iv bolus over 2 minutes) is given; this dose can be followed by another similar bolus if required (advanced cardiac life support protocol). If the polymorphic wide-complex tachycardia is secondary to a prolonged Q–T interval, then overdrive pacing may be beneficial. The patient should be assessed for causes of prolonged Q–T interval, such as hypokalemia, hypomagnesemia, hypocalcemia, and medications. Class IB agents, such as lidocaine, shorten the Q–T interval and may be beneficial. If the agent suspected of causing the prolonged Q–T interval is quinidine, alkalinization of the plasma with sodium bicarbonate may be helpful. Alkalinization increases protein binding of quinidine, thereby reducing the concentration of free quinidine (see Figure 52–5).

Treatment of congenital Q–T prolongation is achieved by decreasing sympathetic activity, either by pharmacological means through the use of β-blockers or surgically by means of left cardiothoracic sympathectomy. If both treatments fail, an automatic implantable cardioverter-defibrillator can be placed (Priori et al. 2001).

β-Blockers are thought to interrupt sympathetic flow. A theoretic risk is that the bradycardia caused by these medications may predispose patients to torsades de pointes. In one study, of 869 patients treated with β-blockers during a 5-year period, β-blocker therapy reduced the rate of cardiac events in probands (0.97 vs. 0.31) (Moss et al. 2000).

Q–T interval prolongation has many causes. Laboratory tests for the presence of hypokalemia, hypocalcemia, and hypomagnesemia are essential. A through family history should be conducted to identify any history of sudden cardiac death, syncope, or deafness. Any medications that may cause Q–T interval prolongation should be stopped. The patient with a prolonged Q–T interval should be admitted to a monitored bed and evaluated with daily ECGs. A cardiology consultation should be obtained. A patient who has torsades de pointes despite medical treatment should be evaluated for automatic implantable cardioverter-defibrillator placement.

Most causes of Q–T interval prolongation are treatable. If a patient has a history of Q–T prolongation, any medications that can prolong the Q–T interval should be avoided. Any electrolyte abnormalities, such as hypokalemia, hypocalcemia, and hypomagnesemia, should be corrected.

Antipsychotics are a known cause of Q–T interval prolongation and sudden death. Therefore, Q–T interval prolongation is one of the many factors that must be considered before choosing an antipsychotic. Occasionally there may be good reasons to use a particular medication that may substantially prolong the Q–T interval. Patients who are taking

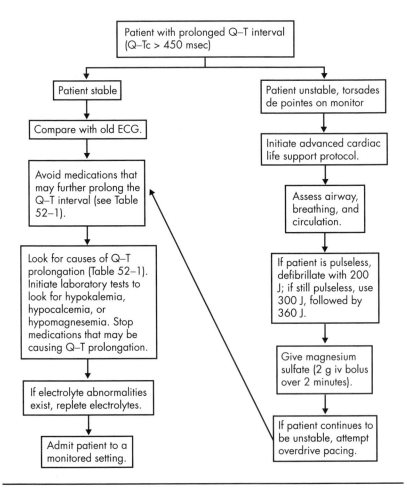

**FIGURE 52–5.**    Algorithm for the approach to a patient with prolonged Q–T interval.

*Note.*    ECG = electrocardiogram.

these medications must be assessed frequently with ECGs and closely monitored for signs and symptoms of cardiac arrhythmias, such as dizziness, palpitations, and syncope. Yap and Camm (2000) outline four key principles for safer prescribing of these medications:

1. Not exceeding the upper recommended dose
2. Restricting the dosage in patients with preexisting heart disease or other risk factors

3. Avoiding concomitant prescribing of drugs that inhibit drug metabolism or excretion, which can prolong the Q–T interval or produce hypokalemia
4. Ensuring that serum potassium levels are regularly checked

# References

Al-Khatib SM, Lapointe NM, Kramer JM, et al: What clinicians should know about the QT interval. JAMA 289:2120–2127, 2003

Garson A Jr, Dick M 2nd, Fournier A, et al: The long QT syndrome in children: an international study of 287 patients. Circulation 87:1866–1872, 1993

Glassman AH, Bigger JT Jr: Antipsychotic drugs: prolonged QTc interval, torsade de pointes, and sudden death. Am J Psychiatry 158:1774–1782, 2001

Moss AJ, Zareba W, Hall WJ, et al: Effectiveness and limitations of beta-blocker therapy in congenital long Q-T syndrome. Circulation 101:616–623, 2000

Pfizer Inc: Briefing document for Zeldox capsules (ziprasidone HCL). FDA Psychopharmacological Drug Advisory Committee meeting July 19, 2000. Available at http://www.fda.gov/ohrms/dockets/ac/00/backgrd/3619b1.htm. Accessed October 5, 2005.

Priori SG, Napolitano C, Diehl L, et al: Dispersion of the QT interval: a marker of therapeutic efficacy in the idiopathic long QT syndrome. Circulation 89:1681–1689, 1994

Priori SG, Aliot E, Blomstrom-Lundqvist C, et al: Task Force on Sudden Cardiac Death of the European Society of Cardiology. Eur Heart J 22:1374–1450, 2001

Richards JR, Schneir AB: Droperidol in the emergency department: is it safe? J Emerg Med 24:441–447, 2003

Roden DM: Drug-induced prolongation of the QT interval. N Engl J Med 350:1013–1022, 2004

Schwartz PJ, Locati E: The idiopathic long QT syndrome: pathogenetic mechanisms and therapy. Eur Heart J 6 (suppl D):103–114, 1985

Wagner GS: Marriott's Practical Electrocardiography, 9th Edition. Baltimore, MD, Williams & Wilkins, 1994, pp 10–15

Yap YG, Camm J: Risk of torsade de pointes with non-cardiac drugs: doctors need to be aware that many drugs can cause QT prolongation. BMJ 320:1158–1159, 2000

Zareba W, Moss AJ, Schwartz PJ, et. al: Influence of the genotype on the clinical course of the long-QT syndrome. N Engl J Med 339:960–965, 1998

Zimbroff DL, Kane JM, Tamminga CA, et al: Controlled, dose-response study of sertindole and haloperidol in the treatment of schizophrenia. Am J Psychiatry 154:782–791, 1997

# PART XIII

# Acute Changes in Mental Status

Section Editors:

Angela Scicutella, M.D., Ph.D.

Peter Manu, M.D.

# CHAPTER 53

# Agitation

Elizabeth M. Sublette, M.D., Ph.D.

Jeffrey Nachbar, M.D.

Howard Hao, M.D.

## Clinical Presentation

Agitation is a psychomotor condition that has been described in a variety of ways. Day (1999) reviewed the difficulties inherent in characterizing agitation and proposed the following definition: "A disorder of motor activity associated with mental distress which is characterized by a restricted range of repetitive, non-progressive ('to and fro'), non-goal directed activity" (p. 89). Haskell et al. (1997) described agitation more broadly as "excessive motor or verbal behavior that interferes with patient care, patient or staff safety and medical therapies" (p. 336). Agitation is a condition that may be viewed more as a group of symptoms (or syndrome), as opposed to a diagnosis (Allen 1999), and that may have a multifactorial etiology.

Agitation has been reported to occur in 10% of patients in the emergency psychiatric setting (TREC Collaborative Group 2003) and in 11%–50% of patients with traumatic brain injuries, up to 67% of patients with delirium, and as many as 93% of patients with dementia (Haskell et al. 1997). In intensive care units, up to 71% of patients may be agitated (Siegel 2003).

Agitation may be presumed to be a manifestation of some underlying disturbance, although its source is not always immediately apparent (Haskell et al. 1997). The overt expression may be goal directed or it may be nonpurposeful: patients may wander, pull out intravenous tubing, refuse care, and become combative, verbally caustic, anxious, restless, or irritable. Because agitated behavior is difficult to interpret, disruptive, and often unsafe, it can create a barrier to the therapeutic alliance between staff and the patient.

## Differential Diagnosis

Medical symptoms, pharmacological effects, psychiatric disturbances, cognitive impairments, and sensory deficits are all possible causes of agitation (see Table 53–1). Combinations of agitation-producing conditions can be confusing. For example, *pharmacological side effects* such as akathisia, serotonin syndrome, anticholinergic symptoms, or neuroleptic malignant syndrome (NMS) in a psychiatric patient may be superimposed on the agitation of *psychosis* or of *delirium*; a medically hospitalized patient may be at risk for delirium and agitation secondary to *infection* or *other illness* or to *medications* that are administered.

### Organic Disorders

Agitation can occur as a result of organic illness and may stem from pain or other physically uncomfortable conditions. Medical problems should be ruled out, including *hypoxia, metabolic disorders,* and *infection,* which have a high degree of associated agitation (Haskell et al. 1997). Elements common to multiple medical illnesses that can potentiate agitation include distress, anxiety, increased sympathomimetic activity, increased arousal, and certain types of pain.

*Neurological disorders* are often accompanied by agitation. For example, almost all patients who have *acute traumatic brain injuries* exhibit hyperactivity, especially during the period of posttraumatic amnesia. This agitation can be dangerous for the patient, because it can increase cerebral metabolic demand, worsening intracranial hypertension at a time when there is greatest risk for cerebral edema (Haskell et al. 1997). Agitation is frequently seen in *delirium*. Until the etiology of delirium can be established and treated, the physician frequently must control associated agitation to prevent injury (Haskell et al. 1997). *Dementia*, a progressive deterioration in cognitive abilities, often presents with agitation. The agitation of dementia may become an emergency situation if the patient becomes violent or has poor self-care. The degree of agitation is often an indication of the severity of cognitive limitations (Falsetti 2000). Some behavioral disturbances particularly characteristic of dementia-associated agitation include aggression or assaultiveness, irritability, disturbances of sleep, abusive vocalization, and wandering (Haskell et al. 1997; Lonergan et al. 2002). Patients with *temporal lobe epilepsy* can be capable of agitated and aggressive behaviors during or after a seizure (Kanemoto et al. 1999; Manford et al. 1998).

**TABLE 53–1.** Differential diagnosis of the etiology of acute agitation

**Drug-related**
Withdrawal symptoms: risk of seizure
Drug reaction
    Prescribed drugs
        Acute dystonic reaction: risk of paralysis of breathing muscles
        Neuroleptic malignant syndrome: risk of renal failure
        Akathisia: risk of exacerbation with further treatment with
            antipsychotic medications
        Anticholinergic delirium
    Drug-drug interactions
    Illicit drugs
    Over-the-counter drugs
    Herbal or other nonstandard "medicines"

**Medical**
Infectious
Toxic-metabolic
Cardiac
Endocrine

**Neurological**
Seizure disorder: risk of falls
Sequelae of head trauma: risk of intracranial bleeding

**Psychiatric**
Psychotic disorder
Manic episode
Agitated depression
Catatonia
Axis II condition (borderline or antisocial personality disorder)
Delirium (a medical etiology should be sought)
Dementia

A critical aspect of neurological difficulties may arise with *problems in the sensory modalities.* A person with dementia may be less able to interpret sensory stimuli and therefore misperceive the environment (Allen 1999). Sensory overstimulation has been hypothesized to contribute to the high incidence of agitation in the intensive care unit, where the patient may experience round-the-clock tactile, visual, and auditory overload, as well as disrupted sleep patterns (discussed by Critical Care Medicine 2002). Patients with cataracts, glaucoma, or missing glasses may misinterpret or miss cues in their physical environment (Allen 1999) and may even experience vivid visual hallucinations, a condition known as Charles Bonnet syndrome (Siatkowski et al. 1990). Patients who are hard of hearing, who are missing hearing aids, or who have ear pain may find it difficult and isolating when they cannot easily understand others.

Agitation arising from frustration may also be seen in those with other communication difficulties such as *aphasia, dysarthria,* or *language barriers.* In patients with dementia, agitation may be an attempt to express feelings and needs that cannot be verbalized, "just as crying in a very young child communicates hunger, fear, or pain" (Allen 1999, p. 37). This same concept of agitation in the context of inability to communicate pain or physical discomfort applies to patients with moderate to severe *mental retardation* or other *developmental disorders.*

## Drug Effects

### Side Effects and Intoxications

Agitation can result from use of illicit substances, over-the-counter drugs, herbal preparations, and prescribed medications, as well as from exposure to toxic environmental chemicals such as pesticides. A thorough medication and substance use history and a toxicology screen are essential in order not to overlook these possibilities. Elderly persons are particularly sensitive to medication-induced side effects in general and to agitation and delirium in particular. This sensitivity is caused in part by decreased water-soluble medication excretion secondary to decreased glomerular filtration rates and by increased retention of fat-soluble medications because of decreased lean body mass (Haskell et al. 1997).

*Illicit drugs* with potential for causing agitation include alcohol, cocaine, hallucinogens, γ-hydroxybutyrate (GHB), and phencyclidine hydrochloride (PCP, angel dust). The latter drug may cause patients to exhibit bizarre behaviors, aggression, and violence, and it confers an insensitivity to pain in high doses. These characteristics are important from a clinical management standpoint because patients who are intoxicated with PCP have been known to seriously injure themselves fighting against restraints (reviewed by Baldridge and Bessen 1990).

*Side effects* of medications are a common cause of agitation. Patients who are taking typical antipsychotics and, occasionally, patients who are taking selective serotonin reuptake inhibitors may experience akathisia, thought to be a form of extrapyramidal symptom. Akathisia consists of feelings of unbearable restlessness and edginess. Agitation may also occur in association with other extrapyramidal symptoms, such as acute dystonia, or in serotonin syndrome, which is caused by the combination of two or more serotonergic drugs. It is vital to keep in mind the possibility of potentially fatal NMS, in which patients exhibit fever, rigidity, autonomic instability, and acute mental status changes. NMS is produced by antipsychotic drugs, but it can also result from use of various antiemetic medications such as promethazine, prochlorperazine, and metoclopramide. Patients who are taking sedatives or hypnotics may become agitated because of paradoxical disinhibition. Medications such as steroids, anticholinergics, β-agonists, dopaminergics, stimulants, caffeine, and levodopa may all lead to agitation due to side effects or toxicity, such as in overdose. The possibility of *medication interactions* and *medication errors* also should be considered.

### Withdrawal Symptoms

The most crucial diagnoses to consider, however, are ethanol, benzodiazepine, or barbiturate withdrawal, all of which can lead to seizures and death if untreated. Six to 12 hours after the abrupt cessation of drinking in an alcohol-dependent person, symptoms of tremulousness, tachycardia, hypertension, nausea, and vomiting begin and can progress to the life-threatening withdrawal syndrome of delirium tremens. Benzodiazepine withdrawal can occur at different times, depending on the pharmacokinetic properties of the specific agent. Clonazepam withdrawal, for instance, can surprise the unwary clinician a number of days after the drug's cessation, because its half-life is 20–80 hours. Cessation of regular use of GHB, an increasingly popular drug of abuse, may lead to a withdrawal syndrome consisting of agitation, psychosis, and delirium with potentially dangerous medical complications (Rosenberg et al. 2003).

## Psychiatric Disorders

Agitation is a nonspecific, nondiagnostic syndrome that can occur in any severe psychiatric disorder, including mood disorders, psychosis, anxiety disorders, and personality disorders. A variety of behavioral presentations, ranging from random repetitive movements to very purposeful actions, are termed agitation in the context of psychiatric illness. Elderly patients in particular are prone to *agitated depression* characterized by pacing or other restless behaviors. An extremely dramatic presentation can occur in the case of *catatonia* due to depression or psychosis, in which the patient may perform repetitive, purposeless movements, such as rocking from foot to foot or from side to side, literally for hours. A catatonic presentation often includes mutism, which makes the patient unable to convey any information to the clinician. Agitation associated with *psychosis* or *intermittent explosive disorder* may include more relatively purposeful movements or verbalizations and can be dangerous at times, for example, in the case of a patient who is screaming obscenities and throwing chairs or suddenly without provocation punches the nearest person. Similarly purposeful actions may be described as agitated behavior in patients with *borderline personality disorder.* These individuals may interpret everyday interactions as terrible rejections and experience overwhelming mood swings and emotional storms that lead to impulsive behaviors, such as screaming, throwing objects, slamming doors, and self-injurious behavior that can reach life-threatening proportions. A person experiencing a *panic attack* or other severe *anxiety* may feel trapped in a particular environment and make frantic efforts to escape. Patients in a manic episode can engage in continuous purposeful behaviors, such as walking for many miles or performing certain tasks ceaselessly for several days.

## Risk Stratification

### Risk of Becoming Agitated

Conditions posing a high risk for agitation include dementia, delirium, receiving treatment in an intensive care unit, major neurological conditions, suspected drug or alcohol withdrawal, and starting new medications. Elderly patients have a much higher incidence of agitation than younger patients.

### Risk of Dangerous Consequences of Agitation

The more severe the agitation and the less controlled the environment, the more likely are sequelae of physical harm to the patient and bystanders.

### Medical Risks Associated With Certain Types of Agitation

It is essential to consider the differential diagnoses of potentially urgent life-threatening causes of agitation, including substance use, substance withdrawal, acute dystonia (can affect muscles of respiration), NMS, head injury, acute infection (such as meningitis), cardiovascular emergencies, and metabolic disorders.

It is also worth repeating that in the agitated mentally retarded or developmentally disabled patient, a very thorough search must be made for occult medical or surgical conditions, particularly in patients with acute-onset agitation.

## Assessment and Management in Psychiatric Settings

It is essential to create and maintain a safe environment for the agitated patient and staff (see Table 53–2). Bystanders should be removed, and potentially dangerous objects should be cleared away. The clinician should call for help with the agitated patient if necessary. For example, a "show of force" may be needed; that is, more personnel may be needed to safely implement the treatment of choice. If an acute medical illness is suspected and the patient is not in a full-service medical environment, an ambulance may be required to transport the patient to an emergency department. Safety is of paramount and overriding importance. Thus, seclusion or restraint, while an unpleasant experience for the patient, is a lesser evil than unchecked aggression or dangerous wandering. The least restrictive restraint device should be used for the minimum necessary time, and the patient should be observed continually while in restraints. The patient's vital signs should be checked periodically, and the patient should be surveyed frequently for comfort and safety, such as adequacy of breathing, tightness of limb restraints, and elevation of the head to prevent choking. A patient who cannot communicate must be assessed scrupulously. A bedbound patient must have the body repositioned at intervals to prevent bedsores.

The clinician should gather essential information as rapidly as possible from all available sources (e.g., staff or other witnesses, the patient's chart, and records of medical assessments) and should make a mental list of possible hypotheses. The differential diagnosis will determine which tests to perform and what treatments to consider. It is always prudent to check whether the patient has just started taking a medication that may have caused the agitation. If the patient may have had access to illicit drugs, a toxicology screen may be useful.

Rapid pharmacological intervention is likely to be necessary. The ideal treatment is parsimonious: it treats both the manifestation of agitation and the underlying illness—for example, intramuscular ziprasidone in schizophrenia and benzodiazepines in a panic attack. Among the safest and most frequently employed calming/sedating medica-

---

**TABLE 53–2.**    Algorithm for assessment and treatment of a patient with agitation

---

1. Prevent injury; call for help, clear the area, and restrain the patient if necessary.
2. Obtain brief overview about what has been happening; use information from the chart, the caregivers, bystanders.
3. Make an initial hypothesis: does the problem seem to be *medical* or *psychiatric*? (See Table 53–1 for differential diagnosis of causes of agitation.)
4. For a medical problem, assess and triage the patient for possible emergency.
   a. If needed, delegate someone to arrange for additional medical help (defibrillator, oxygen tanks, crash cart, ambulance).
   b. Check "ABCs" (airway, breathing, circulation).
   c. Obtain vital signs.
   d. Assess the patient with an electrocardiogram, if warranted.
   e. Test the patient's blood glucose level.
   f. Obtain blood sample for laboratory tests, if necessary.
   g. Transfer the patient to a higher level of medical care, or request specialty consultation, if warranted.
5. For a psychiatric problem:
   Look for the basic etiology (e.g., psychosis, mania, anxiety, rage attack).
   Identify situational stressors that can be mitigated.
6. For either a medical or psychiatric cause of agitation, treat the patient pharmacologically if appropriate.
7. Provide for the patient's ongoing treatment and safety (e.g., maintain a more intensive level of observation, do further medical assessment, stop suspect medications, and issue an order for medications to treat the agitation should it recur).

---

tions in clinical use are haloperidol and lorazepam. They may be given singly, alternately, or in combination; some studies have indicated that the combination works more rapidly and may be more effective than either treatment alone (Battaglia et al. 1997; Bieniek et al. 1998). Both medications can be administered either orally or intramuscularly, and intramuscular administration is often necessary in an emergency when a very agitated patient is not cooperating with oral treatment. Oral/intramuscular haloperidol is typically given in doses ranging from 0.5 mg (for the frail, elderly patient) to 5 mg (for the young, healthy, dangerously agitated psychiatric patient) and has proved well tolerated and useful in treating dementia, delirium, and agitation in a medical context, as well as for treating agitated psychiatric patients. Haloperidol can cause prolongation of the Q–Tc interval and should be used with caution in patients with major risk factors for cardiac instability. Lorazepam is usually given in doses ranging from 1–2 mg (0.5 mg in the frail, elderly patient) and is a medication of choice in suspected withdrawal from ethanol or benzodiazepines and for seizure-prone patients. The predominant risk with lorazepam is oversedation, which in extreme cases could lead to respiratory depression. For example, lorazepam would not be an appropriate choice for treatment of agitation associated with ingestion of another potentially sedating substance, such as alcohol. Lorazepam should be used with caution in the elderly or delirious patient, because it may cause or worsen confusion.

In the treatment of agitation due to akathisia, it is important to decrease and stop any possibly offending antipsychotic medications. The treatments of choice are lorazepam and/or propranolol (if there are no contraindications, such as preexisting hypotension). It is important to bear in mind that akathisia often must be treated for a period of weeks before it resolves.

Other typical and atypical antipsychotics and benzodiazepines may also be useful. For example, ziprasidone (Brook 2003) and olanzapine (Breier et al. 2002) have been introduced in intramuscular formulation. A rapidly dissolving form of olanzapine, which is almost impossible to "cheek," is also very useful in patients who are willing to take it.

Once the agitated patient has been safely contained, it may be necessary to plan further assessment to ascertain the etiology of agitation. Elements of the assessment include laboratory studies to rule out toxic-metabolic processes, electrolyte imbalance, and drug abuse; neuroimaging; and an electroencephalogram. It may also be prudent to reassess the patient at intervals, for example, by performing frequent "neurochecks" for basic aspects of neurological functioning or by administering assessment scales to measure withdrawal symptoms, such as the Clinical Institute Withdrawal Assessment for Alcohol (CIWA-A) (Shaw et al. 1981) or for Benzodiazepines (CIWA-B) (Busto et al. 1989). The patient may need to be transferred to a more secure setting, such as a seclusion area, or to a different medical setting such as an emergency department or telemetry unit.

In the event of a postulated medical or neurological basis for agitation, the clinician may wish to consult the appropriate specialist.

In dealing with a patient with dementia, staff members or other caregivers should 1) provide an environment that is controlled and monitored for safety; 2) redirect and remind the patient as necessary; 3) provide orienting clues in the patient's room, such as familiar objects, a calendar, and a clock; 4) create a reliable routine for activities, meals, medication dispensation, and bedtime; and 5) perform regular vision, hearing, and pain checks.

An easily provoked patient may benefit from fewer stimuli, such as taking meals alone in his/her room or sleeping in a seclusion area. If the patient is frankly manic, psychotic, or paranoid, and there is a danger of violence, the physician may treat the patient more aggressively, which may include sedating the patient preemptively. If the agitated or aggressive behavior is recognized early, a show of force and even seclusion or restraint may be warranted to prevent escalation.

## References

Allen L: Treating agitation without drugs. Am J Nurs 99:36–42, 1999

Baldridge E, Bessen H: Phencyclidine. Emerg Med Clin North Am 8:541–50, 1990

Battaglia J, Moss S, Rush J, et al: Haloperidol, lorazepam, or both for psychotic agitation? a multicenter, prospective, double-blind, emergency department study. Am J Emerg Med 15:335–340, 1997

Bieniek S, Ownby R, Penalver A, et al: A double-blind study of lorazepam versus the combination of haloperidol and lorazepam in managing agitation. Pharmacotherapy 18:57–62, 1998

Breier A, Meehan K, Birkett M, et al: A double-blind, placebo controlled dose-response comparison of intramuscular olanzapine and haloperiodol in the treatment of acute agitation in schizophrenia. Arch Gen Psychiatry 59:441–448, 2002

Brook S: Intramuscular ziprasidone: moving beyond the conventional in the treatment of acute agitation in schizophrenia. J Clin Psychiatry 64:13–18, 2003

Busto U, Sykora K, Sellers E: A clinical scale to assess benzodiazepine withdrawal. J Clin Psychopharmacol 9:412–416, 1989

Critical Care Medicine: The management of the agitated ICU patient. Crit Care Med 30 (suppl 1):S97–123, 2002

Day R: Psychomotor agitation: poorly defined and badly measured. J Affect Disord 55:89–98, 1999

Falsetti A: Risperidone for control of agitation in dementia patients. Am J Health Syst Pharm 57:862–870, 2000

Haskell RM, Frankel HL, Rotondo MF: Agitation. AACN Clin Issues 8:335–350, 1997

Kanemoto K, Kawasaki J, Mori E: Violence and epilepsy: a close relation between violence and postictal psychosis. Epilepsia 40:107–109, 1999

Lonergan E, Luxenberg J, Colford J: Haloperidol for agitation in dementia. Cochrane Database Systematic Review 2:CD002852, 2002

Manford M, Cvejic H, Minde K, et al: Case study: neurological brain waves causing serious behavioral brainstorms. J Am Acad Child Adolesc Psychiatry 37:1085–1090, 1998

Rosenberg M, Deerfield LJ, Baruch EM: Two cases of severe gamma-hydroxy-butyrate withdrawal delirium on a psychiatric unit: recommendations for management. Am J Drug Alcohol Abuse 29:487–496, 2003

Shaw J, Kolesar G, Sellers E, et al: Development of optimal treatment tactics for alcohol withdrawal. I. Assessment and effectiveness of supportive care. J Clin Psychopharmacol 1:382–387, 1981

Siatkowski RM, Zimmer B, Rosenberg PR: The Charles Bonnet syndrome: visual perceptive dysfunction in sensory deprivation. J Clin Neuroophthalmol 10:215–218, 1990

Siegel MD: Management of agitation in the intensive care unit. Clin Chest Med 24:713–25, 2003

TREC Collaborative Group: Rapid tranquillisation for agitated patients in emergency psychiatric rooms: a randomised trial of midazolam versus haloperidol plus promethazine. BMJ 327:708–713, 2003

# CHAPTER 54

# Delirium

Angela Scicutella, M.D., Ph.D.

## Clinical Presentation

Delirium is a neuropsychiatric syndrome that has the following key features: 1) changes in consciousness, 2) changes in cognition, 3) fluctuation over time, and 4) causal relationship with a medical condition. Patients with delirium can manifest elevated or decreased levels of alertness and wakefulness in response to environmental stimuli, such that they can be either hypervigilant or drowsy and lethargic. Attention levels are diminished in delirium, and the patient is easily distracted by competing stimuli and tends to perseverate. Patients with delirium also present with memory deficits, disorientation, or language or perceptual disturbances that are not better accounted for by a preexisting dementia. Delirious patients evidence problems in immediate or working memory that are likely secondary to their attentional problems. In addition, short-term memory and long-term memory can be affected, and disorientation to time, place, and situation is common. Language disturbances can include dysarthria, as well as disorganized, rambling speech marked by tangentiality, circumstantiality, or looseness of associations. Dysnomia, paraphasias, reduced comprehension, and dysgraphia can also be observed. Although the most common perceptual abnormalities are visual hallucinations, other perceptual disturbances, such as auditory, tactile, gustatory, or olfactory hallucinations, as well as paranoid and persecutory delusions, may also be present (Cummings and Mega 2003; Wise et al. 2002). Delirium develops over a short period of time (hours to days), and the disturbance tends to fluctuate during the course of the day. Prodromal symptoms such as restlessness, anxiety, or other behavioral disturbances may develop a few days before the overt manifestation of the full syndrome of delirium. Classically, patients wax and wane between the clinical symptoms already outlined and periods of lucidity. In addition, episodes of agitation known as sundowning occur when darkness falls and patients lose the orienting cues of daylight (Wise et al. 2002). Evidence from the history, physical examination, or laboratory findings suggests that a general medical condition is related to the disturbance.

Associated features of delirium that may frequently be present include sleep disturbances (daytime sleepiness, reversal of the sleep-wake cycle), affective or emotional changes (irritability, fear, depression, lethargy), and neurological abnormalities (tremor, myoclonus, asterixis, reflex or muscle changes) (Cummings and Mega 2003). Delirium may also be characterized by psychomotor disturbances such as motor restlessness or combativeness (hyperactive type); apathy, lethargy and somnolence (hypoactive type); or a combination of the two, known as the mixed state (O'Keeffe 1999).

## Differential Diagnosis

The many potential causes of delirium should be prioritized to rule out etiologies that could lead to irreversible damage if they are not recognized and urgently treated. If these critical etiologies have been ruled out, then the clinician can search for other medical causes to account for the mental status changes (see Table 54–1) (Jacobson and Schreibman 1997; Milisen et al. 1998; Wise et al. 2002).

Virtually any medication can cause delirium, but those with anticholinergic side effects are well known for being associated with this syndrome. Examples of medications that can induce delirium are listed in Table 54–2 (Lagomasino et al. 1999; Simon et al. 1997).

Elderly patients are more prone to delirium caused by medications, because age-related alterations in drug distribution and metabolism and delayed excretion allow toxic levels to build up more quickly in their systems (Carter et al. 1996).

Because of symptom overlap, psychiatric illnesses such as dementia, depression, anxiety, and psychosis should be considered in the differential diagnosis. In contrast to patients with delirium, patients with dementia remain alert and do not evidence wide fluctuations in the severity of their cognitive symptoms over a short time span. Delirium and dementia can be comorbid, and if a patient with a known history of dementia has an acute worsening of baseline cognitive functioning, the likely explanation is that the patient has developed delirium because of a new medical condition. An important pitfall to avoid is the diagnosis

**TABLE 54-1.** Etiology of delirium

| Urgent causes | Additional significant causes |
|---|---|
| Cardiopulmonary | Metabolic disturbances |
| Myocardial infarction, shock, arrhythmias, hypertensive encephalopathy, pulmonary embolus, pulmonary failure, carbon monoxide poisoning | Electrolyte and acid-base imbalances, renal or hepatic failure |
| | Endocrine disorder |
| | Hypo- or hyperfunction of pancreas, thyroid, parathyroid, adrenal, or pituitary glands |
| Neurological | |
| Subarachnoid hemorrhage, subdural hematoma, traumatic brain injury | Vitamin deficiencies |
| | Vitamin $B_{12}$, folate |
| Withdrawal syndromes | Neoplasms |
| Sedative-hypnotics, alcohol | Primary tumor, metastatic paraneoplastic tumor |
| Infections | Other neurological etiologies |
| Encephalitis, meningitis, pneumonia, septicemia, urinary tract infection | Stroke, seizures |
| | Gastrointestinal/genitourinary disorders |
| Toxin exposure | Severe fecal impaction |
| Illicit drugs (cocaine, hallucinogens), pesticides, solvents, medications | Severe urinary retention |
| | Vasculitis |
| Thiamine deficiency | Pain |
| Wernicke's encephalopathy | Unrelieved pain or delirium complicated by analgesics |

of dementia in the context of an acute change in mental status when there is no known history of dementia. The diagnosis of diffuse Lewy body disease (or Lewy body dementia), which is marked by parkinsonian symptoms and visual hallucinations, deserves particular mention because one of the cardinal diagnostic criteria for this illness is a fluctuating level of consciousness in the absence of a medical reason to explain delirium. The distinction between delirium and this category of dementia is especially important, because the administration of neuroleptics used in treating delirium can worsen diffuse Lewy body disease (McKeith et al. 1996).

Symptoms of depression, such as psychomotor retardation, apathy, fatigue, and anhedonia, can resemble hypoactive delirium, but, unlike delirious patients, depressed patients have a gradual onset of symptoms, remain alert, and manifest cognitive and attentional impairments that are less severe (Johnson et al. 1994). An anxious patient can resem-

**TABLE 54–2.**  Some common medications associated with drug-induced delirium

Analgesics: opioids, nonopioids
Antiarrhythmics: amiodarone, lidocaine
Antiasthmatics: theophylline
Antibiotics and antifungals: amphotericin B, ciprofloxacin
Anticholinergics: benztropine, diphenhydramine
Anticonvulsants: phenobarbital
Antidepressants: amitriptyline, imipramine
Antihypertensives: calcium channel blockers, methyldopa, propranolol
Antiparkinsonian medications: amantadine, levodopa
Antipsychotics: chlorpromazine, thioridazine
Corticosteroids: prednisone
Digitalis
Gastrointestinal medications: cimetidine, metoclopramide
Lithium
Sedative-hypnotics: benzodiazepines

ble a patient with hyperactive delirium, as both can evidence increased autonomic arousal and psychomotor agitation. It is important to differentiate between the two conditions, because anxious patients are often treated with benzodiazepines, which can further compromise the delirious patient's clinical status (Milisen et al. 1998). Acute psychosis in the context of a manic episode or a schizophrenic decompensation can also resemble hyperactive delirium. Patients with psychosis secondary to a psychiatric illness are more likely to manifest delusions and auditory hallucinations, whereas visual hallucinations appear to be more commonly associated with the multiple medical etiologies that cause delirium (Webster and Holroyd 2000).

## Risk Stratification

Baseline and precipitating factors contribute to delirium in a cumulative fashion (Inouye and Charpentier 1996; Inouye et al. 1993) (see Table 54–3). Delirium in psychiatric inpatients has been less well studied in this same prospective fashion; however, bipolar disorder (Ritchie et al. 1996), cognitive impairment, and medications such as lithium and anticholinergic antiparkinsonian drugs have been associated with an elevated risk of delirium (Patten et al. 2001).

**TABLE 54–3.** Baseline risk factors and precipitating factors in delirium

| Risk factors | Precipitating factors |
| --- | --- |
| Cognitive impairment | Addition of more than three new medications to patient's regimen 24–48 hours before delirium onset |
| Elevated ratio of blood urea nitrogen level to creatinine level | Malnutrition |
| | Bladder catheters |
| Severe comorbid illness | Iatrogenic complications (medication side effects, infections acquired in the hospital, falls, pressure sores) |

A pertinent history should be obtained either from the patient, if this is feasible, or from a reliable family member, if the patient's accuracy is suspect. The history should assess the time course, acuity, and fluctuation of mental status symptoms. In addition, inquiries should be made about pertinent past medical and surgical history, concurrent medical problems, history of trauma, medications (including any recent changes in dosages), and possible alcohol and illicit drug ingestion. The review of symptoms should proceed with a focus on recent history of headache, fever, sensory changes, motor changes (including gait difficulty or ataxia), changes in bowel or bladder function, nausea and vomiting, and syncope/near syncope. Subsequently, vital signs should be measured, and a careful physical and neurological examination should be performed (American College of Emergency Physicians 1999). A thorough mental status examination is essential and should include evaluation of cognitive functions such as orientation, attention (tested with forward digit span or serial sevens), and memory (recall of three words after a short delay). The initial assessment should also include routine laboratory tests, an electrocardiogram, urinalysis, chest radiograph, complete blood count, urine toxicology screen, and measurement of serum drug levels (Burns et al. 2004).

## Assessment and Management in Psychiatric Settings

In treating delirium, the paramount goal must be to take the appropriate steps to correct the underlying cause or causes of the delirium (see Figure 54–1). The administration of anticholinergics, narcotics, or benzodiazepines should be avoided (Marcantonio et al. 1994). The environment should be enhanced to provide a balance between overstimulation and sensory deprivation, either of which can increase a patient's confusion. Some ways by which this balance can be achieved include having a clock, calendar, familiar token items from home, and the patient's glasses and hearing aids easily accessible at bedside; providing appropriate daytime lighting and dimmer but not absent nighttime lighting; reducing noise by rooming delirious patients separately; and minimizing medical procedures at night. Finally, to reduce the risk of serious injury to a delirious patient, physical restraints, catheters, and intravenous lines should be discontinued as soon as is clinically appropriate (American Psychiatric Association 1999; Wise et al. 2002).

For pharmacological treatment, a high-potency butyrophenone such as haloperidol or droperidol is the medication of choice for managing psychotic symptoms and agitation in patients with delirium for which the underlying etiology is not alcohol or benzodiazepine withdrawal. The benefits of haloperidol, which is considered the first-line drug for delirium, include few or no anticholinergic, cardiovascular, or sedating side effects. Droperidol, a greater-potency butyrophenone, is fast acting, more sedating, and associated with fewer extrapyramidal symptoms, but it has more potential for causing orthostasis and Q–Tc interval prolongation.

There is no consensus on the optimal dosing of neuroleptics in delirium. American Psychiatric Association (1999) practice guidelines suggest that oral haloperidol should be initiated at a dose of 1–2 mg every 4 hours in adult patients; for elderly patients, the pharmacological premise of "start low, go slow" is utilized, and an initial dosage of 0.25–0.5 mg every 4 hours is recommended. In other protocols, the initial dosages are dictated by the severity of the agitation, with 0.5–1 mg every 4 hours recommended for mild agitation and 5–10 mg for severe agitation. Similarly, for elderly patients, the range would be from 0.5 mg for mild agitation to 2 mg every 4 hours for severe cases. More severely agitated patients may require higher doses and may also require parenteral administration of the medication, in which peak serum concentrations are noted within 15–30 minutes. After the resolution of the episode of delirium, the neuroleptic should be tapered and discontinued over about 1 week, depending on the severity of the episode, in order to prevent long-term side effects from neuroleptic exposure (American Psychiatric Association 1999; Jacobson 1997; Wise et al. 2002).

Although the current pharmacological standard is to use the high-potency antipsychotics in treatment of delirium, the newer atypical antipsychotics, which are associated with fewer extrapyramidal side effects, may offer an advantage over the older class of drugs in the future

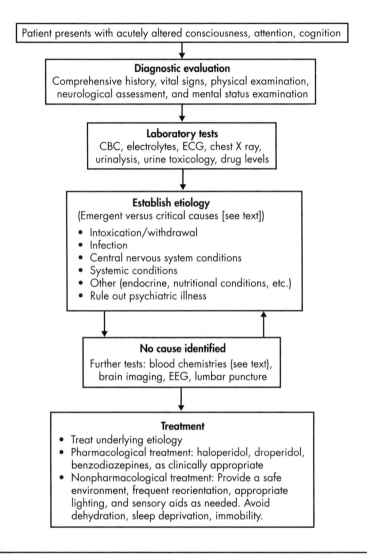

Patient presents with acutely altered consciousness, attention, cognition

**Diagnostic evaluation**
Comprehensive history, vital signs, physical examination, neurological assessment, and mental status examination

**Laboratory tests**
CBC, electrolytes, ECG, chest X ray, urinalysis, urine toxicology, drug levels

**Establish etiology**
(Emergent versus critical causes [see text])
• Intoxication/withdrawal
• Infection
• Central nervous system conditions
• Systemic conditions
• Other (endocrine, nutritional conditions, etc.)
• Rule out psychiatric illness

**No cause identified**
Further tests: blood chemistries (see text), brain imaging, EEG, lumbar puncture

**Treatment**
• Treat underlying etiology
• Pharmacological treatment: haloperidol, droperidol, benzodiazepines, as clinically appropriate
• Nonpharmacological treatment: Provide a safe environment, frequent reorientation, appropriate lighting, and sensory aids as needed. Avoid dehydration, sleep deprivation, immobility.

**FIGURE 54–1.** Algorithm for the assessment and treatment of a patient with delirium.
*Note.* CBC = complete blood count; ECG = electrocardiogram; EEG = electroencephalogram.

treatment of delirium. Thus far, case reports and retrospective studies for risperidone, olanzapine, quetiapine, and ziprasidone indicate that these agents have been effective in treating delirium (Schwartz and Masand 2002). However, more clinical experience and prospective studies, such as the study conducted by Sasaki et al. (2003), are needed before recommendations for specific dosage guidelines can be made.

When the delirium has been attributed to alcohol or benzodiazepine withdrawal, then the drug of choice is from the benzodiazepine class. Side effects of benzodiazepines include sedation, respiratory depression, ataxia, amnesia, paradoxical disinhibition, physical dependence, and withdrawal, as well as the potential for worsening delirium. The benefits of benzodiazepines include effectiveness in decreasing anxiety and agitation, fast onset of action, short half-life, and safety in patients with hepatic dysfunction. The dosing protocols for lorazepam suggest oral, intramuscular, or intravenous doses in the range of 0.5–2 mg every 4 hours. Depending on the level of the patient's sedation, the initial dose can be repeated or doubled every 30–60 minutes in order to achieve the desired effect (American Psychiatric Association 1999; Jacobson and Schreibman 1997; Wise et al. 2002).

When the basic assessment does not reveal the source of the delirium, then further evaluation as guided by the patient's history and physical examination may be warranted. Further evaluation may include blood chemistry analyses such as thyroid function tests, vitamin $B_{12}$ and folate levels, tests for presence of heavy metals, systemic lupus erythematosus screen, antinuclear antibody level, and tests for syphilis, urinary porphyrins, and human immunodeficiency virus (HIV). When the patient's history is significant for falls, trauma, or neurological symptoms, or when there are focal findings in the physical examination, then brain imaging should be performed, and a lumbar puncture may be necessary in a febrile patient in whom no other source of infection can be found (Gleason 2003; Inouye 1994). The electroencephalogram is often considered a standard diagnostic test in delirium, but it is not pathognomonic, because the pattern of generalized slowing can be observed in either delirious or demented patients.

# References

American College of Emergency Physicians: Clinical policy for the initial approach to patients presenting with altered mental status. Ann Emerg Med 33:251–280, 1999

American Psychiatric Association: Practice Guideline for the Treatment of Patients With Delirium. Am J Psychiatry 156 (suppl 5):1–20, 1999

Burns A, Gallagley A, Byrne J: Delirium. J Neurol Neurosurg Psychiatry 75:362–367, 2004

Carter GL, Dawson AM, Lopert R: Drug-induced delirium: incidence, management and prevention. Drug Safety 15:291–301, 1996

Cummings JL, Mega MS: Delirium, in Neuropsychiatry and Behavioral Neuroscience. New York, Oxford University Press, 2003, pp 165–171

Gleason OC: Delirium. Am Fam Physician 67:1027–1034, 2003

Inouye SK: The dilemma of delirium: clinical and research controversies regarding diagnosis and evaluation of delirium in hospitalized elderly medical patients. Am J Med 97:278–288, 1994

Inouye SK, Charpentier PA: Precipitating factors for delirium in hospitalized elderly persons—predictive model and interrelationship with baseline vulnerability. JAMA 275:852–857, 1996

Inouye SK, Viscoli CM, Horwitz RI, et al: A predictive model for delirium in hospitalized elderly medical patients based on admission characteristics. Ann Intern Med 119:474–481, 1993

Jacobson SA: Delirium in the elderly. Psychiatr Clin North Am 20:91–110, 1997

Jacobson S, Schreibman B: Behavioral and pharmacologic treatment of delirium. Am Fam Physician 56:2005–2012, 1997

Johnson J, Sims R, Gottlieb G: Differential diagnosis of dementia, delirium and depression: implications for drug therapy. Drugs Aging 5:431–445, 1994

Lagomasino I, Daly R, Stoudemire A: Medical assessment of patients presenting with psychiatric symptoms in the emergency setting. Psychiatr Clin North Am 22:819–850, 1999

Marcantonio ER, Juarez G, Goldman L, et al: The relationship of postoperative delirium with psychoactive medications. JAMA 272:1518–1522, 1994

McKeith IG, Galasko D, Kosaka K, et al: Consensus guidelines for the clinical and pathologic diagnosis of dementia with Lewy bodies (DLB): report of the consortium on DLB international workshop. Neurology 47:1113–1124, 1996

Milisen K, Foreman MD, Godderis J, et al: Delirium in the hospitalized elderly. Nurs Clin North Am 33:417–436, 1998

O'Keeffe ST: Clinical subtypes of delirium in the elderly. Dement Geriatr Cogn Disord 10:380–385, 1999

Patten SB, Williams JVA, Petcu R, et al: Delirium in psychiatric inpatients: a case control study. Can J Psychiatry 46:162–166, 2001

Ritchie J, Steiner W, Abrahamowicz M: Incidence of and risk factors for delirium among psychiatric inpatients. Psychiatr Serv 47:727–730, 1996

Sasaki Y, Matsuyama T, Inoue S, et al: A prospective, open-label, flexible dose study of quetiapine in the treatment of delirium. J Clin Psychiatry 64:1316–1321, 2003

Schwartz TL, Masand PS: The role of atypical antipsychotics in the treatment of delirium. Psychosomatics 43:171–174, 2002

Simon L, Jewell N, Brokel J: Management of acute delirium in hospitalized elderly: a process improvement project. Geriatr Nurs 18:150–154, 1997

Webster R, Holroyd S: Prevalence of psychotic symptoms in delirium. Psychosomatics 41:519–522, 2000

Wise MG, Hilty DM, Cerda GM, et al: Delirium (confusional states), in the American Psychiatric Publishing Textbook of Consultation-Liaison Psychiatry: Psychiatry in the Medically Ill, 2nd Edition. Edited by Wise MG, Rundell JR. Washington, DC, American Psychiatric Publishing, 2002, pp 257–272

# PART XIV

# The Approach to the Patient With Multiple Medical Problems

Section Editors:

Rosanne M. Leipzig, M.D.

Peter Manu, M.D.

# CHAPTER 55

# Risk Assessment Prior to Electroconvulsive Therapy

Anne Frederickson, M.D.

Peter Manu, M.D.

## Clinical Presentation

Electroconvulsive therapy (ECT) is commonly used as a treatment for depression and other psychiatric illnesses. It has been shown to be as effective as or even more effective than antidepressants (Avery and Winokur 1976; Pagnin et al. 2004). However, ECT is not without risk, particularly in elderly and medically ill patients. Elderly patients are disproportionately represented among ECT patients. Thirty-three percent of patients receiving ECT are older than age 65 years, but this same age group represents only 8% of hospitalized patients (Thompson et al. 1994). Nonetheless, the major morbidity and mortality rates for ECT remain low, at 35 cardiac arrests and two deaths/100,000 treatments (Kramer 1985).

Multiple physiological changes occur during ECT (Table 55–1). The major physiological effects of ECT stem from the stimulation of both the sympathetic and parasympathetic divisions of the autonomic nervous system. During the initial stimulus of ECT, there is a concurrent stimulation of the vagus nerve. The result is a slowing of the heart rate, even in some cases to the point of several seconds of asystole (Drop and Welch 1989). During the subsequent seizure, there is an increase in sympathetic tone throughout the body, leading to increased heart rate and blood pressure. It appears that this increase in sympathetic activation is caused by neuronal stimulation as well as an increased release and circulation of catecholamines (Drop and Welch 1989; Welch and Drop

**TABLE 55-1.**    Effects and complications of electroconvulsive therapy

| Physiological effect | Mechanism | Complication |
|---|---|---|
| *Autonomic activation* | | |
| Parasympathetic effect: decreased heart rate | Direct stimulation of the vagus nerve by electric stimulus | Bradyarrhythmias and asystole |
| Sympathetic effect: increased heart rate and blood pressure | Direct neuronal stimulation and increased release of catecholamines | Myocardial ischemia, hypertensive crisis, arrhythmias |
| *Neurological* | | |
| Increased intracranial pressure | Increased cranial blood flow due to increased metabolic rate of neurons | Possibility of intracranial hemorrhage or herniation in patients at risk (patients with cerebral aneurysm or tumor) |
| *Pulmonary* | | |
| Decreased respiration | Paralysis of respiratory muscles during anesthesia | Apnea, bronchospasm |

1989). In addition, intracranial blood flow increases during ECT. During a seizure, blood flow to the brain increases 300% because of the increased metabolic rate of the neurons, and there is a 200% increase in glucose metabolism and oxygen consumption. This increase in blood flow leads to an increase in intracranial pressure (Nobler and Sackeim 1998). ECT also affects the pulmonary system, because patients undergo anesthesia and muscle paralysis during the procedure, and their effects decrease respiratory drive.

## Differential Diagnosis

### Cardiac Complications

Cardiac complications, the most common type of ECT complication, are most likely caused by the increased autonomic activation resulting from ECT. *Parasympathetic stimulation* can lead to bradyarrhythmias and even prolonged asystole. The increased sympathetic tone is the cause of

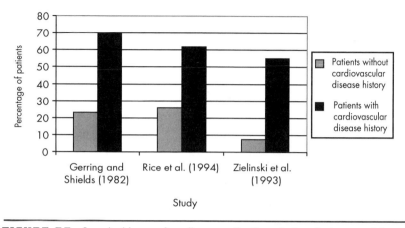

**FIGURE 55–1.** Incidence of cardiac complications during electroconvulsive therapy in patients with and without cardiovascular risk factors in three studies.

many of the other cardiac complications of ECT. In particular, the rise in heart rate can pose potential difficulties for patients in whom there is already a tenuous balance between energy needs and blood supply to the myocardium. A disruption in this balance, such as a sudden rise in heart rate, can lead to myocardial ischemia. In addition, the sudden rise in blood pressure can cause serious consequences for patients at risk, such as those with aortic or intracranial aneurysms. Lastly, the increase in sympathetic tone places the patient at risk for several arrhythmias.

The risk for developing a cardiac complication during ECT is between 7.5% and 26%, but the risk for those with a known cardiac history jumps to 55%–70% (Figure 55–1). The only prospective study to examine this phenomenon was conducted by Zielinski et al. (1993). This group of researchers found that although the rate of cardiac complications was 7.5% in the general population receiving ECT, the rate of complications among those with cardiac disease was 55%. The nature of the cardiac illness was positively correlated with the type of cardiac complication. Patients with coronary artery disease developed acute coronary syndrome, and those with a history of arrhythmias were at substantially higher risk of ventricular ectopic rhythms.

## Neurological Complications

Neurological complications of ECT have not been carefully studied. The main neurological risk for patients stems from the acute increase in intracranial pressure secondary to increased blood flow. In patients who already have an increase in intracranial pressure, either because of hydrocephalus or an intracranial mass, there is the potential risk for herniation and neuronal damage. Isolated case reports of neurological complications from ECT in patients with intracranial tumors have been published (Rasmussen et al. 2002). However, there are also case reports showing the successful treatment of such patients (American Psychiatric Association 2001; Zwil et al. 1990). In addition, there is the risk for prolonged seizure during ECT in patients who are taking medication that lowers the seizure threshold and in patients with electrolyte imbalances (American Psychiatric Association 2001). The acute rise in blood pressure during ECT can also pose a risk for patients with aneurysms. As with patients with tumors, the evidence for or against the use of ECT in these patients is mostly anecdotal (Devanand et al. 1990; Farah et al. 1996).

## Pulmonary Complications

The effects of ECT on the respiratory system appear to be related to anesthesia. The patients most at risk for the development of apnea during ECT appear to be those with impaired metabolism of succinylcholine, an agent often used to induce muscle relaxation (American Psychiatric Association 2001). Bronchospasm may occur in patients already at risk for respiratory compromise, such as those with chronic obstructive pulmonary disease or asthma (Rasmussen et al. 2002).

## Falls

Falls are a fairly common complication that does not have a clear etiology but occurs more often in patients receiving ECT than in the general population. Older patients who receive ECT have a 25.1% rate of falls, compared with 13.1% in older patients who have not received ECT (de Carle and Kohn 2000). The best predictors of a fall were the number of ECT treatments and presence of Parkinson's disease.

## Risk Stratification

Because of the large number of people who undergo ECT every year, in particular the large number of elderly patients, it is necessary to develop a way to assess the risk that these patients incur by undergoing ECT. However, as of yet, there are no risk assessment indices specifically for evaluation of ECT patients. Given that the most common and serious complications appear to be cardiac in nature, it seems reasonable to ex-

**TABLE 55-2.** Risk factors for cardiac complications

Coronary heart disease
Congestive heart failure
Cerebrovascular disease
Insulin-dependent diabetes
Preoperative creatinine level >2.0 mg/dL

*Source.* Modified from Lee et al. 1999.

amine some indices for assessing cardiac risks in other procedures. One such index (Revised Cardiac Index) was based on the examination of patients who had undergone noncardiac surgery (Lee et al. 1999). Lee et al. determined that there are six risk factors for cardiac complication (Table 55–2). The rate of complication was determined on the basis of the number of risk factors present in each patient. Patients with no risk factors or one risk factor were found to have an average rate of complication of approximately 1% (designated as low risk), whereas patients with three or more risk factors had a complication rate of 9% (designated as high risk).

The American Psychiatric Association (APA) (2001) recommends caution in administering ECT to patients with several disease states in addition to the risk factors mentioned in the Revised Cardiac Index (Rasmussen et al. 2002). They include aneurysms (of any kind), increased intracranial pressure, and pulmonary disease states. The current APA guidelines also take into account the patient's American Society of Anesthesiologists (ASA) physical status classification score and recommend caution in administering ECT to patients with scores indicating an unstable or critically ill condition (4 or 5). Lastly, the APA also takes into account any history of serious valvular disease.

## Assessment and Management in Psychiatric Settings

The first priority is to identify patients for whom ECT is contraindicated, after which the psychiatrist must use the Revised Cardiac Index to categorize the remaining patients into high-, moderate-, and low-risk groups (see Figure 55–2). The rate of complication can then be weighed against the potential benefits of ECT and the risk to the patient of not undergoing ECT. It should be noted that patients who would be excluded from ECT at an early point in the treatment algorithm because of a serious condition could be reconsidered for ECT once medical treatment has been optimized and the condition stabilized.

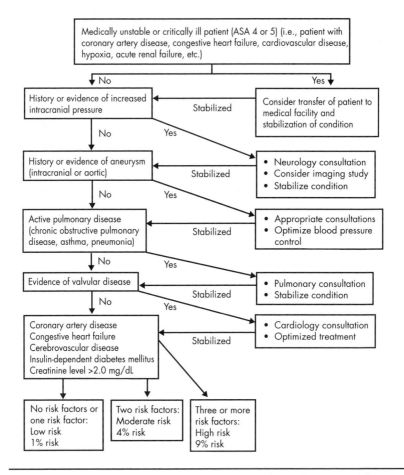

**FIGURE 55−2.** Algorithm for risk assessment prior to electroconvulsive therapy.

*Note.* ASA =American Society of Anesthesiologists physical status classification.

ªAll conditions considered in the Revised Cardiac Index should be stable at the time the assessment is made.

Besides assessing a patient's risk, the clinician can use other strategies before ECT to limit the potential for complications. Many medications should be continued during ECT (Table 55–3) in order to limit the effects of present disease states on the outcome of ECT. The patient's cardiac medications should be continued, especially considering that the risk of cardiac complications is greater in those with a history of cardiac problems. Medications for pulmonary disorders should also be contin-

| **TABLE 55–3.** | Medications continued during electroconvulsive therapy |
|---|---|

Antiangina medication
Antiarrhythmics
Bronchodilators
Hypertension medication
Steroids

ued to optimize the patient's pulmonary condition. Many patients with a history of asthma or chronic obstructive pulmonary disease can tolerate the effects of anesthesia and ECT if they are given their bronchodilators prior to ECT. Medications for treatment of reflux will help patients tolerate the effects of anesthesia. Lastly, as with any patient scheduled for a procedure, corticosteroids should be continued. In patients whose hypothalamic-pituitary-adrenal axis has been suppressed through the chronic use of corticosteroids, it is important to ensure continued administration of the exogenous corticosteroid. An internist should be consulted to help establish the appropriate "stress" dose of corticosteroid before ECT.

Just as there are medications that must be continued during ECT, there are medications that should be discontinued to prevent complications (American Psychiatric Association 2001). As noted in Table 55–3, antiarrhythmics should be continued during ECT with the exception of lidocaine, which has the potential to increase the seizure threshold and may make it more difficult to induce a seizure during ECT. The bronchodilator theophylline should be discontinued as it can decrease the seizure threshold, placing the patient at risk for prolonged seizures during ECT. Many psychiatric medications can increase or decrease the seizure threshold, and their continued use should be carefully examined prior to ECT. In addition, the continuation of any hypoglycemic medications should be carefully examined before initiating ECT, as patients must fast prior to ECT.

# References

American Psychiatric Association: The Practice of Electroconvulsive Therapy: Recommendations for Treatment, Training, and Privileging, 2nd Edition. Washington, DC, American Psychiatric Association, 2001

Avery D, Winokur G: Mortality in depressed patients treated with electroconvulsive therapy and antidepressants. Arch Gen Psychiatry 33:1029–1037, 1976 de Carle AJ, Kohn R: Electroconvulsive therapy and falls in the elderly. J ECT 16:252–257, 2000

Devanand D, Malitz S, Sackeim H: ECT in a patient with aortic aneurysm. J Clin Psychiatry 51:255–256, 1990

Drop LJ, Welch CA: Anesthesia for electroconvulsive therapy in patients with major cardiovascular risk factors. Convulsive Ther 5:88–101, 1989

Farah A, McCall W, Amundson R: ECT after cerebral aneurysm repair. Convulsive Ther 12:165–170, 1996

Gerring JP, Shields HM: The identification and management of patients with a high risk for cardiac arrhythmias during modified ECT. J Clin Psychiatry 43:140–143, 1982

Kramer BA: Use of ECT in California, 1977–1983. Am J Psychiatry 142:1190–1192, 1985

Lee TH, Marcantonio ER, Mangione CM, et al: Derivation and prospective validation of a simple index for prediction of cardiac risk of major noncardiac surgery. Circulation 100:1043–1049, 1999

Nobler MS, Sackeim HA: Mechanisms of actions of electroconvulsive therapy: functional brain imaging studies. Psychiatr Ann 28:23–29, 1998

Pagnin D, de Queiroz V, Pini S, et al: Efficacy of ECT in depression: a metanalytic review. J ECT 20: 13–20, 2004

Rasmussen KG, Rummans TA, Richardson JW: Electroconvulsive therapy in the medically ill. Psychiatr Clin North Am 25:177–193, 2002

Rice EH, Sombrotto LB, Markowitz JC, et al: Cardiovascular morbidity in high-risk patients during ECT. Am J Psychiatry 151:1637–1641, 1994

Thompson JW, Weiner RD, Myers CP: Use of ECT in the United States in 1975, 1980, 1986. Am J Psychiatry 151:1657–1661, 1994

Welch CA, Drop LJ: Cardiovascular effects of ECT. Convulsive Ther 5:35–43, 1989

Zielinski RJ, Roose SP, Devanand DP, et al: Cardiovascular complications of ECT in depressed patients with cardiac disease. Am J Psychiatry 150: 904–909, 1993

Zwil AS, Bowring MA, Price TR, et al: Prospective electroconvulsive therapy in the presence of intracranial tumor. Convulsive Ther 6:299–307, 1990

# CHAPTER 56

# The Patient With Multiple Medical Problems

Cinthya Marturano, M.D.

Rosanne M. Leipzig, M.D., Ph.D.

## Clinical Presentation

Patients with multiple medical problems are a vulnerable population, with decreased reserve and an increased risk of developing adverse outcomes. Most of these patients are either older than age 65 years or have a chronic mental illness. Patients with severe and persistent mental illness have higher rates of physical morbidity (Honig et al. 1989) and mortality (Tsuang and Woolson 1977) and are more likely to die from cardiovascular, respiratory, metabolic, cerebrovascular, and HIV-related diseases than the general population (Corten et al. 1991). Socioeconomic disadvantage (Aro et al. 1995), difficulties in obtaining and maintaining health insurance (Druss and Rosenheck 1998), and symptoms such as cognitive limitations and lack of motivation may limit these individuals' ability to obtain medical care (Druss and Rosenheck 2000; Hall et al. 1982) and increase their likelihood of adverse health outcomes because of poor adherence to treatment, development of complications, poor function, and increased disability (Kane 1985; Keith and Kane 2003).

Chronic conditions, defined as illnesses that last longer than 3 months and are not self-limited, are the major cause of disability and death in the industrialized world (Gill 2002b). The burden of disease and disability is greater for elderly people than for those younger than age 65 years. About 26% of patients over age 65 years have impairments in activities of daily living (ADLs) (bathing, dressing, eating, etc.) or instrumental activities of daily living (IADLs) (shopping, meal preparation, management of money, etc.) (Lawton and Brody 1969).

| **TABLE 56-1.** Basic principles of care for patients with multiple medical problems |
| --- |
| Functional ability and quality of life are critical outcomes. |
| Social circumstances, available social support, and environmental characteristics must be known and considered in care planning. |
| Multi- or interdisciplinary care is the rule rather than the exception. |
| Transitions in care must be carefully planned and monitored to avoid errors and poor patient outcomes. |
| Patient preferences and goals of care must be clarified and periodically revisited. |
| Symptoms and disorders are often multifactorial; small adjustments in several of these factors can result in improved function. |
| Adverse drug events are more common and may resemble age-associated syndromes. |

Geriatricians and psychiatrists share an approach to these patients that is interdisciplinary and focuses on several domains that are not commonly considered in acute medical care (Table 56–1). Geriatric patients and patients with chronic conditions often require care across multiple sites (acute care settings, rehabilitation units, long-term care facilities) (Gill 2002a). Transitions between care settings must be coordinated in order to avoid unnecessary duplication, medical error, and harm to the patient (Boockvar et al. 2004). Goals of care may be multiple, diverse, and conflicting and may require periodic revisiting (Gill 2002a). These different goals reflect the heterogeneity found among chronically ill persons with respect to physiological function, health status, cultural background, values, and personal preferences (Bradley et al. 1999).

The multifactorial nature of many geriatric syndromes, such as urinary incontinence, delirium, and falls, has been demonstrated by studies that identified multiple risk factors for these syndromes; randomized, controlled intervention trials showed that these syndromes could be prevented by amelioration of these factors and that the more risk factors were ameliorated, the lower the likelihood that patients would develop the outcome (Inouye et al. 1999; Tinetti et al. 1994).

## Differential Diagnosis

Care for chronically ill and elderly patients is focused on function. This focus represents a paradigm shift from disease-oriented to function-oriented outcomes and requires knowledge of social, cognitive, and mobility factors that are seldom considered within the scope of traditional medical practice (Fleming et al. 1995).

Problems that are common in geriatric patients, such as hearing and vision loss, lower extremity weakness, malnutrition, cognitive impairment, and affective disorders, are predictors of functional decline (Gill et al. 1995). Functional decline may also be the initial symptom, and in some instances the only symptom, of medical illness in older persons (Pinholt et al. 1987). Evidence that healthcare providers often fail to recognize significant functional impairment and fail to recognize risk factors for functional decline (Bogardus et al. 2002; Calkins et al. 1991) highlights the need for routine assessment of functional status in patients with multiple chronic diseases.

Functional assessment includes various domains, such as evaluation of daily activities, cognition, continence, nutritional status, depression, mobility (gait and balance), assessment of special senses (hearing and vision), and specific social issues (Gill 2002a; Moore and Siu 1996). The degree to which aging or disease may result in disability varies substantially among individuals. However, a systematic approach to screening for impairments in each domain assures that interventions are individualized.

## Functional Assessments

Certain domains of functional assessment, such as evaluation of cognitive function and depression, require the expertise of the psychiatrist. These areas will not be discussed here, except to emphasize that older adults and persons with multiple medical disorders may have significant cognitive impairment that is not evident without formal assessment.

Table 56–2 outlines simple screening tests that can be used to evaluate domains that are important in the function and care of patients with multiple medical problems. The tests reflect ADLs (Katz et at. 1963), including basic self-care functions, and higher-level activities or IADLs (Lawton and Brody 1969). The self-care tasks or basic ADLs are considered essential to independent living. Bathing is typically the basic ADL with the highest prevalence of disability. IADLs include abilities needed to manage one's own living environment. ADLs include the following tasks:

- Personal self-care: feeding oneself, bathing, toileting, dressing.
- Mobility: transferring (able to move from bed to chair or to standing position), ambulating (able to walk with or without an assistive devices), or using a wheelchair
- Continence: continent of urine and continent of feces

**TABLE 56-2.** A practical approach to functional assessment of medically complex patients for mental health providers

| Domain | Recommended screens | Further assessment for positive screen |
|---|---|---|
| Functional status | Do you need assistance with shopping or finances? (IADL) If yes, ask: Do you need assistance with bathing or taking a shower? (ADL) | IADL Scale Basic ADL Scale |
| Driving | Do you still drive? If yes, ask: While driving, have you had an accident in the past 6 months? Any driving concerns expressed by family member? | Vision testing Consider occupational therapy evaluation |
| Vision | Do you have trouble seeing, reading, or watching television (with glasses, if appropriate)? | Vision testing Consider referral to optometrist or ophthalmologist |
| Hearing | Do you have difficulty hearing conversation in a quiet room? Whisper a short sentence 6–12 inches away from the patient (with lips not seen by the patient). | Check cerumen, and remov cerumen if it is impacted. Consider referral to an audiologist |
| Risk of falls | Have you fallen in the past year? Are you afraid of falling? Do you have trouble climbing stairs or rising from chairs? | Administer the Get Up and Go test (see text) Consider full fall assessment Consider physical therapy evaluation Consider home safety assessment |

**TABLE 56–2.** A practical approach to functional assessment of medically complex patients for mental health providers *(continued)*

| Domain | Recommended screens | Further assessment for positive screen |
|---|---|---|
| Continence[a] | Ask: "In the last year, have you ever lost your urine and gotten wet? If yes, then ask: "Have you lost urine on at least 6 separate days?" | Review DIAPPERS (see text, p. 532) Consider urology or gynecology consultation. |
| Weight loss | Weight <100 lb, or unintentional weight loss >10 lb over 6 months | Consider nutritional assessment. Conduct a psychotropic medication assessment. |
| Sleep | Do you often feel sleepy during the day? | Conduct a psychotropic medication assessment. Consider sleep assessment. |
| Pain | Are you experiencing pain or discomfort? | Conduct a pain assessment. |
| Social support | Do you have a caregiver? Are you a caregiver? | Consider social work referral. |
| Elder neglect/abuse | Has anyone ever threatened or hurt you? | Consider referral to adult protective services agency. |
| Advance directives | Do you have a healthcare proxy? Do you have a living will? | Help patient gain access to and complete the proxy forms. Discuss the patient's wishes |

*Note.* ADL=activity of daily living; IADL=instrumental activity of daily living.
[a]Reviewed in Moore and Siu 1996.
*Source.* Modified from Emory University Reynolds Program: Comprehensive Geriatric Assessment.

Functional impairments are identified by self-report and observation. To assess disability, healthcare providers should ask whether patients require the help of another person to complete the task. An informant, ideally a caregiver or family member who lives with the patient, is often required to provide or to verify pertinent historical information about the patient's day-to-day function. If the patient is cognitively impaired, the responses should always be confirmed by a caregiver. Additional information can be obtained at the time of an examination by simply observing the patient's ability to enter the room, sit and stand, undress, etc. This direct observation of physical performance provides an accurate estimate of function and may disclose particular deficits (Applegate et al. 1987). If impairment of ADLs or IADLs is identified, ascertaining the reason for and the timing of loss of function can help determine the underlying cause and the potential for reversibility. Acute and subacute impairments are often symptoms of illnesses (Gill 2002a), and treatment will help to restore function. Chronic disabilities are more challenging, but awareness of these deficits can help in management decisions.

Poor nutrition in older adults may be an indicator of functional decline (inability to cook or shop, inability to feed oneself), financial hardship, social isolation, polypharmacy, dental problems, depression, alcoholism, dementia, or medical illness. Undernutrition is clearly linked to increased morbidity, including prolonged hospital stays, more readmissions, and an increased mortality rate (Sullivan 1995).

Determining undernutrition in psychiatric and elderly patients is difficult (Lipschitz et al. 1992; Reuben et al. 1995). Skeletal height decreases with aging, as does the proportion of lean body mass, whereas the proportion of adipose tissue increases. Therefore, the standard height and weight tables and body mass index (weight in kilograms/ height in square centimeters) are of unproven utility in the evaluation of undernutrition in these populations. No laboratory tests have been validated as effective screening tools for detection of malnutrition in elderly persons. An unintentional weight loss of more than 5 lb in 1 month or 10 lb in 6 months suggests poor nutrition and should prompt further evaluation (Moore and Siu 1996).

The ability of older persons to perform ADLs depends on their capacity to maneuver safely and effectively. Approximately 30% of community-dwelling older adults have a fall each year. Early detection of impairments in mobility can identify those persons at risk for falls and/ or injury. Standard neuromuscular evaluation is insufficient for evaluating mobility. The physical evaluation should focus primarily on the ability to transfer (from a seated to standing position, from a bed to a chair) and to walk and on gait and balance abnormalities (Gill 2002a).

The timed Get Up and Go test (Tinetti et al. 1993), which includes the following steps, can be used to evaluate mobility:

- Seat the patient in a hard-backed chair.
- Have the patient stand while keeping his or her arms folded on the chest. Inability to stand without using the arms suggests lower-extremity, or quadriceps, weakness and is highly predictive of future disability.
- Once the patient is standing, have the patient walk 10 feet (3 meters) with the usual walking aid if one is used, turn around, return to the chair, and sit down. Abnormalities in gait include path deviation, diminished step height or length or both, trips, slips, near falls, and any difficulty with turning.
- Time how long it takes for the patient to complete the Get Up and Go test. Persons who take longer than 15 seconds to complete this sequence of maneuvers have been shown to be at increased risk for falls.

Aging is associated with diminished visual acuity because of physiological changes in the lens, cornea, and pupil, as well as disease-related deficits such as cataracts, glaucoma, and macular degeneration. Patients may be unaware of their visual deficits, particularly of losses in peripheral and central acuity. More than 90% of older adults need eyeglasses. Visual impairment has a major impact on older persons' ability to drive, read, shop, and even walk safely. The combination of visual impairment and hearing impairment is associated with increased risk of falling.

Hearing loss is the third most common chronic disorder among elderly persons. More than 33% of those over age 65 years and 50% of those over age 85 years have some hearing loss (Gill 2002a). Hearing loss is correlated with social and emotional isolation and clinical depression (Maggi et al. 1998). In the geriatric population, presbycusis, or high-frequency hearing loss, is most common. This condition particularly affects the ability to understand women's speech. Initially, persons with presbycusis note that they can hear but not understand speech. Evaluation of hearing loss in elderly patients is important because they may not complain of or even recognize that they have hearing impairment. Hearing loss should be assessed routinely during the history-taking session. Otoscopic examination for cerumen is very important and should be done before any testing for hearing loss.

Urinary incontinence is loss of bladder control that results in leakage of urine. The frequency of urinary incontinence is at least 15% in ambulatory individuals age 65 years and older (Roberts et al. 1998). Of those with incontinence, 25%–35% have daily or weekly episodes. Because of embarrassment and worry about appearance and odor, or perhaps because of the perception that the condition is untreatable or is a normal accompaniment of aging, patients may not report incontinence unless directly asked by the physician.

Many causes of urinary incontinence are transient and reversible. These can be recalled by using the DIAPPERS mnemonic: **D**elirium, **I**nfection, **A**trophic vaginitis, **P**harmaceuticals, **P**sychological, **E**ndocrine, **R**estricted mobility, **S**tool impaction.

Appropriate medication use always requires balancing the benefits of a treatment with its risks and burdens, which are often different in patients with multiple medical problems than in those with a single disorder. To maximize the benefits and minimize risks, healthcare providers need to consider each patient's potential for an altered dose response, an adverse drug reaction, drug-disease interaction, and difficulty adhering to the treatment regimen (Leipzig 1998, 2001).

## Pharmacological Assessment

Patients with multiple medical problems are often more sensitive to medications and have unexpected responses to commonly used doses. This sensitivity may be due to changes in the dose-response relationship, which is made up of the relationship of dose to blood level (pharmacokinetics) followed by the relationship of the blood level to the response (pharmacodynamics).

Age-related changes usually cause elderly patients to have an increased response to a given dose for either pharmacokinetic or pharmacodynamic reasons. Pharmacokinetically, the drug's half-life may be prolonged, increasing the time it takes to reach steady-state drug concentration, or its clearance may be decreased, resulting in a higher steady-state drug concentration. Not only does the drug take longer to reach a steady state, it also takes longer to be completely eliminated after it is stopped. Decreasing the daily dosage can counteract a decrease in drug clearance.

The following key points should be considered when prescribing medications to elderly or chronically ill patients:

1. The dose of renally excreted drugs should be adjusted by using a formula to estimate the glomerular filtration rate (GFR). In older adults, the serum creatinine level does *not* reflect the GFR. Decreased lean body mass leads to decreased creatinine production; thus, the serum creatinine level may appear normal even when significant renal im-

**TABLE 56–3.** Drugs requiring dosage reduction in elderly patients with diminished renal function[a]

| Antimicrobial drugs | Cardiovascular drugs | Other drugs |
| --- | --- | --- |
| Acyclovir | Angiotensin-converting enzyme inhibitors | Acetaminophen[b] |
| Amantadine[c] | | Albuterol |
| Aminoglycosides[c] | Atenolol, sotalol, nadolol | Glyburide |
| Amphotericin | Digoxin | Histamine type 2 blockers (except cimetidine)[c] |
| Cephalosporins (cefazolin, cefepime, cefonicid, cephalexin)[c] | Methyldopa | Insulin |
| | Procainamide[d] | Lithium |
| Imipenem | | Meperidine[d] |
| Quinolones | | Gabapentin |
| Penicillins[c] | | |
| Sulbactam | | |
| Sulfonamides | | |
| Vancomycin | | |

[a]All drugs listed need to be adjusted in patients with a glomerular filtration rate (GFR) ≤50 mL/minute.
[b]Associated with risk of increased nephrotoxicity in patients with severely impaired kidneys.
[c]Adjustment needed in patients with a GFR of 51–70 mL/minute.
[d]Drug is hepatically metabolized to active metabolites that are renally excreted.
*Source.* Adapted from Leipzig 1998.

pairment exists. The GFR is decreased in two-thirds of older adults (Lindeman 1990, 1992) and correlates with the excretion of drugs primarily eliminated by the kidney and so can be used to estimate initial dosing regimens. Several commonly prescribed drugs require dosage adjustments when a patient's GFR is reduced (see Table 56–3).

Most drugs are fully absorbed; however, they may be absorbed more slowly in elderly or chronically ill patients, resulting in a lower peak level and delayed onset of action. These consequences of slower absorption may be important with some hypnotics, anxiolytics, and analgesics.

2. With age, total body water and lean body mass decrease, while body fat increases. These changes may affect the dose. For example, water-soluble drugs such as lithium should be given in lower loading doses, as should drugs that bind to skeletal muscle (e.g., digoxin). Fat-soluble drugs might in theory require a greater initial dose in elderly patients. However, in reality, many of these drugs, such as di-

azepam and fentanyl, are actually given in lower doses because they cross the blood-brain barrier and, for pharmacodynamic reasons, can result in adverse drug reaction.

3. When measuring therapeutic drug levels, a correction should always be made for albumin levels with acidic drugs such as diphenylhydantoin and for $\alpha 1$-acid glycoprotein levels with basic drugs such as tricyclic antidepressants. The albumin level does not decrease with normal aging but can decrease rapidly in acute illness or poor nutrition, resulting in toxicity at "normal" levels of bound drug. $\alpha 1$-acid glycoproteins are acute phase reactants, and their level increases with acute disease, resulting in lack of medication effectiveness at "normal" levels of bound drug. It is noteworthy that, because of pharmacodynamic considerations, toxicity may occur in older adults at drug plasma levels within the therapeutic range (Leipzig 1998; Turnheim 1998).

4. Probably the most important key to prescribing hepatically metabolized drugs is whether there are drug-drug interactions resulting in inhibition or induction of the cytochrome P450 (CYP450) isozyme that is mainly responsible for the drug's metabolism. Age tends to decrease phase I reactions because of age-related reductions in liver mass and hepatic flow (Woodhouse and Wynne 1992). This change results in decreased clearance of drugs oxidized by CYP450 isozymes to about one-half to two-thirds of the usual rate, and so it is suggested that these medications be started at one-half to two-thirds of the usual dose given to younger or healthier adults. There is no age-associated change in Phase II reactions (i.e., conjugation, acetylation, and glucuronidation); however, older or chronically ill adults may demonstrate increased sensitivity to these drugs because of pharmacodynamic effects.

5. Regardless of pharmacokinetic changes, pharmacodynamic changes caused by changes in receptor numbers, affinity, postreceptor cellular effects, or inability to maintain homeostasis can affect the patient's sensitivity to a drug (Turnheim 2003). For example, diazepam produces more sedation and memory impairment in older adults than in younger adults at the same plasma concentrations.

Adverse drug reactions are noxious or unwanted responses that occur with a dose that usually would be therapeutic. Although age alone is not generally an independent risk factor for adverse drug reactions (Routledge et al. 2004), older adults are at higher risk because of pharmacokinetic and pharmacodynamic changes such as those described

**TABLE 56–4.**   Risk factors for adverse drug reaction in elderly patients

Changes in pharmacokinetics and pharmacodynamics related to aging
Polypharmacy (use of more than five drugs increases the risk 50%)
Prescriptions of drugs with low therapeutic index
History of previous adverse drug reaction
Problems with treatment adherence

*Source.*   Adapted from Nolan and O'Malley 1998a.

earlier, the use of drugs with low therapeutic indices, the presence of multiple medical conditions, and the use of multiple drugs (Table 56–4) (Bowman et al. 1996; Nolan and O'Malley 1988b). It has been shown in some studies that 30% of hospital admissions of elderly patients may be linked to drug-related problems or drug toxic effects (Hanlon et al. 1997). Approximately 35% of ambulatory older adults experience an adverse drug reaction, and 29% require healthcare services for the adverse drug reaction (Hanlon et al. 1997).

Toxic effects of medications and drug-related problems can have profound medical and safety consequences. Adverse drug reactions in elderly patients may remain unrecognized because these reactions mimic symptoms and disorders that are known to have an increased prevalence in elderly persons (e.g., delirium, memory loss, dizziness, constipation, urinary incontinence, and falls).

Whenever a new symptom occurs in an elderly patient or a patient with multiple medical problems, the possibility that it may be an adverse drug reaction or a drug-drug or drug-disease interaction must be considered. Both prescribed and over-the-counter medications should be suspected. Herbal preparations and supplements should also be considered. Failure to recognize an adverse drug reaction because of a low index of suspicion can result in misdiagnosis and the prescription of additional medications, further increasing chances for an adverse drug reaction (Leipzig 1998).

Drugs can interact with disease, food, and other drugs. A notable portion of adverse drug reactions result from drug-drug interactions that cause an unanticipated rise in the level of one of the drugs (Montamat et al. 1989) .The likelihood of drug-drug interactions increases as the number of medications the patient takes increases. Cardiovascular and psychotropic drugs are the drugs most commonly involved in drug-drug interactions. Many drug interactions involve induction or inhibition of the CYP450 isozymes. Although each inducing or inhibiting drug does

**TABLE 56–5.**    Inducers and inhibitors of cytochrome P450 isozymes

| Inducers | Inhibitors |
|---|---|
| Barbiturates | Amiodarone |
| Broccoli | Antifungals: fluconazole, itraconazole, |
| Brussels sprouts | ketaconazole |
| Carbamazepine, oxcarbazepine | Bupropion |
| Charcoal-broiled meats | Calcium channel blockers: diltiazem, |
| Chronic alcohol intake | verapamil |
| Cigarette smoking | Chloroquine |
| Glucocorticoids | Cimetidine |
| Insulin | Cocaine |
| Nafcillin | Disulfiram |
| Phenytoin | Divalproex |
| Primidone | Escitalopram |
| Rifampin | Fluvastatin, lovastatin |
| St. John's wort | Grapefruit juice |
| | HIV protease inhibitors: ritonavir |
| | Isoniazid |
| | Methadone |
| | Metoclopramide |
| | Modafinil |
| | Nefazodone |
| | Omeprazole, lansoprazole |
| | Perphenazine, thioridazine, |
| | haloperidol, chlorpromazine |
| | Propoxyphene |
| | Quinolones: levofloxacin, ciprofloxacin, |
| | norfloxacin, ofloxacin |
| | Selective serotonin reuptake inhibitors |
| | (fluoxetine, paroxetine, sertraline, |
| | fluvoxamine, citalopram) |
| | Topiramate |
| | Tricyclic antidepressants (amitriptyline, |
| | clomipramine, desipramine) |
| | Trimethoprim-sufamethoxazole |
| | Venlafaxine |

*Source.*    Adapted from Leipzig 1998 and Sandson 2004.

**TABLE 56–6.** Examples of drug-disease interactions in older adults

| Disease | Drugs | Effect | Mechanism |
|---|---|---|---|
| Heart failure | Drugs with high sodium content (sodium and sodium salts, bicarbonate, biphosphate), nonsteroidal anti-inflammatory drugs | Potential to promote fluid retention and exacerbate heart failure | Sodium retention |
| Hypertension | Pseudoephedrine, amphetamines | Elevation of blood pressure | Sympathomimetic activity |
| Seizures or epilepsy | Clozapine, chlorpromazine, thioridazine, thiothixene | Increased seizure activity | Lowering of seizure thresholds |
| Stress incontinence | $\alpha_1$-Blockers, long-acting benzodiazepines | May produce exacerbation and polyuria | Blocking of contraction of urethral sphincter smooth muscle |
| Benign prostatic hypertrophy | $\alpha_1$-Agonists, anticholinergics, calcium channel blockers | Urinary retention | Contracting of the prostatic and uretheral smooth muscle, impairment of bladder contractility |
| Constipation | Calcium channel blockers, anticholinergics, opiates | Precipitation or exacerbation, including impaction | Decrease of intestinal motility and tone, often receptor mediated |
| Alzheimer's disease | Anticholinergics | Confusion | Increase in sensibility |

**TABLE 56–6.** Examples of drug-disease interactions in older adults *(continued)*

| Disease | Drugs | Effect | Mechanism |
|---|---|---|---|
| Parkinson's disease | Metoclopramide, conventional antipsychotics | Exacerbation of symptoms | Anticholinergic, antidopaminergic effects |
| Depression | Long-term benzodiazepine use, sympatholytic agents (methyldopa, reserpine, guanethidine) | May produce exacerbation | Sympatholytic effect |

*Source.* Modified from Fick et al. 2003.

---

**TABLE 56–7.**  Prescribing guidelines for older adults

- Know your patient's medications (prescription, over-the counter, supplements, and herbal preparations) and medication history.
- Individualize therapy.
- Reevaluate indications for continued drug use.
- Minimize dose and total number of drugs.
- Start low, go slow; use blood levels judiciously.
- Try not to start two drugs at the same time.
- Treat adequately; do not withhold therapy for treatable diseases.
- Drugs with narrow therapeutic window should be monitored closely.
- The indications, duration and discontinuation, and adverse effects of each medication should be clearly explained to the patient and caregiver.
- Recognize that any new symptom may be an adverse drug reaction.
- Know which drugs are available to treat your patient's condition.
- Use agents with caution.
- Anticipate side effects: monitor for orthostatic hypotension, falls, delirium, urinary retention, constipation, syncope.
- Encourage treatment adherence.
- Work and communicate with the patient's other healthcare providers to adjust other drugs that might increase the risk of adverse drug reactions.

*Source.*   Adapted from Semla and Rochon 2002.

---

not affect every isozyme, drugs are often metabolized by more than one isozyme, and many drugs can affect each isozyme. Table 56–5 provides a list of drugs that have been reported to induce or inhibit at least one CYP450 isozyme. Diseases affecting an organ that metabolizes or eliminates drugs, such as the liver or kidneys; the delivery of drugs to those organs; and reductions in the patient's reserve to counteract certain drug effects can also result in an unintended response (Table 56–6).

When prescribing medications to elderly patients and those with multiple diseases, the following considerations can help decrease adverse drug reactions (see Table 56–7):

1. *Know what disorder is being treated.* Establishing a definite diagnosis often permits selection of the proper drug or drugs and treatment period. The choice of medication, dose, formulation, regimen, and the benefits and risks to be monitored should be individualized on the basis of the patient's pathophysiology, psychology, and other medications. A panel of geriatricians and clinician pharmacologists recently identified drugs that should generally be avoided in older adults (Fick et al. 2003) (see Table 56–8).

---

**TABLE 56–8.**    Potentially inappropriate medications for use in older adults

---

**Antidepressants**

*Amitriptyline* and *doxepin* should be avoided because of their anticholinergic and sedating properties.

Daily use of *fluoxetine* should be avoided because of its long half-life and risk of producing excessive CNS stimulation, sleep disturbances, and agitation.

**Antipsychotics**

*Thioridazine* is associated with greater potential for CNS and extrapyramidal effects.

**Sedatives**

*Short-acting benzodiazepines* should be avoided in daily doses greater than 3 mg for lorazepam, 60 mg for oxazepam, 2 mg for alprazolam, 15 mg for temazepam, and 0.25 mg for triazolam. Because older adults have increased sensitivity to benzodiazepines, smaller doses may be effective and safer. Total daily doses should not exceed the suggested maximums.

**Anticholinergics and antihistaminics**

*Chlorpheniramine* and *cyproheptadine* have potent anticholinergic effects.

*Diphenhydramine* is potentially anticholinergic and should not be used as a hypnotic in elderly patients.

**Narcotic analgesics**

*Meperidine* is not an effective oral analgesic and has many disadvantages, compared with other narcotic drugs.

In long-term use, full-dosage, longer-half-life, non-COX selective

**Nonsteroidal anti-inflammatory drugs** (naproxen, piroxicam, oxaprozin) have the potential to produce gastrointestinal bleeding, renal failure, high blood pressure, and heart failure.

*Ketorolac* (both immediate and long-term use) should be avoided in older persons, many of whom have symptomatic gastrointestinal conditions.

**Cardiac or CNS drugs**

Short-acting *dipyridamol* frequently causes orthostatic hypotension in elderly patients.

*Ticlopidine* has been shown to be no better than aspirin in preventing clotting and may be considerably toxic.

*Amiodarone* is associated with Q–T interval problems and risk of provoking torsades de pointes and generally lacks efficacy in older adults.

*Methyldopa* may cause bradycardia and exacerbate depression in elderly patients. Alternative treatments for hypertension are generally preferred.

**TABLE 56-8.** Potentially inappropriate medications for use in older adults *(continued)*

*Long-acting benzodiazepines* (chlordiazepoxide, diazepam, quazepam, halazepam, and clorazepate) have a long half-life in elderly patients (usually several days), producing prolonged sedation and increasing the risk of falls and fractures.

All *barbiturates* (except phenobarbital), except when used to control seizures, should be avoided because they are highly addictive and more adverse effects than most sedative or hypnotic drugs.

**Diabetes drugs**

*Chlorpropamide* has a prolonged half-life and can cause prolonged and serious hypoglycemia. It is the only oral hypoglycemic agent that causes syndrome of inappropriate antidiuretic hormone secretion.

**Supplements**

Doses of *ferrous sulfate* >325 mg/day do not dramatically increase the amount absorbed but greatly increase the incidence of constipation.

The dose of *digoxin* should not exceed 0.125 mg/day, except when it is used in treating atrial arrhythmias.

*Ergot mesyloids* and the cerebral vasodilators have not been shown to be effective in the doses studied for the treatment of dementia or any other conditions.

**Gastrointestinal drugs**

Long-term use of *stimulant laxatives* (bisacodyl, cascara sagrada) may exacerbate bowel dysfunction.

*Antispasmodic drugs* (dicyclomine, hyoscyamine, propantheline) are highly anticholinergic and generally produce toxic effects in elderly patients.

**Hormones**

For *estrogen* only (oral) hormone replacement, there is evidence of carcinogenic potential (breast and endometrial cancer) and a lack of cardioprotective effect in older women.

*Note.* CNS=central nervous system; COX=cyclooxygenase.
*Source.* Adapted from Fick et al. 2003.

2. *Review the patient's drug regimen frequently.* By asking patients to bring all of their medication bottles on a regular basis for review (the "brown bag" evaluation), the healthcare provider can maintain an up-to-date list of all medications taken, including nonprescription medications (over-the-counter medications, supplements, and herbal

preparations) and those prescribed by other physicians, minimizing the possibility of drug overdose and/or drug-drug interactions.

3. *Use the minimum number of drugs needed to deal effectively with the medical condition.* The pharmacological actions and the mechanisms of the drug or drug clearance should be reviewed, and the patient should be monitored for therapeutic and toxic effects of the medications. The minimal effective dose should be used in elderly patients because clearance mechanisms and homeostatic responses may be compromised (Semla and Rochon 2002). Just as medications are prescribed in numbers or doses greater than necessary, they also may be inappropriately omitted or prescribed in doses that are too low to be effective.

4. *Any new complaint or worsening of an existing condition should prompt the consideration of whether it could be an adverse drug reaction or drug-induced effect.* The clinician should avoid attributing signs and symptoms such as weakness, confusion, anorexia, and cognitive impairment to old age rather than suspecting effects of drugs (Bressler 2003; Semla and Rochon 2002).

## References

Applegate WB, Miller ST, Elam JT, et al: Impact of cataract surgery with lens implantation on vision and physical function in elderly patients. JAMA 257:1064–1066, 1987

Aro S, Aro H, Keskimaki I: Socio-economic mobility among patients with schizophrenia or major affective disorder: a 17-year retrospective follow-up. Br J Psychiatry 166:759–767, 1995

Bogardus ST, Richardson E, Macciejewski PK, et al: Evaluation of a guided protocol for quality improvement in identifying common geriatric problems. J Am Geriatr Soc 50:328–335, 2002

Boockvar K, Fishman E, Kyriacou CK, et al: Adverse events due to discontinuations in drug use and dose changes in patients transferred between acute and long-term care facilities. Arch Intern Med 16:545–550, 2004

Bowman L, Carlste BC, Hancock EF, et al: Adverse drug reaction (ADR) occurrence and evaluation in elderly inpatients. Pharmacoepidemiol Drug Saf 5:9–18, 1996

Bradley EH, Bogardus ST Jr, Tinetti ME, et al: Goal-setting in clinical medicine. Soc Sci Med 49:267–278, 1999

Bressler R, Bahl JJ: Principles of drug therapy for the elderly patient. Mayo Clin Proc 78:1564–1577, 2003

Calkins DR, Rubenstein LV, Cleary PD, et al: Failure of physicians to recognize functional disability in ambulatory patients. Ann Intern Med 114:451–454, 1991

Corten P, Ribourdouille M, Dramaix M: Premature death among outpatients at a community mental health center. Hosp Community Psychiatry 42:1248–1251, 1991

Druss BG, Rosenheck RA: Mental disorders and access to medical care in the United States. Am J Psychiatry 155:1775–1777, 1998

Druss BG, Rosenheck RA: Locus of mental health treatment in an integrated service system. Psychiatr Serv 51:890–892, 2000

Emory University Reynolds Program: Comprehensive Geriatric Assessment. Available at www.cha.emory.edu/reynoldsprogram. Accessed June 2004.

Fick DM, Cooper JW, Wade WE, et al: Updating the Beers criteria for potentially inappropriate medication use in older adults: results of a US consensus panel of experts. Arch Intern Med 163:2716–2724, 2003

Fleming KC, Evans JM, Weber DC, et al: Practical functional assessment of elderly persons: a primary-care approach. Mayo Clin Proc 70:890–910, 1995

Gill TM: Assessment, in Geriatrics Review Syllabus: A Core Curriculum in Geriatric Medicine, 5th Edition. Edited by Cobbs EL, Duthie EH, Murphy JB. Boston, MA, Blackwell, 2002a, pp 49–52

Gill TM: Geriatric medicine: it's more than caring for old people. Am J Med 113:85–90, 2002b

Gill TM, Williams CS, Tinetti ME: Assessing risk for the onset of functional dependence among older adults: the role of physical performance. J Am Geriatr Soc 43:603–609, 1995

Hall RC, Beresford TP, Gardner ER, et al: The medical care of psychiatric patients. Hosp Community Psychiatry 33:25–34, 1982

Hanlon JT, Schmader KE, Koronkowski MJ, et al: Adverse drug events in high risk older outpatients. J Am Geriatr Soc 45:945–948, 1997

Honig A, Pop P, Tan ES, et al: Physical illness in chronic psychiatric patients from a community psychiatric unit: the implications for daily practice. Br J Psychiatry 155:58–64, 1989

Inouye S, Bogardus S, Charpentier P, et al: A multicomponent intervention to prevent delirium in hospitalized older patients. N Engl J Med 340:669–676, 1999

Kane JM: Compliance issues in outpatient treatment. J Clin Psychopharmacol 5:22S–27S, 1985

Katz S, Ford AB, Moskowitz RW, et al: Studies of illness in the aged. The index of ADL: a standardized measure of biological and psychosocial function. JAMA 185:914–919, 1963

Keith S, Kane J: Partial compliance and patient consequences in schizophrenia. J Clin Psychiatry 64:1308–1315, 2003

Lawton MP, Brody EM: Assessment of older people: self-maintaining and instrumental activities of daily living. Gerontologist 9:179–186, 1969

Leipzig RM: Avoiding adverse drug effects in elderly patients. Cleve Clin J Med 65:470–478, 1998

Leipzig RM: Prescribing: keys to maximizing benefit while avoiding adverse drug effects. Geriatrics 56:30–35, 2001

Lindeman RD: Overview: renal physiology and pathophysiology of aging. Am J Kidney Dis 16:275–282, 1990

Lindeman RD: Changes in renal function with aging: implications for treatment. Drugs Aging 2:423–431, 1992

Lipschitz DA, Ham RJ, White JV: An approach to nutrition screening for older Americans. Am Fam Physician 45:601–608, 1992

Maggi S, Minicuci N, Martini A, et al: Prevalence rates of hearing impairment and comorbid conditions in older people: the Veneto Study. J Am Geriatr Soc 46:1069–1074, 1998

Montamat SC, Cusack BJ, Vestal RE: Management of drug therapy in the elderly. N Engl J Med 321:303–309, 1989

Moore AA, Siu AL: Screening for common problems in ambulatory elderly: clinical confirmation of a screening instrument. Am J Med 100:438–443, 1996

Nolan L, O'Malley K: Prescribing for the elderly: part I. Sensitivity of the elderly to adverse drug reactions. J Am Geriatr Soc 36:142–149, 1988a

Nolan L, O'Malley K: Prescribing for the elderly: part II. Prescribing patterns: differences due to age. J Am Geriatr Soc 36:245–254, 1988b

Pinholt EM, Kroenke K, Hanley JF, et al: Functional assessment of the elderly: a comparison of standard instruments with clinical judgment. Arch Intern Med 147:484–488, 1987

Reuben DB, Greendale GA, Harrison GG: Nutrition screening in older persons. J Am Geriatr Soc 43:415–425, 1995

Roberts RO, Jacobsen SJ, Rhodes T, et al: Urinary incontinence in a community-based cohort: prevalence and healthcare-seeking. J Am Geriatr Soc 46:467–472, 1998

Routledge PA, O'Mahony MS, Woodhouse KW: Adverse drug reactions in elderly patients. Br J Clin Pharmacol 57:121–126, 2004

Sandson NB: Exploring drug interaction in psychiatry. Psychiatric Times 21:6, 2004

Semla T, Rochon P: Pharmacotherapy, in Geriatrics Review Syllabus: A Core Curriculum in Geriatric Medicine, 5th Edition. Edited by Cobbs EL, Duthie EH, Murphy JB. Boston, MA, Blackwell, 2002, pp 37–44

Sullivan DH: Impact of nutritional status on health outcomes of nursing home residents. J Am Geriatr Soc 43:195–196, 1995

Tinetti ME, Liu WL, Claus EB: Predictors and prognosis of inability to get up after falls among elderly persons. JAMA 269:65–70, 1993

Tinetti ME, Baker Di, McAvay G, et al: A multifactorial intervention to reduce the risk of falling among elderly people living in the community. N Engl J Med 331:821–827, 1994

Tsuang MT, Woolson RF: Mortality in patients with schizophrenia, mania, depression and surgical conditions: a comparison with general population mortality. Br J Psychiatry 130:162–166, 1977

Turnheim K: Drug dosage in the elderly: is it rational? Drugs Aging 13:357–379, 1998

Turnheim K: When drug therapy gets old: pharmacokinetics and pharmacodynamics in the elderly. Exp Gerontol 38:843–853, 2003

Woodhouse K, Wynne HA: Age-related changes in hepatic function: implications for drug therapy. Drugs Aging 2:243–255, 1992

# Index

Page numbers printed in *boldface* type refer to tables or figures.